Young Adolf

An Alternate History

Young Adolf
An Alternate History

Frank Daversa

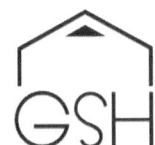

Copyright © 2021 by Frank Daversa.

All rights reserved. No part of this book may be reproduced in any form or by any electronic or mechanical means, including information storage and retrieval systems, without permission in writing from the publisher, except by reviewers, who may quote brief passages in a review.

ISBN: 978-1-956074-57-4 (Paperback Edition)
ISBN: 978-1-956074-58-1 (Hardcover Edition)
ISBN: 978-1-956074-56-7 (E-book Edition)

Book Ordering Information

Phone Number: 315 288-7939 ext. 1000 or 347-901-4920
Email: info@globalsummithouse.com
Global Summit House
www.globalsummithouse.com

Printed in the United States of America

CONTENTS

Chapter 1 1
Chapter 2 30
Chapter 3 66
Chapter 4 93
Chapter 5 118
Chapter 6 152
Chapter 7 185
Chapter 8 200
Chapter 9 244
Chapter 10 288
Chapter 11 269
Chapter 12 294
Chapter 13 316
Chapter 14 330
Epilogue **348**

Chapter 1

SCRIBBLING NOTES ON a small pad was Alois's only distraction from the sounds of his third wife, Klara, struggling with the birth of her fourth child. Her cries were muffled by the heavy, locked, wooden door between their bedroom and his study, where he sat penning notes with his fountain pen, marking the train arrivals that would constitute the amount of work he could look forward to the next day. But he could still hear them. If it were not for some sense of duty, Alois would not have remained at all.

This was the birth of his sixth child, and the process of childbirth had long ago lost the zeal of being one of life's miracles. There was no guarantee this child would fare any better than his or her siblings. Alois and Klara's first two children, Gustav and Ida, died of diphtheria at a tragically young age. Their third child, Otto, had passed in his first few hours of life. However, Alois's legacy was secure in his eldest child, born of his second wife, Franziska. He had even given that boy his own name.

Alois Hitler, Sr. sat in a large, high-backed leather-bound chair in the small study outside his bedchambers. By the crude light of a smoke-sullied oil lamp, he read the newspaper he had purchased on his way home from the office that day. He did not read political articles or editorials. He was not interested in the headlines or classifieds. Instead, Mr. Hitler reviewed the train tables for April 20, 1889, and noted the number of freights that would be arriving that night, which gave him an idea of the volume of work he could look forward to the next day.

His work was always the best distraction from his family.

Klara would name this latest addition to the Hitler clan. Really, the only reason he sat outside the room, enduring the sounds of a difficult birth, was his promise to his young wife.

As another agonized cry squeezed through the space beneath the richly stained door, Alois sighed and folded the newspaper. How much longer did he need to wait? He could not help but wonder if he had enough time to leave his post and visit the inn's common room downstairs, where he might enjoy one of the town's Mai bock ales. The malted spring brew would certainly take the edge off the proceedings within the bedchamber, but just as he thought to stand, the heavy door opened and the town's attending doctor beckoned Alois inside.

"It was a difficult birth, perhaps for how early it came. But there were no complications, and both mother and child are healthy enough. I will send you a bill in the morning, of course." The doctor was already replacing clamps and scissors back into a black leather bag, the only sterilization a quick wipe with the same damp cloth that had cleaned the newborn of birth fluid. "Oh, and congratulations, Mr. Hitler

The afterthought was wasted on Alois, who only gave the doctor a simple nod of acknowledgement. He was still unhappy that the doctor's presence had been necessary at all. A midwife could do the same job—and cheaper. Given the mortality rate of Klara's other three children, he had paid the extra expense, just to appease his wife. However, hearing both mother and child were healthy, Alois could only think the doctor's presence had been a waste of his money after all.

The expense of a doctor did not save Alois the cost of a midwife. Klara had wanted the older woman's experience as much as the doctor's medical expertise. The midwife would be there to comfort the laboring mother as much as to assist with the actions that followed the birth. Alois rarely bent his own will to accommodate that of his wife, but when it came to their children, he was content to allow her the expense.

The midwife, who had been swaddling the newborn, made the inadvertent mistake of first offering the child to its mother. Perhaps if Alois had held the babe first, he might have felt a stronger affection for the child. Instead, Klara took the boy, cuddling him to her breast. Alois looked at mother and child and felt no swell of joy or pride.

The entire process felt worn to the older man. He was twenty-three years Klara's senior; the boy might as well have been his grandchild.

Klara, no less wary than her husband by the deaths of her other three children, was still a mother and possessed a mother's love. She held her boy and cooed at him and tickled his pink nose, never thinking to offer the child to his father. Alois never asked to hold him. He gave his young wife a kiss on her forehead and told her she had done well. "He is handsome, Klara. Perfect in every way a babe can be."

Through her exhaustion, Klara smiled at her husband, and then down at her son. "He takes after his father, I think."

Alois looked at the newborn in his arms and shook his head, "No, he has far too much hair!"

Klara managed a feeble laugh. Alois must be happy with pride to make any sort of joke about himself. He was normally such a stoic man.

"What do you think, Adolf? Do you look more like your mama, or your papa?" The cooing of Alois's normally commanding tone sounded strangely to the mid-wife who was still present.

"Yes, definitely your mama." And there returned that certain authority that made the decision absolute. He gave the child back to his tired mother's arms after he had made his pronouncement.

He then sat on the side of the bed, watching his youngest boy, whose fine black hair was still damp. He waited for mother and baby to fall asleep, and then rose, making his way downstairs to the inn's common room. He would have that beer after all.

Alois was a man of average build and average taste in clothing. His most striking trait was self-importance, a likely result of working as a civil officer. Alois was responsible for collecting taxes on trade items. There were seven freights expected that night, but judging from their places of departure, they would be rather boring: food stuffs and textiles. No chance to make a little extra coin in looking away from an extra bolt of silk or a box of precious stones.

At least the birth had gone well, which was one less worry on his mind, but he could not help but dwell longer on the children he had lost than those that now lived. He could hardly be called a family man. A bastard, Alois felt that providing his name to his children was enough. Passing along the Hitler name was the reason he had married his second wife—and his third, for that matter. His children would not endure the hardships of a bastard's life.

He drank his Mai bock ale in silence, his mind empty of significant thought.

Finishing his ale, in a melancholy mood, he instructed the barman to charge his tab, and then returned to their apartment on the top floor of the inn. As he sat on the edge of the bed, where Klara slept, the newborn still resting on her chest, he sighed deeply, grunting as he pulled off a dust-worn boot. The sound or movement must have awakened the child, for he began to wail, and the sound cut straight to the center of Alois's already dark mood. Few things were more irritating than the incessant wail of an unhappy newborn.

Awaking at her babe's cries, Klara tried to soothe the child back to silence. The crying continued as Alois stripped off his trousers and shirt, folding them neatly over the back of a chair for use the next day.

"If you cannot keep the baby quiet," he said, "then take him into the den. I need my rest, and he is probably hungry."

Klara, having just given birth to the boy hardly more than an hour ago, needed her rest as well, but she knew better than to raise her husband's ire. With very shaky steps, she left her side of the bed and took the child into the small sitting room that lay beyond the study. Alois watched the pair go, and then pulled back the comforter to make sure the midwife had changed the sheets before she left. As the door closed behind them, the baby's cries were as muted as his mother's had been, and Alois soon drifted into a deep sleep that was beyond the child's crying.

Rocking in the chair Alois had bought her as a gift after their second child, Klara fed her newborn. She sat in darkness, her own dark eyes drifting shut not long after she had begun the feeding. She did not sleep, but in the relative void, thought about how she had come to be there.

Klara was not a particularly attractive woman, being large of frame and plain of feature, but she was very kind. Her husband, also her uncle, employed her as his housekeeper. Grateful for her position, she had been too trusting of Alois—which is not to say she found him unattractive. He had possessed the defined looks of an older man, and his confidence, or perhaps, more accurately, his dominance, had piqued her interest. He had been her first, and once she was with child, she knew he would also be her last. But he had not gotten her with child, she would never have married him—he was certainly no longer the man who had seduced her under the closed eyes of his second wife.

Most times, she was grateful for the life he had given her. She had three other children by him already, and it was no fault of his that they had passed so suddenly. He was a hard man, who demanded respect and obeisance, but she could have married worse. No, what worried her was the fact that he seemed to be growing harder as he grew older; he had almost come to blows with her already. She was certain that the issue was her own failure at keeping his household the way he wanted it. Perhaps now that there was another baby, he would soften and be the stern, but fair, man she had married.

Klara caught herself dozing, and found that the babe had unlatched himself at last. She rose and took the already sleeping newborn back into the bedroom, where she lay him in a crib that glimmered softly in the moonlight with its fresh white paint. The crib that had held for her previous three children had been burned after young Otto's sudden death.

The young mother tucked a small fleece blanket around her baby boy and smiled. She still had not decided on a name for the child, but that would not matter for some weeks to come. The boy would need to live long enough to earn a name. That had been Alois's decision after Otto's death.

Klara thought her husband's mandate was harsh at the least and cruel at worst, but she also recognized that her husband, older than she, had lost even more children than she had delivered. It hardly made his attitude right, but it did at least serve to mitigate it.

She kissed her fingertips, and brushed them over the baby's scalp, smoothing his fine black hair. Then she carefully climbed into bed with Alois, hardly closing her eyes before she too, was asleep.

The days after the baby's birth passed without particular importance. The Hitler household returned to the normalcy of Alois tenuously balancing his profession against his domestic practices. Klara enjoyed no particular routine, as the baby refused to abide the schedule of feeding and sleeping she had been able to impose on her previous children. His behavior disrupted her own resting habits, and she found herself with far less energy than was normal for her; as she slept fewer hours, but found herself accidentally napping for many more minutes. Her household chores had become an almost impossible task. Alois had struck Klara in the past, and she had noted well the whiteness of his knuckles when he found her dozing instead of cooking the dinner meal.

The baby was happy enough. Once he had learned to smile, the expression balanced equally with the horrible face he made when crying. He was very light in his complexion, but his face would turn quite red when he balled his fists in miniature imitation of his father's own displeasure.

She had hoped to recruit the assistance of Angela, Alois's second child from his second wife. The girl would be six years old in July, but she was the only help Klara could enlist. Alois Jr., though older, was a male, and Alois Sr. would never allow his son to partake in "women's business." To his credit, Alois had offered to hire a house servant to assist Klara in her domestic responsibilities. However, given Alois's record of bedding his servants (it was how he came to marry not only her, but also his second wife), Klara, was quite against the offer of aid from a housekeeper. Instead, she continued her struggle to accomplish the cooking and cleaning while caring for her fickle baby.

The months passed, and the baby grew beyond the immediate

risks of infant mortality. Klara herself became ill on more than one occasion, but she was a robust woman and always recovered after a day or two of rest.

The baby became ill around his third month, developing a cough and a low fever. The family feared whooping cough or some similarly common malady, but another visit from the town's doctor put that fear aside, and it was decided that the child had simply contracted a summer cold, blaming the change of weather from cool to warm. He suggested that the child be provided with opportunities to experience the fresher air of the outdoors, thus acclimating him to the changing seasons.

When the cold had passed, Alois deemed the boy of hearty enough constitution to at last receive his name. Klara had spent all those months debating what the infant's name should be, and now that the time for a decision had come, she named him Adolf. Names beginning with the letter A were already prevalent in the family, and Klara liked very much the sound of "Adolf." Alois agreed without debate, though it seemed a stronger name than the small child deserved.

After earning his name, young Adolf seemed to become more content in general and at last agreed to the schedule his mother set for him. Klara finally found respite from sleepless nights—which in turn enabled her to keep house better and to suffer less from an aggravated husband. She did not like a disorderly household any more than her husband, and she now had the energy to perform her duties, while still finding time to take baby Adolf for strolls in his carriage. Walking with her stepmother and stepbrother, Angela often picked wildflowers in the fields surrounding Braunau Am Inn.

This was, by the accounts of all parties involved, the happiest times in the Hitler household. Alois spent his days in the customs office, being very official and rather well respected. He came home to the smells of his laundry hanging on summer clotheslines and dinner almost ready on the stove. There was little reason for him to become angry, and what cause for anger there was, Klara was able to deftly soothe with womanly charm before that anger could percolate and boil over.

By the time Alois Jr. was enrolled in grade school, his marks were sufficient, if not extraordinary, befitting for a civil servant in the making, or so his father believed.

Alois Jr. paid even less attention to Adolf than Alois Sr. The father had little time for domestic concerns that did not require his administration of discipline. Alois Jr. on the other hand, simply had no interest in having a younger stepbrother. Alois Jr. was an independent lad, and when he was not studying, he was often away from home playing with friends in the countryside.

His sister Angela, however, paid a great deal of attention to Adolf. When her stepmother was doing chores, Angela took care of Adolf. She was only his half-sister, but she was a very good sister and delighted in amusing the baby boy. She would make funny faces or playfully tickle the child. He would grab at her fingers with his soft, chubby hands. Angela had been very young when her other siblings had perished and thought of them rarely. This child, however, was healthy, and much more entertaining to play with than her dollies. She would often hold him and softly sing songs her mother had taught her.

"Be gentle with him, Ange," said Klara, watching Angela bounce the boy rather vigorously on her knee, just as she had seen her father doing the night before. Young Adolf seemed to enjoy the motion immensely. He squealed and smiled as his already long and dark hair bounced in the air.

"I will not drop him, Mother," said Angela. Her own mother had passed away a year after Angela's birth—and her older brother, Alois Jr., reminded her often that Klara was not truly their mother—so she and her brother always used the formal address of "mother," rather than the familial "mama" that most children adopted.

"Certainly not, but you do not need to give accidents a chance, do you?" Klara's lap was occupied with folding the day's laundry. "Set him down, and leave bouncing to your father or brother."

"May I hold him, then?" Angela never left the baby alone for very long and released him only for the purposes of feedings and changing. It kept the baby relatively content to receive such constant attention.

"Of course, just be gentle."

Angela, a child herself, entertained Adolf with silly stories that Klara did not understand. Adolf seemed to enjoy the tales as much as he did his sister's songs, which often times were equally foolish. If Angela could not remember the words as her mother sang them, she did not hesitate to simply make up her own.

A knock at the door, sounding fast and thrice, was a signal that Alois Jr. had returned from school, and so Klara laid aside a pile of clothes and unlatched the bolt on the door. "Hello, Alois, you are home early."

"Hello, Mother," said Alois as he swung his tied stack of books onto an empty chair. "There is an exam tomorrow."

"You should be more careful with your books, Alois. They are expensive, and young Adolf may need them some day. You must think of your brother as well as yourself, now."

Alois narrowed his eyes somewhat at his mother's reproach, but only nodded. He did not see the younger brother as any particular threat to his future inheritance or his standing in the family hierarchy, but he was most definitely a nuisance. He did not understand why his father needed more children, especially children by Klara. He had been old enough to understand the deaths of Klara's first three children, and he was convinced that the same fate awaited this latest addition to the family. As such, he kept his distance from the baby more often than not.

On top of that, Angela, his true blood sibling, did not seem to fawn over him half as much as she had before the baby's birth. He had often been cruel to the sister that followed his every footstep, and now it seemed the baby held all of her attentions. Alois Jr. was too surprised to acknowledge he felt a degree of jealousy.

"An exam?" Klara said. "That has never been reason enough in the past for you to return straight home. It must be a very difficult exam.

What is the subject?" Having been the housemaid for the previous Mrs. Hitler's household, Klara had known the children almost since they were born. "Geometry, which is not my strongest field of study. I did poorly on the last quiz, and Father will be very cross if my score does not improve." He would likely feel his father's hand, if not his belt, if the score did not *vastly* improve.

"You are right, and I will not blame him, as I will be cross as well. I am glad you are responsible enough to understand that, at least. Go to your room for your studies. I will be busy in the kitchen soon enough, so you will not want to use that table." Klara looked to the large wooden clock that hung on the den's wall, noting that the iron-wrought hands were already pointing past four o'clock. She would need to begin dinner very soon indeed if it was to be ready by Alois Sr.'s arrival.

Alois Jr. disappeared into the kitchen briefly, returning with a glass of water and an apple. He gathered his books, and then retreated into his small bedroom in the corner of the apartment. Angela had her own room, though it was smaller still than Alois's. Adolf slept in his parent's bedroom, but in a year or so he would be moved in with Alois Jr.

Yet when her husband returned home from the customs office, dinner had barely been started. Young Adolf had insisted on being fed first, and, like most babies, his needs came before those of the rest of his family.

His father gave no credence to that excuse. "Another hour? What have you done all day? Folded clothes and swept a floor?"

Klara had known that Alois would be upset, but she did not expect the open fury with which he spoke. She could not help but become defensive in her own tone. "I did much more than that. Time simply got away from me, and just as I was starting dinner, Adolf wanted his. I thought you would have more patience than your infant son."

Alois had worked through his lunch hour. His hunger added to his temper, and he was in no mood for Klara's insolence. "You dare speak to me that way!" his hand was swift, and fell with a crack against her cheek. "You will apologize for your words." The back of his hand then struck her other cheek. "And you will apologize for dinner."

Klara, who still held Adolf, had no way of defending herself from either blow. She was as stunned by the second as the first, and though she possessed a strong will, she could not help the tears that fell wetly onto young Adolf's forehead as she fell backward into a chair.

"Monster." she whispered, her throat choked with emotion.

"Do not ever take such a tone with me again," said Alois, his eyes still large with anger.

Upset by the volume of his father's voice and his violence of his actions, Adolf began to cry. His mother tried to calm him while she stared through her tears with little else than genuine hurt at being treated this way. Alois had struck her before, but never for something as mundane as having a late dinner.

Alois did not wait for confirmation of her understanding. The wailing sound of his youngest son only irritated him further. "I am going downstairs for my supper."

Klara kept her eyes on the man as he left, slamming the door behind him, all the while hugging young Adolf to her closely, making soothing sounds that were as much for her as they were for her baby. She let the tears continue to flow over still-stinging cheeks, and waited for that pain to subside.

Angela, who had been sitting on the floor during the entire exchange, continued to sit with saucer eyes in scared silence, her dolly abandoned on the floor. She did not say a single word. Alois Jr. had heard the fight through his closed bedroom door, but he dared not emerge to see what exactly had transpired.

After a few minutes, Klara recovered herself enough to stand. Adolf had stopped crying by then as well, and his mother had sense enough to show more concern for the children than she did for herself. "Are you all right, Angela? Here, take your brother, and play with him. Dinner will be ready soon."

Angela did not speak, but held her arms out to receive Adolf. He was getting heavier and heavier, but she could still hold him easily enough. With the baby in his big half-sister's care, Klara returned to the kitchen to put the sauce on the pork chops broiling in the stove. The water for the rice had not yet begun to boil, so she built up the fire.

Downstairs, in the inn's common room, Alois had failed to calm his temper. He ordered himself a particularly dry glass of wine, rather than the smoothly malted beer he would normally drink at this hour. The wine would go well with the club sandwich he had ordered for dinner.

Klara had been so meek and subservient when they were first married. He remembered all too well her propensity for calling him "Uncle" throughout their wedding day. Maturity and years of marriage had apparently emboldened the girl to foolery. How dare she compare his patience to that of the baby's! How dare she not have dinner ready to begin with! His rules were few, and certainly simple. He expected them to be followed, and having dinner on the table promptly after his return from the office was second in importance only to having his breakfast ready before he left for the day.

He hoped her cheeks still stung and hurt until whatever dinner she had been making was finished. The barman brought his sandwich to the small wooden table at which Alois sat alone. A few other men were in the common room, most at the bar, where they washed the day's dust away with ales or pilsners. Alois was the only man drinking wine, and his face soured as he took his first sip.

"Keeper!" Alois called across the room. The room was filling rapidly as the men who lived alone in their apartments sought an easy meal after their hard day's work, and the barkeep was already sliding pints across the bar top. The barrel-bellied man looked up from the tap and gave a flick of his head to show Alois he had his attention.

In the official tone he used around the customs office, Alois raised his glass and swirled its contents for effect. "This wine has passed. Check your corks, and bring me a new bottle." He had not wanted the contents of an entire bottle, but in an establishment such as this, where a man might order a single glass in a week, the next bottle the barkeep tried was as likely to have soured as this one had.

Wine was not particularly popular in Braunau Am Inn. The region was not conducive to growing Spätburgunder, or the relatively new and surprisingly popular Müller-Thurgau that was becoming so loved in Germany. Braunau Am Inn was too far south and east, and relied mostly on beer for its alcoholic beverages. Just the same, drinking wine distinguished him from the commoners who populated this inn.

The barkeep did not appreciate Alois announcing to
the room that he was selling soured wine, especially in the tone Alois had employed. Who was he to be ordering wine, anyway? It was usually reserved for high-ranking military officials, not a low-ranking civil official. Everyone in town knew Alois was a customs officer—those who knew him at all, at least.

Still, he paid his tab every week, which was better than most of the inn's clientele. The barkeep poured the last pint from a barrel that could tip no further, and then instructed one of the two barmaids, who would begin their shift soon as the room filled with the onset of darkness, to watch the bar as he made his way into the inn's wine cellar.

The barkeep at last returned from the wine cellar, even redder in his jowls from the exertion of so many stairs. "Apologies, Mr. Hitler. You were correct. One of the girls must have failed to press the cork tightly into that last bottle. I believe this one will be more to your liking."

It would not be an expensive bottle; the barkeep knew Alois better than that. He catered as much to Alois's ego as much as he did to his customer's thirsts. Alois raised the glass and made a show of swirling its contents to release whatever aromas this vintage had to offer. Whatever berries had been added to the fermentation had mostly succumbed to the overpowering tannins of the drink, but the wine was not sour, and it went very well with his sandwich indeed.

His meal finished without further event, and as he sat and made his way down the bottle, he was disappointed that no one approached him for either conversation or favor. He had never had many friends in his life. Being a bastard, he had seen it as a major accomplishment just to become a customs officer.

As another swallow of wine bit his palate, he began the reflective introspection that is the miserable companion of men who drink alone. He thought of his first wife and the official whose favor he had sought to gain by the marriage. It had worked, to an extent. He had earned a promotion, but it was as much for his talents as his relations. Still, it was unlikely he would not have had the opportunity to display those talents if it had not been for the notice the marriage had gained him.

He had not loved Anna in any true sense of the word, but then, he was not sure he truly loved any of his wives.

Anna had been fifty years old when they met, and if not for her money, there would never have been any marriage at all.

That of course made Franzisca all the more appealing to Alois. In Anna's sickness, Alois had hired Franni as a housekeeper to help care for the household and the rapidly deteriorating health of his wife. Infidelity followed shortly after: Anna's age was such that Alois had a lustful eye for younger women. Being a bastard, perhaps it was in his genes to propagate his line similarly. Franni was soon pregnant with Alois Jr., and that had been a hard time indeed for Alois Sr.

Knowing his own struggles as a bastard in such a rigid society, he decided the boy must be legitimized, much the way he himself eventually had been. So he had married Franni, and she was good enough to give him both a boy and a girl. He had never had much interest in children beyond siring them and had left their rearing to their mother. Once he had made Franni his wife, Klara had replaced her as housekeeper, and Alois had repeated the pattern.

Another sip, and Alois relived the arguments with Franni over the young and moderately attractive Klara's presence. Franni, all too aware of Alois's lack of commitment to wedding vows, did not appreciate the younger girl's presence. There was little in Klara's figure to attract him, given that she was tall and somewhat boxy in her stature.

At the memories, he smiled into the bottom of his glass. Sediment that Alois had stirred in a particularly violent pour now stained a ring in the glass. He had the presence of mind to wipe the glass clean with his napkin before pouring the final third of the bottle.

When the doctor had told Alois that Franni should move to Ranshofen for fresher air, Alois had been left in Braunau Am Inn with his work and two children. He sent for Klara almost immediately, and she was eager to return.

She had been eager in many things, and despite her lack of Franni's innate beauty, Klara proved herself a more than adequate replacement as a female presence in the household. It was a tragedy when Franni died. She was only twenty-three, and the idea of having both wife and mistress had always appealed to Alois. Now he had buried two wives (though he had separated from Anna long before her death), and he was left with Klara, who technically had become his niece when he himself became legitimized.

It was a tangled affair he had caught himself in, made even more complicated by the fact that Klara was soon pregnant herself, and Alois again faced the issue of siring an illegitimate child.

A long, long sip for that memory.

There had been such fear in the young girl's eyes when she told him. If Franni had recovered from her illness, Klara would surely be sent away again, and already being with child, it would be difficult to find employment elsewhere. But Franni eventually succumbed to her illness, dying of a lung hemorrhage.

Alois finished the glass's contents, his head feeling hot and cotton-stuffed. His thoughts were blurring with increasing intoxication.

The courts had not wanted to marry them, for they were first cousins, but he submitted an appeal to the church, and they provided him with a humanitarian waiver after Alois explained the circumstances of his own birth.

If not for Klara's larger frame, she might not have been able to hide her five months of pregnancy by then, and the church would never have granted the waiver. But, they did, and Alois now had his third wife, and despite the passing of his first three children by the girl, he now had yet another baby boy.

He pushed himself away from the table, but did not rise from his chair. Instead, he leaned back against the wall and fixed his bloodshot eyes on the ceiling. He would not allow himself to be publicly inebriated, despite the presence of countless other drunks in the room. While he waited for the alcohol to return him to the calmer level of a somewhat sleepy buzz, he wondered if he should apologize to Klara when he returned. He had allowed his temper to flare too hotly. He should not have struck her twice—once, perhaps, for it was still her fault for not having dinner ready.

He had his foibles, and he was aware of them. His temper had only increased as he aged, and his desire for younger flesh had never matured, but he still considered himself a family man. He worked a respectable job, and though he lacked the education to rise beyond his current title, it was still an accomplishment to have come this far. He put a roof over his family's head and provided food for his wife to put on the table. He had given his children a name. Alois decided he was doing well indeed.

He remained alone at his table for the balance of the night, the other patrons filing out long before he chose to rise and make his way up the long flights of stairs to his apartment on the top floor. His key was loud in the lock, mainly due to his initial difficulty of finding the proper angle of attack for the hole. The hinges needed oil, but the sound was not enough to wake the baby, and for that Alois was entirely grateful. His head was beginning to pound, likely due to the combination of alcohol and exertion of climbing so many stairs.

He was pleased to find a shuttered oil lamp still burning, and, while making his way to its dim light, he found Klara asleep in the rocking chair. She seemed to have made an effort to remain awake, waiting for his return. The baby was not with her; presumably he slept in his cradle.

"Klara, dear. Come to bed" his words were soft, lacking all the anger and violence he had felt earlier.

Klara woke, and though startled at first, offered him a sleepy smile. He bent and kissed her cheek, tasting the makeup she had likely applied to cover the bruise his palm had left. He regretted striking her, and made the effort of helping her up from the chair. He then took the shuttered lamp, opening the window enough to allow a smoke-dulled shaft of light to illuminate the path to their bedroom.

"I am sorry, Alois. Tomorrow will be better, I promise." Her voice was gravelly with sleep, but utterly sincere and almost heartbreaking to the remorseful Alois.

"Yes," he said, "it will. I am sorry, too. It was a hard day, and instead of having patience, I made it harder." But even in his apology, he could not avoid a hardening of his tone. "But this had better not become a habit. It is time Adolf began obeying a stricter schedule. That will allow you to follow a better schedule yourself."

Klara knew he was right and could hardly be mad at him. She kissed him and promised again that tomorrow would be better. The other effect of wine then seized him, and despite the hour—or the proximity of his youngest son—he coupled with Klara. As she performed the majority of the work, he decided that he did not miss Franni so much after all.

The next day was better. Klara accomplished her chores quickly, despite her lack of sleep the night before. When she had finally fallen asleep, she had slept very well indeed, at least. When she had woken, she remembered looking at Alois in the early morning light, wondering if he would ever allow his hair to grow beyond the dark, fuzzed stubble that gave harshness to his countenance. All his hair was on his face, in the form of a giant mustache that extended like a walrus's tusks, long enough to brush his chest. He was not a particularly heavy man, bearing the belly of most his age, but otherwise quite fit.

In the morning, she had left the bed well before he had so that his breakfast would be waiting on the table after he had donned his uniform. With a dozen buttons down its front, cinched at the waist by a thin white belt, matching his fitted white trousers, it was far more handsome than what most military officers wore. He was very attractive in that uniform. Her own attire was simple by comparison, a white blouse that buttoned snugly over her ample bosom and a common dress of light-blue that hung loosely from her post-pregnancy frame. She kept her brown hair in a tight bun, as much for style as functionality. She was young and did not need to pull the hair tight enough to remove
wrinkles, as women of Alois's age might.

The children were soon up and dressed as well, Alois Jr. wearing a collared white shirt and a short brown coat that matched his brown trousers and shoes. His hair was cut as closely as his father's. Angela wore a simple dress, dyed green to hide the stains children could never avoid acquiring.

So Alois Sr. went to work for the day, and Alois Jr. went to school, leaving Angela, Adolf and Klara to themselves in the apartment. It was a fair-sized apartment for a growing family. Alois had inherited money when he had been legitimized, and his first wife had been wealthy—though he forfeited the majority of those sums when they separated. Franni, having been a housekeeper like Klara, had little more to offer financially than Klara herself had, but at the end of the day, Alois supported his family well enough from his officer's salary. Though they did not live extravagantly, they lived comfortably.

With the addition of Adolf, Alois and Klara both decided to put off the redecorating project they had planned a year before. The couch needed to be reupholstered, and the pillows needed to be stuffed. A new carpet might brighten the room and soften its wooden floors. The lamps could likely suffice with a simple cleaning, but Klara was tiring of oil lamps and wanted Alois to have lines run for the usage of the electricity she had heard so much about. Lines had been set in Braunau Am Inn, and though the innkeeper swore the inn was connected, no one had seen a bulb in use yet.

Alois had already begun talking about his retirement and insisted that they begin saving for that event. Electricity would likely cost more than he was willing to spend, whether or not they could really afford it. He would agree to minor projects, like a new carpet, but electricity? Well, perhaps she could convince him during the rare moments of agreeability that came when she had particularly pleased him.

She smiled, realizing she should have asked him last night. Not only had she applied herself to their reconciliation with fervor, but he had obviously been drunk, which would have made the task even easier. Well, there was always tonight or tomorrow. Last night had been the first time since Adolf's birth that she had accommodated him, and he would likely be all the hungrier for such when he was sober.

Breakfast was still waiting to be cleaned up, but Klara was already busy cutting vegetables for a stew that could sit and simmer all day. Dinner would most definitely be ready when he returned home tonight.

Angela's cry from the sitting room startled Klara so much that she almost sliced her finger instead of the end of a carrot.

"Mother! Mother, come quickly! Mother!"

Klara dropped the chopping knife and hurried from the kitchen. As she made her way into the sitting room, she saw the reason for Angela's distress. Young Adolf was coughing violently, tears forming in his dark, infantile eyes.

Klara swooped down on her baby, lifting him to her chest so that she could pat his small back firmly. "Did he swallow something?"

Angels was very frightened and did not answer straight away. Angela did not know for certain. She was usually very good at watching the baby, but she was only six, and her attention did wander from time to time. She had been fixing her dolly's dress when the baby began coughing.

"Well? Angela, answer me! Did you give him something small?

Did he swallow something?"

Angela began to cry herself, very scared for her stepbrother and at the anxiety in her stepmother's tone. "No Mother! I did not give him anything! I do not think he swallowed anything. There was not anything to swallow!"

As the child spoke, Adolf's coughing subsided, replaced instead by the wailing of a scared baby. In between cries, he still coughed, but not as violently as before. Klara sat in the rocking chair and soothed the baby as best she could. Laying her hand on his forehead, she found he was running a fever. Unlike electricity, the telephone was a modern invention that the inn provided. Individual apartments did not have dedicated lines, but shared a party line. With Adolf still crying, Klara made her way to the phone. Before she lifted the receiver, she looked to Angela, "Take your dolly and play quietly in your room. I am going to call the doctor, and I do

not want you to distract me."

Angela obeyed her stepmother, still fearing she had done something to cause the baby's distress. Yesterday had been stressful enough for the young child, seeing her father hit her stepmother so violently. Now the baby was sick, and Angela felt very much alone and scared. She wished her older brother were home, but he would not return from school for a few hours still.

Klara, with the sound of Adolf still crying into her chest, wondered if she should set the child down in his cradle before making the call, but she had already lifted the receiver, so she put it to her ear. The voices of two women came through clearly, obviously annoyed by the intrusion of a babies cries on the open line. "Who is this? This is not your hour. Hang up now!"

"This is Klara Hitler, in room 219. I am very sorry to intrude, but I have an emergency with my baby, and I need to call the doctor. Would you mind clearing the line? This will not take long . . ."

Adolf's cries were proof enough to the two other women, and they each promised to call the other back in a few minutes, after the crisis passed, and then hung up their ends of the line. Klara dialed a number she had memorized from her four pregnancies and the illnesses of her other three children.

The girl on the other end of the line had not even had time to go into her usual speech of having reached Dr. Ramsfeld's office, as Klara simply began speaking as soon as the ringing tone ceased.

"Dr. Ramsfeld? Is this Dr. Ramsfeld's office?"

"Yes, this is Dr. Ramsfeld's office. Who may I ask is calling?"

"Klara, Klara Hitler at the Gustof zum Pommer Inn. My baby is coughing violently and seems to be running a temperature. Is the doctor available?"

"He is with a patient right now. Can I take a message?"

"I just told you the message!" Klara said rudely, but amended herself. "I am sorry, but will the doctor be available shortly?"

The girl, who did not make a show of being spoken to in such a tone, calmly answered, "The doctor has other patients waiting and will not be making house calls until Friday. I can put your name on that list or you may bring your child to the office, and the doctor will see you by the order of your arrival"

If she had not been trying to become a proper Christian, Klara would have sworn. The deaths of her first three children had surely been punishment for her premarital relations . . . especially with a man who himself was married. Two sins in one act, and she was very much afraid that God's punishment would be to take all her children from her.

"Yes, yes thank you. We will be down right away." She hung up the receiver and set Adolf back in his cradle. He had been fine when she had fed him earlier that morning. She could hardly believe he had become so sick so quickly. Calling for Angela, Klara hurried back to the kitchen.

The child appeared shyly, half behind the kitchen's door, still afraid she had done something wrong, still scared for her baby brother's welfare.

Klara spoke kindly. "Can you get your coat and shoes on Ange? And get Adolf's as well. We need to bring him to the doctor's office."

Angela nodded and disappeared back into her room. Klara was thankful to have the intelligent child at home with her. She now had time to finish cutting the flank of beef into cubes she tossed carelessly into the large stew pot. She did not bother cutting the other vegetables, throwing in potatoes, zucchini, carrots, tomatoes and stalks of celery whole. The stew would be cooking long enough that it would not matter, and it would be just as easy to cut those vegetables later as it would be now. She took no time to add salt or spices, but at the very least, dinner would be hot and ready for Alois, no matter how long she spent waiting at the doctor's office with Adolf. Alois would be in a bad enough mood when he learned Adolf was ill again.

She took just a few more precious minutes penning notes to Alois Sr. and Jr., noting where they had gone and the respective conditions of the stew and the baby. She found Angela struggling to reach through the bars of the tall cradle. She had actually managed to get one sleeve of the baby's coat on already.

"That is a very good job you are doing Ange. You are a big help to Mama right now."

Angela paused to look at her stepmother, recognizing genuine appreciation. "You are welcome, *Mother*. I am trying!" She always made a point to correct her mother when she referred to herself as "Mama." Her older brother had insisted she do so, and even though she enjoyed pestering him, she listened to him far more than she did her real father or her stepmother.

Klara paid no attention to Angela's correction. It was somewhat irritating, even disturbing, given the child's age, but now was not the time to chastise the girl. Klara simply went on dressing herself in a long black frock that would keep the threatening rain from her shoulders. It was early summer, but the storm clouds had brought an unnatural chill to the air.

Dr. Ramsfeld's office was almost four blocks from the inn, but Klara had already spent her weekly allowance on extra groceries and hard candies for Angela and Alois Jr. She had no funds remaining to pay a coach. The doctor would have to bill Alois for whatever services he rendered to young Adolf.

Klara did not bother lugging the heavy baby carriage down the long two flights of stairs, and instead carried Adolf while leading Angela by her hand. The girls' small legs slowed Klara, who, with her large frame, also had a long stride.

"Come along Angela—the sooner we get to the doctor's office, the sooner he can help your brother."

She hoped . . .

It had already rained earlier that morning, leaving the streets pocked and puddled. Despite the dreary weather, the town was busy with commerce. Although Braunau was not a city, it was not a small town by any means. After unloading their fruits and vegetables, farmers drove their empty wagons down the rutted cobbled streets, while workers loaded other wagons with casks of beer or possibly fortified ports. Karla and her children passed a variety of markets as they made their way to the doctor. Klara, worried as she was about Adolf, still had the presence of mind to remember she needed to visit the cheese shop tomorrow, and the bakery, as well. The butcher could wait until Friday, which would give them fresh steaks for Saturday and perhaps a chicken for Sunday dinner. Alois would appreciate her careful planning.

Feeling Angela's grip tighten, Klara took notice of a particularly mangy looking dog cantering toward them with a diagonal gate. In town, stray dogs were as prevalent as stray cats, but they reduced the number of mice and rats, so most were simply ignored as a necessary nuisance.

"Get! Go on! Get away!" At Klara's shouts, the dog changed direction, reversing instead into a dark space between two houses.

But then Adolf began crying again, drawing the eyes of the other women on the street, who stared just to see what the commotion was about. Seeing Klara's pace, young Angela trailing somewhat in tow, they whispered, their heads close together, knowing well where the young mother was bound. Many of them knew the same losses as

Klara—, not a few children had been lost to diphtheria that autumn. The children had joint funeral services, mainly because the town's priest had not had time to bury them with separate rites.

Klara did not look back at the faces that watched her, instead spending her efforts on coaxing her stepdaughter along. "Come along, Angela, try to keep up."

"I am trying, Mother. My legs are tired."

"You are doing very well," Klara encouraged. "We are almost there,"

Adolf stopped crying, but resumed coughing, and Klara grew worried. The cough sounded dry, so she did not fear he had any fluid in his lungs, but she could not imagine what had brought on this cold. The weather had been mild until today; even now the temperature was comfortably in the lower sixties. If the clouds ever broke, it might turn into a pleasant day.

A little less than half an hour after setting out, they at last reached Dr. Ramsfeld's office. The sign read such, but there was also the depiction of a stethoscope for the many citizens of the town who could not read. Klara led Angela up the short flight of granite steps and opened the heavy wooden door to the doctor's office, juggling Adolf carefully. The bell affixed to the door rang, and the eyes of other patients turned to Klara and her children. There were two other women in the waiting room.

The older woman had two boys sitting beneath her outstretched wings, one with a bandage around his head that was already stained with the brown of dried blood. The other woman, closer to Klara's age, also held a baby in her arms. That mother exchanged a fearful look with Klara as she noticed young Adolf. Yes, the tragedy of diphtheria was still fresh in many minds.

Klara swallowed the worry that came in the unspoken understanding of the other woman's eyes and approached the receptionist's desk. "Hello, my name is Klara Hitler. I believe I spoke with you on the phone?"

"Yes, and you can see Dr. Ramsfeld is as busy as I warned." She gestured to the two women already waiting. "Please, take a seat, and the doctor will be with you as soon as he can."

Klara nodded her understanding and led Angela to a pair of empty seats in the small room. She laid Adolf on the shelf of her bosom. His dark eyes were open, looking with interest at the strangeness of these new surroundings, and Klara was thankful that her baby was still alert. He began another coughing fit; there was little Klara could do besides gently pat and rub his small back.

The other woman's baby sneezed, and then sneezed again. Klara could not help but look expectantly, and when the other mother's gaze caught her own, Klara broke the silence. "Forgive me for asking, but does your baby have a fever?"

The other mother seemed somewhat relieved by the question, which had eased the relative tension in the room. "No, not that I have noticed. He has been sneezing like that quite frequently, and he seems to have lost his appetite.

I hope he does not develop one . . ."

Klara nodded, "And I hope Adolf does not start sneezing. These coughs trouble him enough. His appetite was fine this morning, though. This all came on rather suddenly."

The other woman wiped her baby's nose, which had begun to run. "Interesting. My child has been sneezing for the past day or two. I did not think it serious enough to come here, but when he refused to eat last night or this morning, I knew something was wrong."

"Sounds to me as if they both have a cold." The woman with the two boys encircled in her arms smiled. She was the oldest of the three, lines of worry long worn into her broad features. "Be thankful they are not old enough yet to try killing each other." The woman pinched the ear of the boy who had caused his brother's injury. He yelped, and the other managed a weak smile.

"I certainly hope so," answered Klara, echoed by the other infant's mother.

The receptionist rose from her chair and poked her head beyond the counter separating the waiting room from the doctor's practice. "Dr. Ramsfeld will see you now, Mrs. Hinkler."

The woman stood, helping the one boy with a gentle guiding hand, pulling the other through the door by his ear.

"I do not think that woman has ever lost a child," said the other young mother.

Klara looked at her. "You know her?"

"No, but she would not speak so dismissively of a cold if she had lost a child."

Klara only nodded, and then sighed gently. "Well, just the same, she is probably right." Klara patted Angela's head, as much to show the other woman she did not want to upset her girl as to reassure her stepdaughter that Adolf would be all right.

The two mothers then sat in silence. Adolf coughed, and the other woman's baby sneezed, and Klara began to hope Angela would not catch whatever germs must certainly permeate a waiting room such as this.

It was perhaps ten minutes before the receptionist called the other woman and her sneezing baby into the office. As she went into the examination room, the older woman came out with her two sons, offering an encouraging smile to Klara, for which Klara felt oddly appreciative. The woman's confidence was beginning to restore some of her own.

Time passed as Adolf continued to cough. Another patient came into the waiting room while Klara waited. The newcomer was a younger girl, who, by a few inconsistencies in her figure, Klara guessed would soon find out she was going to be a mother herself. Klara had looked very much the same when she learned she was carrying her first child. Somehow, Klara doubted this girl's man was married, as hers had been. Then again, given Alois's record, it was just as likely he was the father of the other woman's babe. The thought was amusing at first, but rapidly soured in her heart.

After what seemed an impossibly long time, the woman and her still-sneezing baby reemerged. She also offered Klara a smile in her departure, which reassured Klara further. Both children would be all right.

"Dr. Ramsfeld will see you now, Mrs. Hitler."

Those were the most relieving words Klara had heard since Angela first called for her that morning. She led the girl by the hand as she had through the streets, entering the office, Adolf coughing as they went.

The doctor was a small man of advancing years who grew his white hair around the baldness of his scalp and wore his thin, rectangular glasses hooked around his large ears, as if they might fall off the bulb of his nose at any moment.

"Hello Mrs. Hitler. I understand your baby is running a fever? And he obviously has a nasty cough. If you could, remove his clothing, and lay him on my table there."

The table was covered with a fluffy white towel, which Klara hoped had been changed since the other sick baby had lain upon it. "It came on him very suddenly, Doctor. He was fine when I fed him this morning, but then he was struck with coughing. I had thought Angela let him swallow something until I felt his temperature."

The doctor nodded, scribbling Klara's account into a leather-bound notepad. "Mmm, and has he shown any other symptoms? Diarrhea, unusual frequency of spitting up or vomiting? You say he ate this morning, so his appetite is intact."

"Yes, and no, he is had no other symptoms that I know of."

"Mmm, good. That is good to hear. Well, Let us have a look at him."

The doctor lifted Adolf, setting him on a baby scale to make note of his weight and length, and then proceeded to subject the child to a full battery of tests and checks, looking down his throat, into his ear, up his nose and into his eyes. He listened to the baby's chest with a stethoscope, to his back and to his belly, the doctor's vein-riddled hand scratching notes onto his pad.

There were murmurs of "hmm" and "ahh" or "mmm" and, of course, "mmhmm"; all the while, Adolf progressed through cycles of crying, coughing, screaming and back to crying again. As there were only two chairs in the office, Klara held Angela on her lap, while the Doctor sat down, made a few notes, and then stood up again. She held her arms about the girl's middle, hugging her gently, more in nervousness than with any intention to comfort the child.

"Well, he does have a low temperature, but this is not his first coughing episode, right? He went through a similar period a few weeks ago, if I am not mistaken. He may have a cold, or he may have asthma. I do not believe it is whooping cough or the croup. So long as the coughing does not become particularly violent, I should think he will recover in a few days at the most. Try soothing his throat with honey, jelly or jam. Keep him hydrated, and watch his temperature. That aside, I am not sure there is much else I can do for him."

Klara nodded, relieved to some extent, but not entirely satisfied, either. "Thank you, Dr. Ramsfeld. You do not think it could be an allergy to something, do you?"

The doctor shook his head in the negative. "Doubtful, not with the fever present. It is the same reason I do not believe asthma is the proper diagnoses. I am afraid the child simply has a weak constitution and will need to be watched diligently for signs of illness more severe than a simple cold. He is not old enough for me to be certain of that entirely, but we will see how he does in the coming days. If his fever rises significantly, or if he develops other symptoms, be sure to let me know. I know it can be difficult for you to bring both him and your girl this far from your apartment, so if he does not improve, call my office, and I will schedule a house call with you, even if I must come after my normal hours."

"Thank you very much, Dr. Ramsfeld. You do not know how much I appreciate such kindness." And truly, whether her relative relief was just striking her, or the culmination of the stresses of the past 24 hours was catching up to her, she needed to wipe tears from her eyes.

"There, there, Mrs. Hitler, I have come to know your family far too well these past few years. It is the least I can offer. I do not mean to rush you, but I am certain there are other patients waiting on me.

I will have a bill sent to your husband, as per usual. Best of luck to you and young Adolf."

Klara thanked the doctor again, and then dressed Adolf. He continued his coughing even as she exited the office, but there was nothing to be done for it, so she would return home and see that he had as much rest as was possible. If Alois chose to raise his voice to her tonight and upset Adolf's sleep, he would sorely regret doing so.

As she returned to their home, she noticed shops were packing up. The doctor's visit had taken most of the day, and she was very glad she had decided on a stew for dinner that morning. Angela was even slower in her walk back, tired from such a long day without her dolly. Klara was sure Alois would be home before she was.

She hoped he would not worry too much as she realized that her note had been incredibly vague, obviously written in a hurried script. Then again, knowing Alois, he would read the part concerning the status of the stew and be content enough to simply eat while he waited for her to return.

Chapter 2

ALOIS SAT BEHIND his immaculately ordered desk, kept so as much out of necessity as personal prerogative.
The desk occupied the majority of his small office, and what little room that remained was given to various file cabinets that held paperwork dating back to the first day he had been given the key to this space. His chair, a sturdy, wooded piece of furniture that in no way catered to comfort, was disproportionately large to the desk it sat behind. It had no arms, as Alois rarely sat back but he had no need for resting his elbows on anything besides his desk, as he wrote reports for his superiors or tickets for violators who thought to circumvent the Austrian government's taxes.

He did not slouch as he worked. His uniform would not permit relaxation of his body, which kept his mind rigidly self-aware. How else could a man focus for hours on series of numbers and associated items that varied anywhere from the amount of cucumbers arriving by wagon to the number of Italian-made shoes that arrived by freight?

As Alois looked over the latest shipping manifest, he recognized the name of the merchant who had arranged this particular shipment and decided he would offer the man one of his special discounts. Italian shoes rarely appeared this far north. Most merchants would bring such wares so far as Switzerland, but this enterprising fellow had a knack for understanding the bohemian culture that was spreading down from Austria's nobility to its middle classes. The shoes arriving that day would be cheaper imitations of the shoes offered to the noble class, but Italian leather was still a great deal better than any found in Austria. The shoes would outlast many of those made by his countrymen.

So Alois sat, tumbling numbers in his head and wondering if overlooking a single crate's worth of shoes would be enough to obtain the shoes that happened to "fall off" the train in transit to shoe his family with the footwear for the rest of the year.

The import tax on such items was relatively low, nothing compared to the tax on wine, which currently ran around fifteen percent a case. No, the tax on these shoes would be somewhere between six and eight percent, and that percentage would be dependent on Alois's inspection of the merchandise and his assessment of its quality. His authority was not so grand as that of an officer commanding troops, but, like any good officer, he knew how and when to use the authority he had.

He would offer the merchant the lower end of the tax and provide the additional favor of overlooking the presence of one crate. In return, he would have new shoes for Klara and the children. For himself, he would find a particularly fine pair of boots, and while he would not dare to ever wear them to this office, he would have them for social occasions. People always took notice of men with fine boots.

A self-satisfied smile had managed to break his normally austere manner. Klara would think he was being so very generous to the family, and his eldest son would no longer need to complain about the tightness of his current footwear. Best of all, the money he might have had to spend on new shoes he could instead transfer directly to his personal retirement fund. What money he did not spend on feeding, housing or clothing his family, he saved for the farm on which he one day hoped to retire. It would be a fitting end to his life of civil service, eventually leaving city life behind to rule a plot of land. It would be a welcome change from the apartment he now rented.

When the door to his office abruptly swung open without so much as a knock, Alois slowly looked up from the manifest, trying to appear as if he were just concluding some calculation.

"Excuse the intrusion, Mr. Hitler, but Mr. Eckhel would like to see you when you have a moment."

Alois laid down the manifest and sat back with straight posture. He did not bother hiding his displeasure. "Thank you, Mr. Faerber, but the next time you barge into my office without first announcing yourself, I will have you working the midnight shift for a month."

The young officer flushed in embarrassment as he made a swift and short bow from his waist. "Of course, Mr. Hitler. How rude of me. I have been in such a rush this morning with the—"

Alois rose from his chair and held up his hand to silence the younger man. "Mr. Faerber, make your apology first. Save the excuse for when you are asked to provide one. None is necessary right now—simply remember not to do it again. "Now then." Alois lowered his hand and gave his uniform coat a short tug to ensure neatness and absence of wrinkles from having sat so long. "I do not want to keep Mr. Eckhel waiting."

"Yes, Mr. Hitler. I am sorry sir." The junior officer turned and walked out of the small office in almost the same step. His face by then was redder than the sash he wore to denote his rank, which kept foreign merchants from mistaking him for a senior customs official. Alois decided that the scatter-brained lad would never mature enough to leave that sash behind.

As he walked down the hallway to his superior's office, Alois wondered if he had ever appeared so foolish in his career as the junior officer. The heels of his state-issued boots clapped loudly on the tiled floor as he walked with the measured and precise steps befitting a senior official—never in a rush, but always timely in his inspections.

At last he stood before the office of Flavian Eckhel, the only official permitted to close the curtains over the window of his office door. Those curtains were closed now, which, despite being Mr. Eckhel's prerogative, was something of an oddity. Alois generally enjoyed seeing who walked his halls, and rarely did someone have the confidence or arrogance to peek into his office window.

Alois wondered what the man could want and sincerely hoped he would not be asked to work another Saturday. Such assignments should be beneath his status by now. Though the pay was good, Alois would be just as happy spending his Saturday morning with the bees he had taken an interest in keeping and his afternoon in the tavern.

His knock at the door was quick and precise. The voice that

answered from within was no less official, so Alois opened the heavy door and entered. The office was spacious, vast in comparison to his own. Mr. Eckhel's desk was nearly twice as large as his, and two cushioned chairs sat before it, whereas Alois had none—nor the room for such.

"Thank you for coming, Mr. Hitler. Please, close the door, and have a seat. Would you care for a drink? I have a bottle of cognac from that last shipment of French grapes. It may help to warm our conversation."

Alois closed the door and chose the chair to the left, putting himself to Eckhel's right, where he always believed he should be. Almost always in control of his emotions, Alois was as surprised by his superior's offer of the cognac as he was the butterflies taking wing within him. "Yes, Mr. Eckhel. Very generous of you to offer."

Mr. Eckhel opened the bottom drawer of his desk and produced a bottle that Alois would never have guessed was kept so close to hand. Eckhel then provided two snifter glasses and poured a fair four-fingered measure in each. Very generous indeed, given the cognac's value. Alois accepted the libation with a nod of gratitude and waited for Eckhel to taste first before lifting his own glass.

Alois had never been a man for liquor, as he usually enjoyed ales or wines. The cognac was stronger than he anticipated, and he could not help a small cough at the sweet liquor's strength. "That is very good," he managed in the somewhat strained voice of a man unused to proofs beyond thirty.

The older man took another, somewhat longer, sip and smiled. "Yes, it is." He set the glass down on his desk, keeping his hand on it. "Alois, I asked you in here to inform you that you are being transferred. Your new office will be in Passau, Germany."

The words reversed the flushing in Alois's face from the liquor; instead the color seemed to drain into his hands, where they turned red, except around the white of his knuckles for the grip on his glass. "Transferred, sir? Not for any deficiency in my performance here, I hope."

"Not at all, Mr. Hitler." The reversion to formal titles had a calming effect on Alois.

Eckhel went on. "No, your performance has been exemplary, despite the occasional—and of course entirely minor—discrepancies I have sometimes come across in your reports. Nothing more than I might have accidentally committed in my time at your position. No, I am afraid the transfer is more due to the politics of things than anything else." Eckhel paused. "You must know that you have climbed as high as you can. Your lack of proper education excludes you from ever obtaining my position. But, even if you could, I am myself not yet thinking of retirement, and so you would be transferred anyway."

Alois only nodded, and then finished the last of his cognac in a deep swallow. The color was returning to his face, as much from his anger as the drink. "I see." There was little else he could think to say.

"You should be happy enough. Passau is at least twice the size of this town. With three rivers feeding it, it is a veritable hub of trading. You will have plenty of work to occupy yourself with, which I know you have always enjoyed. Your experience will be a true asset to our office there, and while your position may be more diplomatic than you are used to, being in a foreign country and such, I am sure you will find your niche as quickly as you did here."

Alois nodded again. He had hoped he was old enough to be passed over for transfers such as this. They had been common enough in his early career, but he had known for some time he would rise no higher and had hoped to finish out his days in this office, in this town in which he had worked so hard to build his reputation. Now he would be dealing with entirely new merchants, new underlings and new supervisors. He wondered if he had the energy to start fresh again, especially in another country.

"I am sorry to lose you . . ." offered Mr. Eckhel at last somewhat awkwardly. He finished his own drink.

Alois recovered his wits and rose from his chair. He set his glass on the desk and offered his hand. "It has been an honor and pleasure to work under you, Mr. Eckhel. I thank you for your praise and for this opportunity to travel. I have never been to Passau, but you paint a promising picture."

Mr. Eckhel rose with Alois, taking his hand while listening to the man's humility. He had heard Alois was a man of great temper, but he had always been nothing but professional in their relationship. It was a true shame to see him go. But Faerber was the son of some minor Baron, and he was due a promotion, even if he were not deserving of one. Eckhel was glad Alois had the sense not to ask who his replacement would be.

"I will write a letter of recommendation for you to carry to your new superior. If there is anything else I can do to help, let me know. Feel free to use the remainder of the day to clean out your office, and tomorrow as well, if need be. I will see you are paid for both. You have the rest of the week to arrange lodging in Passau, but be sure to report to the office there by next Monday morning. Good luck, Mr. Hitler."

Alois thanked Mr. Eckhel a last time, and then returned to his office. There was not much to remove. His personal effects hardly filled a small brown box that had been storing extra sheets of paper. He took his letter opener, a fountain pen, a pot of ink, an almanac, an extra pair of reading glasses and the desk lamp he had brought from home. Looking at the mostly empty box, he could not help but wonder if it was even worth the effort of carrying all the way back to his apartment.

But he wound up making use of the box; he remained at the office late enough to find the merchant and his shoes. The deal went as smoothly as he had known it would, and Alois could not help but chuckle softly to himself as he replayed the conversation with Mr. Eckhel in his head. "Minor discrepancies" indeed; the old badger had known all along about Alois's dealings and had all but admitted having done the same.

He walked back to his apartment by lamplight, the tops of his new boots sticking up above the edge of the box. Klara would likely be worried about him by this hour, but with any luck, his children would already be asleep. It had been three years now since Adolf's birth, and though he was still a child of delicate constitution, the doctor's visits had so far proven to be an expense that was worth the boy's life. No doubt the doctor would come to regret the family's move to Passau even more than the Hitler family.

The key was as loud in the apartment door's lock as always, but the inn's handyman had at least come around and oiled the hinges earlier this year, so the effort Alois made in slowly opening the door was actually rewarded with relative silence. Klara was indeed waiting for him in her rocker, trying her hand at a new stitch, it seemed. The children were in bed, if not necessarily asleep.

Klara looked at the box her husband carried and smiled softly. "Presents?" But she regretted the question when the single lamp in the room cast its light on his face.

"Yes and no," was Alois's reply. His voice was tight, but not stern, as it usually was. "My dinner?"

Klara set aside her needlework and stood, "I can reheat your sausage and beans while you change and get comfortable. Is everything all right?"

Alois could not blame her for not having a hot dinner ready for him and simply dropped the box onto an empty chair. "I have been transferred. We will be moving by the end of the week."

"Transferred, to where?" Concern in her tone was evident, along with obvious surprise.

"Passau, Germany." Alois began unbuckling his belt.

"But why you? Why so suddenly?" Klara was cautious now not to sound at all disappointed in her husband. His temper would be even shorter if the man's pride was wounded, and Klara was very careful to only show support. "They must need your qualities badly in Passau."

Alois, undoing the buttons of his coat, did not look up at his wife. "Yes, my experience is needed there, they say." He would not admit that his inability to gain promotion was the primary factor. "My dinner?" he said again, his patience now beginning to slip.

Klara, understanding that she would have to ask questions after he ate, left him to change into his nightclothes while she lit the stove.

The news was as much a shock to her as it was to him. She had grown very fond of their apartment. Just last year, they had finally put down a new carpet. Now she doubted it would be worth the cost of shipping it to Germany. Germany! She had never been to Germany, and though its culture was in many ways similar to Austria's, she had always seen Germans as a barbaric people when compared to her fellow Austrians. Perhaps it was due to the legends and myths that came out of Germany. Germans were proud warriors, with legends about gods and gold and many other things to which Austrian folk did not pay half as much attention.

Alois changed. For the first time since receiving his uniform, he did not fold it or hang it neatly in his wardrobe, but cast the garments into a crumpled pile on the bedroom floor, nearly kicking his boot through one of the windows in his effort to remove it. The resulting thud against the wall was enough to wake young Adolf, who cried out in his fright. He now slept in the same room as his older stepbrother, Alois Jr., who could be heard yelling at the child to be quiet and go back to bed. This, of course, made young Adolf cry all the more, and though Klara hurried herself from the kitchen to quiet the children, Alois reached the door first.

He opened the door violently, the anger and stress of the day's events combining with his exhaustion and lack of dinner to fire his temper into a quick intensity. "Both of you be quiet! Stop yelling at your brother, Alois! And you, Adolf, stop crying and go back to sleep!"

Klara put a calming hand on her husband's shoulder. "Alois, please, you will wake Angela and the neighbors, even."

But Adolf continued to cry, though Alois Jr. was now deathly silent as he pulled the covers over his head.

"By God, I told that boy to stop crying, and he will, or I will give him a real reason to cry!"

Adolf was old enough to understand his father's words, but he could not stop crying, and began calling for his mother in between choking sobs.

"Alois, go and eat," Klara said, hoping to sooth him. "I will quiet him. He just needs to be held a moment or two. He will calm down."

"He will do as I say! When I say it!" The older man took a step forward.

"Alois, please!" Klara begged, her hand holding his arm as tight as she could.

With a backhanded gesture meant only to gain release from his wife's grasp, Alois instead accidentally struck the woman, who fell sideways into the doorjamb. Adolf, frightened, cried louder. Alois, now free of his wife's grasp, advanced swiftly on the crib in which the three year old slept.

The father grabbed his son and turned him over, preparing to pepper the child's rear until he stopped his crying. But when the boy's cries became coughs, Klara was quick to recover from the shock of being thrown aside and rushed to her youngest child's defense, snatching him from the other side of the crib and taking the truly terrified boy into her arms.

In a voice trembling with fear and anger, Klara said, "Shhhhh, shhh. It is okay, Adi, Mama's here. It is okay, just breathe. You are okay Adi, calm down." She stared at her husband with hard tears in her eyes; he stared back, but said nothing.

When it became apparent that Klara would not flinch, he at last said, "You coddle that child. It is why he is so weak." And with that, he left for the kitchen and his dinner.

Passau was very different from Braunau.

The German city was at least twice the size of the Austrian town, and Alois encountered difficulty in adjusting to the new customs office. His role was essentially the same; he had been neither promoted nor demoted. The difficulty resulted primarily from the fact that he had no reputation here. He could not bully underlings or merchants. He had no idea who could be trusted to provide him with things such as the fine Italian boots he now wore without fear of reprisal.

Alois's work had always given him refuge from his family, but this new small office was an alien place. Because the volume of trade was so much greater here in Passau, he spent far less time pouring over manifests in the solitude of his office and far more walking the loading docks and train yards. His work went largely unappreciated, no matter how long past the closing bell he stayed, and his mounting frustrations were leading to sharp confrontations with his family and co-workers.

At least the confrontations at home were eventually resolved. Klara took upon herself the blame for Alois's anger, doing her best to assuage his ill-temper with intimate pleasures and submissions. And, indeed, because work in Passau's Customs House was far more stressful than it had been in Braunau, it was no surprise when Klara became pregnant again.

Five years after Adolf's birth, Alois again sat outside his bedchamber, reading a newspaper while his wife labored to deliver another son. The arrival added more stress to the Hitler household that could no longer be remedied by Klara, alone. This led to sharper conflicts with merchants and fellow officials alike.

Hardly a month had passed since little Edmund Hitler's birth before Alois received word that he was being transferred yet again. Without a meeting with his superior or any other explanation, he was being sent back to Linz, Austria, where he had worked earlier in his career. He learned of his transfer by way of an official order, stamped in triplicate, without so much as well wishes, and certainly no thanks for his service. The reassignment was almost a reward for the aging man, for he saw it as such. Linz was a city of culture, of commerce he understood better than the hectic traffic of Passau.

It was decided that Klara would remain in Passau with the children for the time being. She did not have the strength to follow her husband to Linz and, given the children's predilections for contracting illnesses, it seemed wise to allow Edmund to remain in the home of his birth until he was old enough to endure the long train ride back across the Austrian border to Linz. There would be weeks, perhaps months before the family could be reunited again.

Fearful of his propensity for infidelity, as well as a number of other factors, she did not want to be separated from her husband, "You will be all right without us?" By "us," of course, Klara meant herself.

"I will endure, as you will." Alois had come to see much of his life as an endurance of some thing or another, but his stoic sentiment could not entirely prevent a tender element from entering his tone.

Klara could not help but feel suspicion for the housemaids or servants Alois might employ in Linz. Someone must launder his shirts and uniform and darn his socks and small clothes, so there was sadness for Klara. She had been a maid herself.

Having given birth to Edmund only a month ago, Klara's ability to soothe Alois's stress was greatly diminished. Was he being transferred because of her failure? Had his transfer been a sham—was he really plotting an escape from his burgeoning family, even if only for a short while?

"It will not be long before Ed is teething," Alois said. "If he is not old enough to travel by then..." but seeing the intense look of denial that flashed across his wife's face, he did not finish his sentence. He should not have even thought of saying what he had almost said. Instead, he shrugged, "Well, I will send for you when I can. You can decide then if the boy is fit for travel."

Klara would have had a very difficult time caring for a newborn and the other children by herself. Although Alois rarely changed diapers, when he was home, he was another set of hands and eyes. Angela also helped a great deal, but she was hardly into her teens herself. Klara needed real help, so she sent for her younger sister, Johanna. Johanna was only three years younger than Klara, but she had much less worldly experience than her older sister. Klara had first left their home town of Spital when she was 16, when she began her job as a house servant during Adolf's first marriage.

Johanna was not given the same opportunities as Klara. She suffered from a cruelly hunched back and was known for her sour disposition. She did not have many friends. This trip to Passau was the first time she had left Spital.

For days after she arrived at the family's modest apartment, Adolf's aunt complained of how long and uncomfortable the train ride had been. How terribly the coach from the train yard had bounced and bumped over the rutted spring roads. She went on about how cramped the apartment felt with so many children underfoot.

Adolf could not help but look at his aunt with a shy curiosity; he was embarrassed about her ailment, which made her hideous in his eyes. He did not know how to look into his aunt's face, and not bear the sight of the horrible curve of her back. He avoided her gaze when she looked at him and ignored her attention entirely when he could.

Johanna settled quickly into her role of babysitter and maid, but seldom left the apartment. Passau was a bustling hub of commerce compared to Spital's farmland. Even without her physical deformity, the young woman would not have had the confidence to venture out on her own in a foreign city. As it was, she only walked the city streets in Klara and the children's company.

"Adolf, hold your auntie's hand," Klara instructed as she shifted Edmund in her arms.

Adolf did not look in Johanna's direction. Instead, he moved to Angela's side. "I want to walk with my sister!"

His sister looked at Johanna, and then at her stepbrother. "Adolf, don't you think you should stay at your aunt's side? She may need your help, you know."

At her step-niece's comment, Johanna made a disapproving "tssk" sound between her teeth.

Adolf looked at his aunt at last, and then back at his mother. "Can't I walk with Angela?" he asked with trepidation.

"Let the child walk with whomever, if it'll stop that whining sound from him." Johanna would not allow her nephew to be coerced with guilt into taking her hand. She knew her appearance frightened the child. There was no reason to embarrass herself by coaxing the child into walking with her. He would either grow used to her appearance or mature enough to hide his fear of her. In any event, pushing the child into her company would only deepen Adolf's fear. Klara could hardly believe her sweet Adolf could behave with such prejudice. Perhaps it was only the strange situation of having Johanna suddenly move in with the family, which would somewhat excuse the child's behavior. Still, it could not continue. Adolf would have to learn to tolerate differences in people. His attitude toward poor Johanna was

not fair to her at all.

"I am sorry, Jo. I do not understand what has gotten into Adolf lately, but I am sure it is just a phase. He will warm up to you soon enough." Klara tried to keep pity from her voice, as she knew her little sister would not accept pity from anyone.

"He is only a child, Klara," Johanna said. "I have dealt with children before. Come, let us get moving before the market closes on us and we waste the entire day." Though Johanna spoke in a matter-of-fact tone, she was hiding her true feelings. She had dealt with children before, and as well as with adults who were not mature enough to either politely ignore her disfigurement or avoid staring at her awkwardly. She would never have children of her own, though. What man would ever ask her to dance?

But her personal problems were nothing to dwell on in the middle of the street. Perhaps later that night, in the lonely darkness of her bed, her insecurities would rise and seize her thoughts, her misfortunes breaking her heart.

The very thought brought a solitary tear to her eye, but she quickly wiped it away with a handkerchief. Not even Klara knew how often her sister sobbed in silence when she was in the privacy of her room.

Johanna had learned that the only way she could be treated as an equal, rather than an invalid, was to speak with clarity and confidence. Her body and her emotions might be subject to her deformity, but her intellect remained strong and sharp. She did not go frolicking through the fields as other young girls might. She did not pick flowers for her hair and sit by the village well, waiting for some young man to meet her. Instead, she sat in her room and read books, which had made her eloquent in speech, despite her farm-girl upbringing.

There were times when Klara found herself jealous of her sister's demeanor. Oh, Johanna could be bitter, even caustic, in her blunt appraisals of other people's behavior, but she had a definite strength in her opinions. "If you don't buy a ham along with that roast, we'll be having beef leftovers for the rest of the week. It is going to rain hard tomorrow. You won't have a chance to go out again."

"How do you know that, Aunt?" Angela should have known better than to question her step-aunt, but she could not help herself. Aunt Jo must have used some strange magic to predict the weather: She was seldom wrong.

"I feel the rain coming," would be Johanna's answer. Almost reflexively, she would reach up to rub the soreness in her hump, but even that instinctive gesture brought attention to her condition out here in public, and so her hand soon fell to her side again.

Adolf looked at his aunt and cocked his head to an inquisitive angle. "You feel the rain coming? How? I feel the breeze, and the sun, but there are not many clouds today."

Klara was grateful for her sister's advice. "Then we'll have to buy another loaf of bread, as well." She ignored Adolf, which was a mistake.

"We'll be all wet!" exclaimed Adolf, concerned by his mother's lack of concern and by his lack of an appropriate coat or footwear. "Mama I don't like rain! It's cold and wet, and I don't like getting wet!"

Johanna shook her head at the boy. "Coming, Adolf. I said I feel the rain *coming*. It will not be here for another day. Calm yourself, your mother is not so foolish as to take you out in a storm."

Adolf considered that statement, and felt embarrassment rising in his young cheeks. "I want to go home." he announced at last.

"After we finish shopping, we'll go straight home." His mother's answer was hardly satisfying.

"I want to go home *now!*" And with that pronouncement, Adolf stopped walking. He crossed his arms over his chest as he had often seen his older stepbrother and sister do. "Now, now, now!"

Klara could hardly believe the tantrum Adolf was throwing in public. Her little boy had never acted up like this before. Why was he being so petulant now? "Stop that. Stop that right this minute. Hold Angela's hand, and keep walking with the rest of us like a good boy. It is not far now to the butcher."

Rarely denied anything by his mother, Adolf could not believe his demands would be answered by his mother's chastising tone. She spoke that way to Al, not him!

Johanna spoke up. "Do as your mother says, child. Walk along with us. Your young legs cannot be tired. Come along." Because his aunt's tone was even stricter than his mother's, Adolf rooted himself to the street and refused to say another word. Instead, he stared with defiant anger at his aunt.

"Adolf!" was Klara's surprised reaction. "Stop acting like that. Stop it I said! Don't you dare glare at your aunt like that."

Adolf blinked at his mother's reproach, shocked at her rising anger. The surprise was too much for his young emotions to handle, and he began to cry.

"Mother would have taken to the strap to him by now," Johanna said.

"Oh, come on, Adi. Stop your crying and act like a big boy." Angela felt some measure of responsibility for her young stepbrother. "Come on, you wanted to walk with me. Let us stop this foolishness and keep walking. The sooner we get our errands done for the day, the sooner you can go home and play with your toy soldiers, okay?"

Adolf wiped his tears as his stepsister's words calmed him. Eventually, he took her hand and began walking again.

"Thank you, Angela," Klara said with no small amount of relief, as she shifted a now-fussing Edmund to her other shoulder.

Johanna, on the other hand, watched Adolf as he began walking with his stepsister. She could hardly believe the intensity that had been in the boy's eyes. They were almost frightening in their determination. She had never seen a child act like that before—of course, she had not seen many children at all, but she knew this behavior was unacceptable. Adolf was very young, but Johanna knew this would not be the last altercation between her and Adolf. The child was just too willful.

In time, the family grew used to Johanna's presence as much as Alois's absence. Adolf would still steal looks at his aunt when her attention lay elsewhere, and he continued to contest her authority in mundane events around the household. He would not help aunt clear the table, but he would help Angela, or even Al.

For his part, Al was able to disguise his feelings for his disabled aunt. He was old enough to understand his aunt's handicap better.

He did all that he could to escape the attention of his family, using his father's absence as an opportunity to break away from what he had begun to consider his family's tyranny. Without his father hawking over his schoolwork and grades, the eldest Hitler son roamed the streets after school, running with a crowd of German boys who found no serious trouble, but enjoyed flirting with it. They made games of stealing from markets or, on one particularly brazen occasion, a wine shop. Although he was never caught, rumors of his illicit activities eventually made their way back to Klara.

She was a powerful woman, but she could not bring herself to strike her children as Alois did. She tried imposing curfews on her stepson, threatening to send him to Linz for his father's discipline, but Al never listened to his stepmother, and his father's authority had left the moment his hand was too far away to swing a belt at the boy.

Taking care of a newborn and three other children was no easy task for Klara, but she was a dedicated mother. She maintained her mild manner despite sleepless nights before Edmund fell into a regulated schedule. It was an immense help to Klara that Angela was old enough to perform a variety of household tasks, such as sweeping carpets or cutting vegetables for dinner. Her stepdaughter showed no increase of affection for her, but Angela's kindness toward her brother and stepbrothers was sincere.

But despite Angela's willing aid, Klara still found herself feeling overwhelmed. Her energy levels had not returned as quickly as they had when she had birthed her other children. She could not make the time to brush her hair in the mornings, instead coiling it into a loose bun that began fraying almost immediately thereafter. She dressed in her simplest skirts and found that without her husband, life was dull and listless.

Alois sent letters that expressed a genuine concern for her welfare and the state of their family, but she did not have many friends in Passau, where people saw her as just another immigrant from Austria's mountainous countryside. Alois's uniform gave her social status, and with his transfer back to Austria, his reputation had gone with him.

Although Klara worried that her husband would be unfaithful, she daydreamed about him during the quieter hours of the day, while Edmund and Adolf napped and Angela and Al did schoolwork. She greatly missed being the object of her husband's desire.

As the weeks passed, Klara noted that other men in Passau had begun to look at her differently. Not as a stranger at the train yard or the grocer from whom she bought her vegetables, but in a way she should only see in her husband's eyes. At first, Klara wondered if she were imagining the eyes fixed on her figure, still full from her most recent pregnancy. Was she secretly hoping a man would still find her attractive? Did she exaggerate the sway of her otherwise-boxy hips when she went to post letters back to Alois?

Edmund had been a healthy baby at his birth and remained so throughout his infancy. They had only needed to summon the doctor once since Alois had left, and that visit had been on Adolf's behalf. The boy had somehow acquired an inner-ear infection, and his subsequent cries

and whimpers would not be remedied without a physician's narcotic tincture. But the Hitler family was otherwise healthy, and Klara waited eagerly for a reunion with her husband. Despite Alois's infidelity and often-abusive nature, she missed her husband. Did he dream of her at night? Did he think of her at all throughout his day?

He must. And yet when she had taken a letter to Alois to the train-yard post office, her thoughts had been as much about the postmaster as they were about the letter in her hand. Was it was sinful to enjoy the complimenting stares of men such as Passau's postmaster? They were only glances.

The postmaster was not the only man to follow Klara's figure, even when she wore the simplest of skirts. Her eyes held the majority of her beauty, for she was kind, and intelligent in her looks. She knew her girlish figure, such as it had been, had long been sacrificed to the births of her four children. Tragedy had bereaved her of the two oldest, but she was still young, and when Alois at last sent for her, she would hope for another child. Perhaps a daughter of her own, since Angela was so insistent of reminding her that Klara was not *her* mother.

Despite her repeated requests about when she and the children could join him, Alois only wrote of how terribly he disliked his new position. Everything was different from when last he had served in the Linz office. New faces, new titles, new regulations and new taxes all made Alois's life even more stressful than his service in Passau had been. He had been searching for an appropriate apartment for Klara and the children, but had not yet found anything suitable for the Hitler clan's needs.

So Klara was left with her worries over Alois's fidelity, and her own need to be wanted and appreciated in that manner. Her fantasies grew in detail and extravagance, soon forgetting the attention of older men for those who might even be younger than she.

A butcher's apprentice, perhaps, less than twenty years if he was surely older than ten, had been less discreet in his looks of interest than more experienced men might have been. And Klara found herself actually smiling at the youth! She encouraged his wayward glances from her eyes to her chest, and she leaned with a certain exaggeration over the glass-countered display of sausages and salami, beef shanks and quartered lambs.

Whatever the reason, the butcher boy's attention quickly became the highlight of her week, for he was very handsome, possessing a broad jaw that might have been too large for his young face if it were not for his broad shoulders. She rarely spoke more than a few words, relating the quantities of shaved bologna she required. And yet, in Alois's absence, Klara could not help but wonder what life might have been like if she had not married her uncle.

Alois was so much older than her. She never allowed much consideration of what her life might have been like if she had married someone closer to her own age. More than one doctor had suggested that the age difference between Klara and Alois might account for Adolf's proclivity for illnesses. Oh, many children suffered ear infections and the like, but few suffered from the frequency that Adolf did.

So what if her lashes may have batted the butcher boy's smile? Weeks had passed since Alois shared her bed. How many maids had kept Alois cozy in his apartment in Linz? The man had surely found an inn at which to stay. He usually sought inns of prestige wherever he dwelt, and Klara knew that even living by himself as he was, Alois would have purchased the finest room there was to rent. That appearance of wealth would attract any number or manner of women to make his acquaintance.

While Klara never actively engaged men such as the butcher boy, she could not restrain herself from privately fantasizing about such dalliances that might lead to more erotic confrontations if she were not so faithfully married. The young butcher-to-be had such sure hands. He made such firm, fluent motions with his blade . . .

"And will you take a cut of the veal as well?" the young butcher said. "I can tell you myself how tender this calf is. It is on special." It was the first time the boy had recommended anything. His voice wavered as he asked, but his hands remained constant in their measured cuts of Genoa salami. Klara was startled from her observations and flushed beneath the powder she had begun applying before going out. She may have an infant at home, and perhaps she was too lazy to comb out her hair in the evening or control it

when it became willful, but she was always presentable.

"I . . ." Klara's startled response was quickly tempered with a kind smile. "It has been a long time since I made wienerschnitzel. Tender, you said? Very good, then."

And the butcher boy only swallowed. Klara felt no shame for her tame insinuation, but she did feel a little sinful. His hands on the young calf meat were very firm, and she would remember the concentrated expression of the young man as his arms flexed against the flesh his knife angled to trim the fat.

So she paid for her purchases, and carrying the wax-paper-parcels of various meats, a mildly flushing Klara began the walk back to her apartment. She resolved she would no longer flirt with the butcher's apprentice, which would be a greater sin than the one her imagination was committing all that evening, while she was enjoying the quieter peace of Edmund's midnight feeding. No, she would be the dutiful housewife, even if her husband was likely to take his own fantasies further than she. She would keep her thoughts private, and in time, become even more powerful because of it.

It was not until early spring of the year following Edmund's birth that Alois began to insist that Klara and the children join him in Linz. By then, Edmund had grown into a healthy baby boy, suffering none of the maladies that chronically troubled Adolf. Perhaps the German doctor, who suggested the family's tensions were the cause of Adolf's illnesses, had been correct. Since Alois had been in Linz, five-year-old Adolf had only suffered one ear infection and a minor case of the flu since. Alois would surely insist that the mild winter was as likely the reason for the boy's improved constitution, but Klara thought the doctor had been right.

As Klara read Alois's letter by the window, she could not help the tear that rolled down her cheek. The man was no poet. His writing possessed the same austere manner that ruled his life as a civil officer, and yet there was a definite loneliness to the words. Klara was certain that the older man had truly missed his family over these past few months. Part of her still feared that he had taken another mistress in her absence, but words almost managed to put such fears from her mind. He was entering into his golden years, and it seemed that his ambitions for promotions were as far from his mind as acquiring new women.

The letter explained that he had submitted his application for retirement, and that he had purchased a handsome parcel of land in the rural highlands outside of Linz. The man may not have a poet's ability to romanticize the new home's appearance, but his work as a civil officer had honed his perception for detail. The letter described a farm that looked out from a high ridgeline toward the Salzkammergut Mountains, where orchards grappled with rocky ground, but produced full and excellent fruit for pies and ciders.

After these past few years of life in the hectic city and the bustling town of Braunau, Klara was convinced her husband had found a piece of heaven. Alois had always spoken of retiring to a farm for a simple, quiet life for the rest of his days, but Klara had thought those were only idle daydreams. She had never believed he would retire from the job in which he took so much pride.

He had clawed his way up from society's dirt. He had been a cobbler's apprentice. He worked long hours, and then studied late into the night to educate himself. He was self-driven, self-regulated, and to no small extent, self-possessed.

But Alois had worked hard his entire life, and at last his dreams had been fulfilled. After forty years of civil service, he finally owned nine acres of farmland in the rural village of Hafeld. Soon he would retire and pass his final years working this land his dedication had bought him. He had his own home, his own land and his own name to pass on to his sons.

The house was surrounded by apple and pear orchards, trees that grew stoutly on a broad ridgeline. The air was sweeter here, open and filled with the scent of over-ripened fruit rotting where it fell. There was so much fruit that they could not use it all.

Adolf flourished in this higher, cleaner air. He spent many of his childhood hours romping over hills and climbing trees. Although no one would call him robust, the rural atmosphere infused him with a certain hardiness, not only to his constitution, but also to his character. He suffered from half as many ear infections and sore throats as he had while living in the city.

Alois Jr. did not fare as well as his younger stepbrother. There was simply nothing for a boy his age to do in this hamlet. He missed his German friends and the mischief they managed to find or create. Worst of all, he was again under his father's roof, and the man's scrutiny of his schoolwork was more severe than it had been before.

"You will never pass the service exam if you do not improve your marks in geography and mathematics, Alois." Al hated it when his father called him by his birth name,

for it was his father's name, and with each passing day, he was becoming more and more convinced that he wanted no part of that man's legacy.

Adolf sat before the hearth, playing with a pair of toy soldiers that cast long shadows from the flickering firelight, but his father's tone distracted him from the battle.

"I am doing the best I can, Father. You see me come home each night and study for hours on end." Al's defensive reply perhaps held too challenging a tone.

Adolf continued to knock the wooden soldiers' bayonets together, but was listening closely to the exchange between his father and his older stepbrother. He would be starting school himself soon, and he wanted to be prepared for encounters such as this.

"You do now," Alois Sr. said. "If you had not neglected your studies in Passau, you would not be so far behind your classmates. You will simply have to work that much harder to catch up. Improve your scores, or you will learn the hard way. My belt will no doubt smarten you with all haste."

Al gritted his teeth, wanting to show what his own belt might accomplish, but his father possessed a man's strength, while he was still years from growing into any measure of challenge for the older man.

"Do you understand me, Alois? Speak so that I am certain. Then we will not have need of this conversation when your next grades are issued. If you do not improve, I will simply punish you first, and we can discuss how you will improve after. Now answer me!"

Adolf had stopped the pretense of playing with his soldiers. He now sat with wide, dark eyes fixed on the older males. He was old enough now to know the vessel which throbbed above his father's right eye meant the man could lose his temper to violence at any moment. He could also see his stepbrother's fists, clenched tightly at his sides.

At last Al let out a breath and slumped his shoulders, bowing his head in subservient defeat. "Yes, Father, I understand, and I will do better."

Alois Sr. narrowed his eyes, forcing the vessel to protrude even further against the tightened skin of his brow. Adolf was certain his father would strike the eldest boy anyway, and Al flinched instinctively as the older man's hand rose. But it did not strike with swift ferocity. Instead, it settled on Al's shoulder and squeezed it firmly. "You have a good future ahead of you if you work for it now. You will not have to climb from the bottom up, as I did. You will start in the middle, and think where you might rise from there."

Al's face was flushed with fear and an emotion akin to hatred, but he nodded and eventually stepped from his father's grasp. "I have a lot of work to do," he mumbled with a strained voice.

Alois watched his eldest son retire to his bedroom, and then looked to young Adolf. "And you," he said, settling into his armchair before the fireplace. "You will soon start school yourself. I know you heard my words just now. I hope you listened to them closely."

Adolf smiled with a child's eagerness to please his parent. "Yes, Papa. I will study hard too. I will get good grades!"

Alois managed a rare smile and patted the child's dark head of hair. "Very good grades, I hope."

Adolf began school on the first of May, when he was six years old, at Fischlham Grammar school. He walked just over two miles, holding Angela's hand the entire way. He never felt the fear that many children experience when they first begin school. He felt very smart in his navy-blue sailor suit. It reminded of him of his father's uniform, though its buttons were painted wood instead of glittering gold. Bedecked in his miniature uniform, he attempted to emulate the self-important, authoritative air his father used in public

Adolf presented himself to his teachers as a very well-mannered boy. He distanced himself from the children his display of authority had forced into roles of inferiority, quickly making as many friends as enemies. These friends were either appreciative of his stoic presence or sycophants that fed their own self-esteem by associating with someone who radiated it. Because his family was not from the region, he had enemies, as well, children who punished intruders.

Although his teachers initially found him shy, many came to learn that he was simply discerning and somewhat elitist in forming relationships with the other students. It was a rare personality to find in a boy so young, but knowing who the boy's father was answered whatever questions that might have arisen. Simply put, the apple had not fallen far from the tree.

As the year progressed and summer replaced spring, it became clear that Adolf was not the smartest boy in class, but he was not a dunce, either. His largest deficiency was his attention span. He had a poor habit of looking out the classroom window more often than at the slate board behind his teacher. The screeching sound of hard chalk on the blue-grey board sent shivers down Adolf's spine, causing him to cringe, both with apprehension and embarrassment. The other students of the classroom did their best to stifle their laughter. Adolf, caught entirely by surprise by the muffled sound, feared for a moment that the laughter was directed at his reaction, rather than the action itself.

"Quiet yourselves." said Mr. Hoff, the teacher. A few students continued to chuckle until Mr. Hoff cracked his yardstick on his desktop. "I said quiet!"

The last boy to stop laughing was Axel Berkowitz, a boy whose horribly pinched face and ridiculously large ears made him the homeliest boy in the class; he also had a speech impediment that gave a gurgling lisp to his speech. With a tremendous nose to match the size of his ears, the boy looked like a great rat. His personality only added to the rodent comparison, as he often tattled on classmates and took whatever opportunity he could to ridicule them.

Adolf disliked him greatly, as did most of the class. Axel was Jewish and claimed friendship with the three other Jews in the class. Adolf and his own friends avoided social civility with the boy.

Mr. Hoff adjusted the small spectacles that balanced precariously on his nose and took out a new piece of chalk. "Mr. Berkowitz, since you are so amused by the chalk's sound, perhaps you would care to solve this mathematics problem for the class?" Raising his eyebrows, he gestured to the chalkboard.

Axel stood, an arrogant smirk already affixed on his narrow face, took the chalk and broke it in half. Mr. Hoff's ruler was even faster than the class's laughter, which was quickly silenced by the sharp crack of lacquered wood striking the boy's hand, still holding the larger piece of chalk. Axel dropped it, the larger half breaking when it landed on the hardwood floor.

"Pick up the smallest piece, Mr. Berkowitz, and stop wasting our time."

Axel, clasping his smarting hand, did his very best to hide the tears that were forming in his sunken eyes, hunching over to pick up the chalk and recover himself. Fumbling with the smallest piece—hardly more than a centimeter long—Mr. Hoff's ruler lashed out again, this time catching Axel on the small of his exposed back.

The boy cried out and could not hide the tears that followed this time. Sniveling, he rose and began solving the long-division problem that loomed before him on the board.

"Remain after class today, Axel. You will carry a note to your parents tonight explaining why they now owe this school a piece of chalk."

Those words broke what little concentration the boy had managed to summon for the problem, and as he forgot to carry a three, the ruler lashed out one last time, this time striking his thighs, just below his buttocks. "Wrong. Utterly wrong, Mr. Berkowitz. Return to your seat."

Head down, the Jewish boy moved gingerly back to his seat. Even with his trousers to protect him, the blow would leave a welt.

Adolf could not help but grin malevolently at his classmate's misfortune. He disliked the boy's appearance as much as his attitude and could not help but feel some degree of satisfaction at seeing the boy dressed down before the entire class. But Adolf's indulgence in Axel's failure was cut far too short.

"Mr. Hitler, perhaps you think you can do better?" Mr. Hoff, however, like most of his kind, possessed a pair of keen eyes in the back of his head.

Adolf's confidence in mathematics was low. He rose, and chose the smaller of the two pieces of chalk Mr. Hoff now offered in his mottled hand.

Adolf erased the Jewish boy's work. Cunning might suffice when intelligence is lacking, but Adolf possessed a certain pride in his youth that dissuaded him taking advantage of whatever portion of Axel's work might be correct. Instead of leaving even a faint smear of the other boy's work, Adolf scrubbed furiously, making sure he truly began the problem with a clean slate.

When Mr. Hoff cleared his throat, Adolf finally laid the eraser on its narrow tray. Then he put the chalk to the board, and with only the faintest sound Adolf began the problem in a very precise hand.

It was not a horribly difficult problem, or else Adolf would have had little chance at solving it. Even at this early stage of his academic career, Adolf was more suited to the arts of drawing and painting than he was to math or sciences.

His concentration was divided between working through the problem and ignoring the eyes of the thirty classmates behind him, who were as eager to see him fail as he had been when watching Axel make his mistake. Worst perhaps was knowing Axel's reddened eyes were also on him. At least his friends would be hoping for his success.

The answer suddenly revealed itself, and what was better, it proved to be the correct one.

"Well done, Mr. Hitler. I think Mr. Ramsden might have solved it twice as fast, but with practice, you will do well."

Adolf took the half-praise and returned to his seat with the full satisfaction of having at least outdone Axel Berkowitz. He tried to catch the other boy's eyes in triumph, but the Jew kept his head down, as if studying the contents of his book to discover where he had gone wrong in the problem.

The weather was still mild enough to allow the students to eat on the school's grounds, so Adolf sat with his back against an old Alder tree while he unpacked the egg sandwich his mother had so lovingly prepared for him that morning. He was soon joined by the few friends he had managed to make at school already.

Albert Mae, a healthy lad, was only a few inches taller than Adolf, with blond hair that seemed like spun gold in the sun. He loved games of athleticism, whether it was trying to swim the narrow part of the river or seeing who could climb highest into the tree Adolf now sat against.

As he sat down across from Adolf, Albert said, "We are going for a swim after school, Adolf. Want to come?"

Adolf looked up from his sandwich. The other boys made no comment about the bow Adolf's mother had tied around the wrapping, as they had learned already that poking fun at his mother's thoughtful actions would only arouse his violent temper.

Adolf was not a particularly strong boy, and still possessed by a relatively weak constitution, it seemed unlikely he would ever grow into anything like a strapping young man. All the same, his dark eyes held an intensity that was his truest inheritance—his father's temper.

The air had warmed while the children were in class—it would prove to be one of the warmer days of summer—but Adolf disliked showing his poor athleticism to his peers. Swallowing a bite, he said, "I do not think so, Albert. I promised my mother I would be home, and it is getting too cold to swim." Unlike his older brother and sister, Adolf almost always called his mother "Mama," in private, but he had realized that doing such would earn the scorn of his peers, no matter how threatening his temper, so he referred to her as "Mother" in public.

"It is a good day to swim." said Berthold Schlage, a child of similar physique to Adolf, but with blond hair, as opposed to Adolf 's dark brown.

Adolf just shook his head. "I promised Mother. There will be other days, I think."

A cow bell rang the children back into the school, and the afternoon's lesson went quickly, though Adolf's attention waned long before Mr. Hoff released his pupils. Adolf had little to look forward to, and so the dismissal surprised him from a daydream of what he might have been doing otherwise that afternoon if his mother did not require him to return home from school straightaway.

The walk home always felt shorter than the walk to school, though in his wandering ways, it often took him twice as long to arrive. Today, he was hurrying as quickly as he had on his way to school that morning. He was not trying to beat the school bell, but rather his stepbrother Alois. He wanted to make his mother happy, and despite Alois's longer legs, Adolf was committed to being the first one home. Given his stepbrother's tendency to ignore his mother's wishes, he would likely be home long before Al, even if he took his most meandering route, but Adolf did not risk that today might actually be a day that Al listened and obeyed.

Despite this commitment to being the first through the door, Adolf could not help but pause to pick a few of the cattails that grew along the riverbank. Most wildflowers had bloomed already, but the cattails were pretty in their own quiet way. He was sure his mother would appreciate them. It was not every day he brought her flowers of any sort, but then again it was not every day that he came straight home as she requested, either. Today she had demanded he be home directly, which was unusual.

"Are those for me?" asked Klara, not more than a moment after Adolf opened the door. She was sitting in a rocker with Edmund tiny and asleep on her lap. Adolf was too old for his mother's lap, but that did not stop from feeling a twinge of jealousy that he was not there himself.

"Yes Mama, I could not find any flowers, but I thought you would like these."

"Well, that was very sweet of you to look, and these are very pretty. Put them in the kitchen, and I will find a vase once your brother wakes."

Alois Jr. soon returned from school, one of the rare occasions that he had actually listened to his mother. Klara then set Edmund in his cradle, and called Angela from her room.

"Children, today was your father's last day of work. Tomorrow he will officially be retired. That means we will see him a great deal more, and while he assures me that he will keep himself quite busy working this farm of ours, I expect there will be no small number of changes in the days to come. For the peace of this household, please be sure to come home from your classes at a reasonable hour. He will be hawking over your studies more than ever, and he has worked very hard for you all to have your education. Make him proud, and take your schooling more seriously than ever. It will make things better for all of us, but for each of you especially."

Adolf smiled with the good intentions of a boy his age, but Al, being older and more experienced, understood that his stepmother was offering not an inspirational speech, but a warning. He had known his father's career was coming to an end, but he had hoped it would not be for another year or two. He very much wanted his own freedom, and with his father home every day, it would be impossible for him to do as he liked. The man's strict adherence to schedules would demand his eldest son to return promptly after classes were dismissed and spend many more hours on his studies.

Hafeld was not half as much fun as Passau had been, but he had just found a circle of friends who enjoyed capers similar to those he had been involved in while he had lived in Passau, without his father's supervision. But now he would have no fun with his new friends. While he waited for his father's final return home from the office, he sat, and instead of studying, he plotted.

Months passed, and life was indeed harder for the Hitler children now that Alois was home throughout the day.

Peasant farming was very different from his dreams as a civil servant He soon understood how backward his retirement dreams had been. Most people want to retire to the life of an apartment in the city, not the long hours of a farm—and for good reason. While he made his own hours and followed his own rules, the actual work was difficult and tedious. The poor quality of the soil effectively spoiled his agricultural efforts, so he never truly reaped the fruit of his labors. So instead of farming his land, Alois spent his hours tending to the bee hives he kept at the far end of the fallow fields, wearing no protection and using only the smoke of his cigar to calm the tenants of his hives.

He spent the rest of his hours either reading the paper and enjoying a glass of wine at the local tavern or peering over his children's shoulders as they endeavored to live up to his academic expectations. Adolf and Angela were both still doing quite well and received high marks. Alois Jr. was not, and did not. In fact, despite their previous father-son conversation, the boy's grades had continued to decline. Alois blamed his son's lack of discipline for his poor grades, but the cause was something else entirely.

The boy had come to guess when his father was likely to be at the tavern instead of waiting for him at home. The few times he had guessed wrong and returned home to find his father nearing belligerence, he had thought quickly on his feet and explained that he had either stayed after class to receive tutelage from another student or stopped at the town's small church to pray for help in his studies. Alois Sr. was not nearly as religious as Klara was, and although he did not discourage his children from practicing Catholicism, he did not visit the church himself frequently enough to ever ask the priest if his son's alibi checked out.

The more Alois tried to influence his eldest son, the more Al seemed to balk at the idea of taking the civil service exam at all. Only Klara had been able to calm his temper the night Alois Jr. proposed he move to Linz to pursue his studies as an independent young man. Alois Sr. refused the very idea, believing his eldest son was still too young and immature to be allowed such freedom. He was only fourteen, after all.

Klara's efforts to pacify her husband's wrath that night eventually produced another member of the Hitler clan. On a bitterly cold night toward the end of January, Alois again sat outside his bedchamber, this time waiting for a baby girl, Paula, to be born.

With this addition, the family seemed complete. There was much of the tension that existed at Adolf's birth. When Adolf was born, Alois Sr. had worked late to distract himself from infantile cries and smelly diaper cloths. Now that he was retired and home for most of the day, the baby was just another source of irritation to the aging man.

Soon, Klara's disfigured sister, Johanna, would also come to live at the family farmhouse. The house seemed that much smaller with these new additions, and Alois's temper became shorter and shorter. When a letter arrived by post in the family's second spring at the farmhouse, Alois's anger might have given him an aneurism.

> To the parents of Alois Hitler, Jr.:
> Your son is hereby suspended from attendance of this institution for the duration of two weeks for having played truant a third time in this early semester. We cannot teach a student who does not display the commitment of, at the very least, presenting himself to class on time each day. Please discuss this issue with your child and instill in him a sense of importance regarding both his education and his

responsibilities to himself and this school. This letter is a final warning. The next unexcused absence will result in immediate expulsion.

>Sincerely,
>Armin Van Yuren
>Head Principle

The letter tore in Alois's hand as his fist clenched on the condemning article. His eyes, reddened and straining in an expression of anger not yet known even to Alois's temper, began searching for an instrument appropriate for disciplining such insolence. His hand first dropped to his belt, but remembering his own teacher's yardstick when he was a boy, he left the belt at his waist, grabbed a knife from the kitchen and proceeded out of the house to the nearest apple tree. There, he took a cutting that was perhaps as thick as the width of his thumb, leaving many of smaller, scragglier branches on for effect. He then quickly stripped off the leaves and a few small, still-green apples, and then returned inside.

He sat before the low fire that was kept in spring's cooler days and there whittled a firm handle into the branch. With plenty of time to spare, the work was slow and meticulous; for Alois knew his son would be late in returning from the classes he never attended.

"Praying, indeed. He had better pray," Alois muttered as he smoothed the handle.

"Who had better pray? What are you doing there?" Klara, having just come from baby Paula's room, did not see the ire etched on her husband's countenance before she asked the questions. Even still, she had heard his tone, and without looking, knew she should have known better than to ask at all.

"That ungrateful son of mine! He has been skipping out on his classes to do who knows what. He is been lying to us, Klara! He has been lying straight-faced to me!"

"Alois . . . he is only a boy. What are you making there?" Klara knew too well and was becoming all the more frightened.

"He is my son, and he will obey me! If my belt is not heavy enough to teach him that lesson, then maybe this cane will!"

Klara shook her head. Nothing she said would calm the man. She was more likely to exacerbate the problem, and so she moved into the kitchen and began to weep softly for the violence she knew was to come.

Adolf and Angela returned home from school first, and Adolf 's dark eyes were full on his father's features as the still-livid man continued to craft his punishment tool. Klara took both children by their shoulders and led them to their rooms.

"Your father is very angry with Al tonight. Al did a very bad thing. He skipped school and lied to your father. Stay in your rooms tonight, and focus on your studies. I will bring you your dinner, but I do not want you to see the punishment Al deserves."

Adolf and Angela nodded in understanding, muted by fear such punishment excites in any child. Angela went to her room and closed the door tightly behind her. Adolf waited for his mother to leave, and then left his door just barely ajar.

At last Alois Jr. opened the door. Outside, dusk was settling, early as it did with the mountains fencing their backyard. All the same, the boy was at least two hours later than he should have been. So concerned with the state of his dinner, he failed to notice the flushed, strained face of his father. He simply dropped his leather-bound stack of books onto a chair and began making his way into the kitchen, from whence the smell of roast chicken with potatoes and rosemary wafted throughout the home.

"Alois . . ." The name was spoken without fury, without heat, without emotion at all. Alois Sr.'s voice was cold, calculated and sterner than the boy had ever heard his father be. He stopped in the kitchen doorway, managing to catch his stepmother's tear-stained face before turning to his father.

"Yes, Papa?" He could not help using the more familiar, almost placating, word. A lump had lodged itself in his throat, while a stone twice its size settled in his gut. His eyes went as wide as his father's after he had read the letter, but the expression on Al's face was sheer terror, not anger.

At last Alois put down the knife with which he had been whittling. The branch now had two hand grips carved into it, with a place for every finger, carved as smooth as a woodsmith might turn a table leg. "I received a letter from your school today. Should I read it to you?"

Al swallowed hard, knowing the letter could only say one thing. He had been able to intercept the first letter sent home after his second absence. He had not expected this one to arrive for another two or three days.

Alois did not wait for his son to respond. "No, no, I did not think I would have to." The man's tone was still frozen and grating, terrible. "Well, what do you have to say for yourself?"

"I . . . I wanted to tell you . . ."

His father stood, hefting the long branch as if testing its weight and balance.

"But I could not!" Al cried. "I wanted to surprise you with my news." The boy's fear was cracking his teenage voice. He was thinking furtively, desperately, for an excuse that would assuage his father's anger.

His father frowned. "What news?"

The words were so deliberately spoken, so heavy from his tongue, that Al stuttered his answer. "T-t-th-that I am going to apprentice, with a . . . a chef."

"What? What chef? What nonsense are you speaking? Your excuse for skipping three days of classes is that you are going to be a chef?!" The words were no longer as cold as absolute zero, but heated into an impossible inferno. The volume of Alois's voice rattled the decorative bronzed plates that adorned the fireplace's mantelpiece.

"You are lying!" Again you are lying, and to my face! You ungrateful, insolent, idiot!" The apple branch Alois held like some medieval claymore now whistled through the air, twisted ends of scraggly branches feathering its end, catching the boy across his cheek, cutting deep scratches into that tender flesh.

Al cried out at the sudden stinging pain, twisting away and falling into a protective crouch that offered only his back to his father as his arms covered his head.

"How dare you disobey me?" The branch swung again, this time held in both hands, the branch's thicker end striking across the small of the boy's back. The resulting crack sounded almost as if it was the boy's back that had broken, rather than some of the smaller twigs.

"How dare you disappoint me?" Again the branch descended, this time on the boy's rear, as the last blow's force had toppled him, so that he now lay prostrate on the farmhouse floor.

"How dare you embarrass me? My name!" With strikes that were as fluid as if Alois was swinging an axe, the punishing branch rose and fell across the boy's buttocks and lower thighs.

"You will not go running off after school now, will you!" Spittle was frothing on the man's lips as he landed the branch against the boy again and again, each time leaving bruises and welts that would be as painful in days to come as if the father had broken the boy's bones instead.

"Will you!" screamed Alois again.

Alois Jr. could do nothing to protect himself; he curled into a ball and cried harder than he ever had in his life—or ever would again.

Klara stayed in the kitchen, knowing there was nothing she could do to help the child. She knew that this one time, Alois's anger had to run its course. She only hoped the father did not murder the son in that process.

Adolf, who was supposed to be studying himself, instead stood a few inches from his hiding place behind his slightly opened door. From that sliver of perception, he witnessed his father's most violent display of abusive punishment. Clenching his small fists, he swore he would never become such a man, would never allow his anger to make him into such a . . .

He would never be such a monster.

"WILL YOU!"
And the branch broke in two.

Chapter 3

"HE IS DEAD to me."
Klara kept her eyes lowered, staring into a cup of black birch tea. Her husband's mood had been even darker ever since Angela had shown her parents the note Alois Jr. had left for her, which explained that he could no longer exist within the confines of his father's tyranny. Since then, Klara had felt very cold, fearful of her husband's wrath.

"Not a single penny of inheritance! Nothing! I would strip him of his very name if I could! Ungrateful wretch! How dare he rebel so openly! I gave him a home. An education. A name!" Alois was staring at his wife, despite her refusal to meet his eyes. They were bloodshot, straining in his face, which looked like an over-ripened tomato, bulged and splitting where his veins pulsed. "I gave him a life! Gave what I had to work for, and he repays me by running away!"

"You gave him everything, Alois." Klara spoke quietly, in no effort to calm the man, but because she had felt overwhelmed and powerless since Alois had punished his son two short days before.

"I wish I would have broken his legs before I broke the branch!" Alois was standing behind his chair, hands gripping the spindle backing so tightly that his knuckles cracked. If he strained any harder, he might snap the hand-turned chestnut dowels.

At last Klara looked up from the teacup and met the horrible visage of her irate husband. "You hurt him enough," she said flatly.

Alois clenched his teeth. He seemed ready to immolate himself in a moment of spontaneous combustion if the heat of his emotion should somehow be converted to an elemental energy. He continued staring at Klara, even as he remembered the severity of his punishment. But he knew no other way of disciplining the child. He had no wages he could garnish from the boy. No miserable shifts to which he could assign the lad, as he did with subordinates who disobeyed him at work. There were no fines or harsher taxes he could impose, as he did with merchants who lied to him.

Perhaps the most difficult issue was that he had not had a father of his own to discipline him. He had learned to discipline himself, as it was the only way he was able to advance his education and his career as a civil servant. His children had not inherited his work ethic, and he did not know how to teach it. He did not know how to reprimand shortcomings, other than using the fear of his corporal punishment. Now even that had failed.

Klara watched her husband as the truth of her words settled within him. She saw his anger replaced with a feeling that was neither despair nor acquiescence. He did not feel regret for his violence, but the void of numbness that is felt once anger has simply exhausted itself. It was resignation.

Klara said, "Remember the Lord's book, Alois. Remember the prodigal son. Al might be gone a week before he discovers how hard life is on his own. He may learn the very lessons you did and become the well-respected and accomplished man you are. Do not hate him, Alois. He is only a boy, after all."

Although his wife's words reached him within his void, they were so distant, so unable to offer true consolation for his earlier anger, shame and disappointment in his namesake, that eventually he was only able to repeat, though in a much calmer, quieter tone, "He is dead to me."

Adolf, like most children, had been jealous of his brother, Edmund, when the boy was born. His mother's attentions were now focused on the baby, and Adolf, no longer as sickly as he had been in his infancy and toddler years, was given less of his mother's concern. And he was jealous. Very jealous, in fact, but he was also intelligent and understood that since Edmund could do nothing Adolf had learned to do for himself; the baby simply required his mother's attention more.

When Adolf learned his older stepbrother had run away, he experienced a different kind of jealousy. He had always loved Angela, for she was as kind and caring for him as his mother had been. She had proven herself in that role even more since Edmund had been born. And yet when Adolf learned that Al had left a note for her and nothing for him, he was very jealous of his stepsister, too.

He was too young to truly understand what step-anything meant. Al and Ange were his big brother and big sister, and just as close to him as he expected Edmund would one day be. He was genuinely hurt by his big brother's failure to leave any parting words for him. What was worse, he could not help a growing sense of guilt for his passive surveillance of the punishment that had driven the elder boy from home.

He could have defended his brother. While the branch rose and fell with methodized rage, he might have burst from the crack in his doorway. He might have grabbed something to strike back at his father with, or perhaps, more realistically (and pragmatically), begged his father to stay his hand.

Instead, Adolf had watched in rooted terror as the branch rose and fell, until it broke. He had only thought of himself, swearing he would never allow anger to move him to such violence. He remembered closing the door quietly once the branch broke and sitting at his desk, staring at his schoolbooks. But he could not study. All he heard were his brother's sobs in the next room, until his anguish must have given way to exhaustion.

The next day, Al had hardly left his room. He had visited the kitchen briefly just before lunch, while their father was again working in the field with futile determination. Adolf had again been plotting battles for his toy soldiers, but his brother's tender, wooden steps were too noticeable not to draw Adolf's dark eyes to stare. Al did not notice, and with a plate of pear slices and a cheese sandwich in hand, gingerly made his way back to his room.

That would be the last time Adolf saw his older brother.

From that point on, Adolf was the eldest male child in the Hitler household. His father's relentless scrutiny of schoolwork and overall behavior was now focused entirely on Adolf, who knew all too well what awaited him if he should fail to meet any of his father's expectations.

Grades would not be an issue while Adolf attended grammar school. He received high marks and even some praise from his teachers for his intelligence and demeanor. He was distant from most of his classmates, but seemed to be the leader amongst the small group of friends he chose. In a small town such as Hafeld, people came to know Alois Sr. rather well, rather quickly.

Once the household had returned to a semblance of normalcy after Al's departure, the new topic for conversation became just how long the family could afford to dwell on a farm that failed to produce crops of any kind. Farm life suited Adolf very well, but it was not as good to his father, who performed all of the farm's chores. After forty years as a civil servant, a peasant life had seemed an ideal dream, but the land was terra firma, not as soft as a daydream. Much of the land was rocky, which might have been obvious, given its proximity to the mountains. What soil there was had long since been exhausted, and might as well have been blighted.

Alois was stubborn at first, flatly denying Klara's suggestion that the family move back to a more urban setting.

"I have never quit at anything I set my mind to, Klara. I do not see why I should now. This was a bad year. Farmers have bad years."

Klara nodded as she rocked Edmund by the fire. "You are right, of course. This may have been a bad year, but bad land does not help. I tried planting my flowers along the walk the other day, and I spent more time digging up stones than I did digging dirt."

"But there was dirt," insisted Alois from his armchair. "The land needs work. Adolf will be old enough next year. He can help me turn the field and fertilize it. A wagonload or two of manure, and we will have radishes and peppers as big as my fist next harvest."

Klara smiled kindly at her aging husband. White had replaced any lingering hints of gray that had endured for so long in his mustache. His head was as bald as it had ever been. "You have the heart, my dear husband, but you do not have the years. This farm needs young hands and a young back to work it."

"Precisely why A—"

Klara cut him off in a louder tone, "And when do you expect Adolf to study if he is working with you in the field? There is a reason farm children grow up to be farmers, Alois. Rarely does it work the other way around. And besides, the young back I spoke of should be in its twenties. Adolf is not yet in his teens."

Alois was quiet then, letting his eyes move from his wife to the warming flickers of the fire. She was right. Though he was stubborn, he was not a fool. His efforts in the field were sincere, but their results were less than encouraging. What was worse, a day in the field left him sorer than had his entire career as a civil official.

"So the Hitler family moves again," Alois said at last. "I wanted to put down roots once I retired. No more being ordered to transfer from one town to the next, all that aggravation. I am sure the children would rather stay here as well."

Klara lifted a sleeping Edmund and kissed his brow. "I know at least one who will not mind."

But Alois was still gazing into the fire, and did not see his wife raise their youngest child. Instead, he could not help but think of the son that was dead to him. At least in leaving here, he might become free of that ghost.

The family sold the farm and left Hafeld for the nearby town of Lambach. The family's new home was set on a small hill that provided a view of Lambach Abbey, but the market town did not offer the panoramic vistas they had enjoyed from their farmhouse. What the town lacked in natural beauty, it provided instead with medieval architecture. Lambach Abbey dominated the town's aesthetics with its size and Gothic motifs. The Abbey was a monastery for a sect of Benedictine monks, who, despite their Catholic alignment, were often be accused of purveying Gnostic ideologies.

Adolf was awed by the sheer size of the Abbey, easily the largest piece of architecture he had encountered in his young life. With stone spires that seemed to pierce the clouds overhead and rows of high-arching windows about its long walls, the Abbey aroused in the boy a sense of importance emanating from the very structure. It was nothing like Passau's city hall, and certainly nothing like the church in Hafeld. The stone and stained glass dominated the town from where it overlooked the Ager River. The Abbey was as awe-inspiring as a medieval castle would be to boys his age. He spoke of it often during the first few days after the family had arrived in the market town. His excitement was so prevalent that his father decided he should attend the monastery's school, and so Adolf continued his grammar school education under the tutelage of the Abbey's Benedictine monks.

There were forty one boys in his class, far more than at his last school. He was given less individual attention at first, but his grades did not suffer. He was an exemplary student, though his demeanor still distanced him from his fellow classmates. Making friends always created instances of vulnerability, where trust was required without having first been earned. For Adolf, offering or accepting such trust was difficult. He had forged bonds with his small group of friends in Hafeld, but already knew he would not see any of them again. Even his relationship with his stepbrother had been betrayed. So when Adolf came to the formality of the monastery's school, he isolated himself in his studies and in the school's rigid protocols. He was, by all accounts, a copy of his father's tenacity and ability.

His self-discipline served him well. He focused his interests in his intellectual love of history and his creative hobby of drawing. He often sketched the surrounding countryside, and even began attempts at recreating the Abbey itself.

One day, Adolf had stayed late after school and sat in the grass outside the Abbey while he penciled a depiction of the Abbey's upper edifices. His artistic eye was already developed enough to recreate the shading that played within the stone's etchings from the afternoon shadows. He had been so immersed in his work that he failed to notice the soft whisper of Friar Roald's robes in the long grass.

"You have a keen eye for details, Adolf. A good mind for proportion, as well."

Friar Roald knelt beside Adolf, and his hand touched the boy on his shoulder. "God has given you many gifts, and you please Him by using them. Do you have any other artistic talents? Music, perhaps?" The Friar's voice spoke with a musical lilt of its own that was gentle, and disarming. "You have a strong voice, and Brother Dominic has commented that students take notice of whatever you say in class, though he admits that such performances are a rarity for you."

Adolf flinched almost imperceptibly as the Friar raised his hand, an instinctive reaction so slight that Friar Roald had not seemed to notice. "I do not like to speak unless I am sure of what I should say." Adolf's words contained no trace of nervousness that his body language might have otherwise just betrayed.

"Wisely said, Adolf." Friar Roald patted the boy's shoulder, and then withdrew his hand. "Well," the Friar's hazel-green eyes narrowed at their edges, as if he were himself considering with care just what he should say next.

At last he smiled and clasped his hands together in his lap, now sitting cross-legged instead of kneeling. "Do you like to sing, Adolf? A voice such as yours is surely as much a gift of God as your talent for drawing. I would like it if you joined the monastery's choir."

Adolf's nervousness was usurped by the Friar's praise. He sought his mother's approval before any other. His desire to make her proud was founded in his love for the woman. His father, of course, came next, but not only for the man's love, but also for fear. Adolf enjoyed the respect of his peers, but he did not always respect them, so their opinions counted for less. To hear praises from Friar Roald, though, a man he neither loved nor feared, but certainly respected greatly, was one of the greatest experiences of his young life.

"My mother and sister both sing beautifully." Adolf spoke as he began to smile, "I would very much like to learn to sing as well."

"Excellent. Your parents will be very proud. The choir rehearses for performances in the Sunday mass three times a week. You may attend your first rehearsal practice tomorrow, an hour after your classes dismiss. Inform your mother that you will be late from school, and perhaps see if she will pack you a snack. Rehearsals generally last an hour and a half, so you may be late for your supper." Friar Roald reached out again, this time to pat Adolf on his thigh.

Adolf normally hated to be touched by anyone. His brother had often beaten him as older brothers tend to do, and of course he was the recipient of his father's abuse often enough, but he did not flinch again when the Friar patted his thigh. He only listened to the man's words and smiled with unbridled excitement. His parents would be very proud indeed, but his beloved mother especially. She was always humming some tune or another around the house when his father was not home and demanding silence.

"Perhaps you will come to find you like singing even more than you like drawing," Friar Roald continued. "I cannot help you to draw any better, but I might help you sing. If you find you enjoy the choir and would like further instruction, come to my office after class on the days you do not have rehearsal. I can give you more individual attention, there."

Adolf smiled broadly and closed his notebook, leaving the sketch of the Abbey unfinished. "Thank you, thank you very much, Friar Roald. I can hardly wait to tell my mother!"

Friar Roald at last stood. He was young by comparison to most of his brothers in the Abbey, but the top of his dark head had just begun to bald, and hints of gray peppered his sideburns. The wrinkles at the edges of his eyes and brow were shallow, and his belly had yet to develop the paunch that most holy men acquired from brewing ales within the Abbey's walls. He smiled back to Adolf, again looking down at the boy. "You are deserving and so very much welcome. I look forward to our future meetings. For now, I think it is time you headed home."

Adolf stood and offered the Friar a formal bow of respect, and then another smile of gratitude. The Friar continued to smile, and then gave a small wave of his hand before turning and walking back to the Abbey's high-arching doors.

Wasting no time, Adolf ran through the broad, cobbled streets, up the hill, to where the family's new home overlooked the Abbey.

He arrived just as his father was returning from the nearby tavern. Alois had been drinking a glass of wine or two more than was his usual while reading the day's paper, and was somewhat unsteady as he made his way into the kitchen for the dinner. He rarely drank beyond a glass at a time these days, but the paper had proven to be an inadequate distraction from his thoughts that day. Seeing Adolf run through the streets, and with thoughts of his eldest son swimming in his sloshed mind, he instantly assumed the worst.

Adolf had no idea that his father had been brooding over his stepbrother's desertion, and was excited, though out of breath still, when Alois entered only a few steps behind him.

"And just what are you running from, boy?" Alois slurred, moving toward Adolf.

Adolf, bent double with his hands on his knees as he stood in the kitchen, still trying to catch his breath, lost the excitement and elation that had propelled him with such alacrity up the steep hill. Fear at his father's tone and state instead seized him, and his attempts at catching his breath quickly became coughing, and then choking for air.

"Answer me, boy! What were you running from?" Alois took a step forward and faltered, needing to catch himself for a moment on back of one of the dining chairs. His face was red from the wine and the added pressure of his unwarranted anger.

Klara was again caught in the confrontation, seeing that Adolf was experiencing the sort of attack he had not suffered since having left Passau. "Stop it, Alois! You are scaring him!" She undid the bow of her apron and removed the garment so that its stains did not transfer to Adolf's school uniform as she hugged her boy to her, putting herself between Adolf and Alois, with her back to the man.

She held Adolf to her, gently rubbing his back and patting it with her hand, the way she had when he was a baby and unable to regain his breath. Adolf had no idea why his father was so angry, but in his mother's embrace he relaxed and calmed enough to at least breathe again. Had his mother not reached him when she did, he would have passed out entirely.

"Step away from him, Klara." Alois's voice had taken on a different tone, no longer slurring, but possessed of the searing clarity of a man whose frustration was not in the moment, but fueled by past transgressions: the absence of his eldest son and the cumulative frustrations of children who continued to be disobedient.

Klara, feeling her boy's breaths even out, at last released him from her arms and turned to face her husband. "Be calm, Alois, and let him speak now that he is able. He was smiling when he came here so out of breath. I doubt he would smile if he had done a wrong."

Alois was still thinking of his departed son and how that boy had lied so easily to his face. Would Adolf not have the same capacity? "I asked him a—" Alois swallowed hard and closed his eyes against the sudden stab of pain the pressure of his blood put in his temples. "I asked him a question, and I will have my answer."

Klara saw the older man's discomfort, but she had little sympathy for him. Ever since they had left the farm, Alois did little else besides spend his days at the tavern, and while he hardly ever returned drunk, he certainly never returned happy. They had been in Lambach only a few weeks now, but already Klara wore longer sleeves to hide her new bruises.

"I have good news, Papa." Adolf at last spoke, a hint of a smile returning to his face now that he remembered the Friar's words. "Friar Roald complimented me today. He also asked me to join the monastery's choir. We practice three times a week and perform in the Sunday mass!"

Klara forgot her husband for a moment and gave Adolf a great tight hug that was very different from the soothing embrace in which she had held him moments before. "That is wonderful!" She kissed her boy on the top of his head. "You have a very fine voice. I am sure you will sing like one of the Lord's angels."

Alois regretted his own foolishness, but his ego allowed for no semblance of an apology. Instead, he focused on what he considered the more pragmatic issue. The heat was still in his face, flushed by the wine and emotion, but now at least his anger had passed. He had reverted to that feeling of being within a void. At least he had recovered enough sense to avoid slurring his words. "Three times a week? What of your studies? Singing will not find you a job, Adolf. Your studies will."

"You have seen my marks, Papa. I could not do any better unless they created a grade above best. Even Friar Roald commented on my ability. He thinks I have a strong voice and said the choir will be good for me. I will still have plenty of time for my studies at night. I will stay up later at night if I must."

Alois pushed his bottom lip into the upper and sighed through his nose, which was as much of a blessing as Adolf would get from his father. The boy was disappointed that the man had not reacted with the pride Adolf had hoped the news would elicit. At least his mother was as pleased as he expected she would be, and so he smiled all the same.

"When do you start?" Klara asked as she began setting dinner on the table.

"Friar Roald says I may attend tomorrow's rehearsal." He did not mention the Friar's offer of private lessons, only because he was not himself yet sure he would like singing at all. He thought it best to wait until he attended such a lesson before mentioning what the Friar had said.

"Well, I will have to pack an extra sandwich for you tomorrow, then. I would say we could have late dinners, but that is not fair to your father or sister, and soon Edmund, too." He had not even needed to suggest a snack as Friar Roald had instructed. His mother knew to include the extra contents from her own motherly care.

Adolf shrugged. "I will eat the leftovers whenever I get home." He looked between his parents and, At last smiled, saying. "I like it here."

Alois looked at Adolf, but then dropped his eyes and began eating the chicken pie that was tonight's dinner. The boy might be happy in this town, but he had not been happy since leaving Hafeld. He had not been really happy since leaving the customs office.

And, as much as his namesake was dead to him, he had not been happy since Alois Jr. had run away.

As the months passed, Adolf continued to do well in his classes and his singing, in which he had soon found himself adept. His grades ranked him in the top fifth percentile of his classmates, and he discovered in the choir an artistic joy that was very different from his drawing efforts. His drawings were so self-concentrated, so private to him, for simple lack of a larger audience. His singing, by contrast, was a very public affair.

Each Sunday, he was given the opportunity to display his talent for the pleasure and approval of the entire town, attention that was both pleasing and empowering. Adolf felt exhilarated by the performances. In the moments between songs, he would look out at the audience, imagining himself in some grand opera hall. He dedicated himself so thoroughly to singing that the day came when Friar Roald asked if Adolf would like the opportunity to sing a solo.

He had not met with the Friar for private lessons very often. The time he spent at choir rehearsal detracted from his schoolwork, time that Adolf was not willing to sacrifice, lest he disappoint his father. He was quite certain that his father would forbid him from participating in the choir if his grades ever slipped. Just the same, he did meet with Friar Roald occasionally, and those meetings had always taught Adolf a great deal about music. The Friar had taken a special liking to Adolf, as he often singled out Adolf's harmony for praise. This only increased the distance Adolf placed between his fellow classmates and himself.

"Yes, Friar Roald, I would be very happy to perform a solo."

Friar Roald smiled broadly. "Wonderful. You will do your parents and the entire town very proud, Adolf. But," he added quickly, "you must agree to visit my office more regularly for private instruction. I do not have time to teach the entire choir the things a soloist must know. Come to my office after class on Thursdays, and we will have you ready to perform for the Easter masses."

The first of such meetings did not last long. Friar Roald complained of a headache that had been bothering him all day, so Adolf was only given a set of breathing exercises to improve his overall lung capacity. Without ever singing a note, a mildly disappointed Adolf returned home to work on his studies.

The next meeting was very different. Adolf entered Friar Roald's office and found the man smiling softly behind his desk. A bottle of wine was open, a pair of glasses sitting next to it.

"Adolf!" said the Friar. "Come, have a glass of wine with me. It will help to warm and relax your throat."

Adolf set his books on the Friar's desk and sat in the stiff, walnut-stained chair that offered very little comfort. Rarely did anyone visit the Friar's office, unless it was for punishment or repentance, which the stark furniture reflected. "Yes, Friar, I would like that."

The Friar continued to smile, emptying the bottle with the measures he poured for Adolf and himself. If the Friar had been drinking previously, as the bottle might have suggested, only his smile might have betrayed such, and Adolf believed it was genuine enough. The Friar was probably as excited to teach as Adolf was to learn.

Friar Roald sipped and made a sound of satisfaction. "That is very good." He set down his glass and settled his hazel eyes on Adolf. "I trust you will not tell your classmates I offered you this glass. In fact, it is probably best if you do not tell anyone of what we do here. Private lessons are private for a reason. Some people would not understand why we do some of the silly exercises I am going to show you. Do you understand?"

Adolf looked over the brim of his glass as he took another sip. The wine had already worked color into the corners of his cheeks, and his throat was indeed warmer. He could feel the wine draining into his belly and beginning to warm that, as well. He set down the glass and nodded. "Yes Friar, I understand."

Friar Roald smiled again. "Good. So long as I have your word,

I think we will both enjoy these meetings a great deal. Now then, finish your wine so we can get to work."

Adolf still had more than half his glass left, and the strong wine was difficult to drink. He did not particularly like the taste or the warmth that was spreading through him. Under the Friar's scrutiny, however, he drained what remained in his glass before setting it back on the table.

"Excellent. Now then, have you been practicing the exercises I showed you last week? Let me see you do them."

Adolf had indeed been practicing. He breathed in slowly and steadily for a measured count of four, keeping his lips formed in the shape of an o. He then breathed out for the same measured count, and then repeated the process, this time breathing in for a count of five. He continued the cumulative repetitions until his count reached ten. By then, he was taking very long, very deep breaths. With the wine coursing through his system, he soon felt light headed, almost giddy.

Friar Roald watched the boy. His eyes were first on the perfect o Adolf's mouth made, and then he focused more on the steady rise and fall of the boy's chest as his breaths deepened. "Mm, that is good. Very good, Adolf." The Friar finished his own wine.

Adolf then sang his scales for the Friar, and when he finished those he felt very good indeed. He found that the wine had given him confidence to his pitch that in the past he might have tried to compensate for by sheer volume. He then sang the hymn in which he was supposed to solo, though the Friar stopped him before he reached what would be his entrance.

"Well sung, Adolf. You are singing as you do with the chorus, which is how you should. Save your unique voice for your solo, so that your sound will be all the more profound to the audience."

"My unique sound, Friar?" Adolf did not have any idea what Friar Roald could possibly mean.

The Friar rose from his chair and came to stand in front of Adolf. "Yes. When you sing with the rest of the choir in the chorus parts, you have been taught to blend your voice to those around you.

Now, you must stand out. Stand apart, and reveal your unique voice. Sing with inflection. You must sing with a personal passion. Raise up your voice to the Lord, and he will listen with joy. Your family will listen with joy. Now, sing your solo as I have described."

Adolf did his best to follow the Friar's instructions. He sang with passion for the words and notes alike. He anticipated notes to add emphasis to them. He managed his crescendos without straining or over-singing the notes of fermatas. He sang without being flat or sharp, and used every skill he had learned over the past few months since joining the choir. Those skills, combined with his natural talent and recently discovered keen ear, made his voice impressive and beautiful as it resounded in the Friar's office-space.

The Friar smiled warmly as Adolf finished his solo. "Excellent. Very well done, Adolf. Your parents will be very proud indeed, but we have work to do still. You must use your diaphragm more to reach the higher notes, instead of relying on your vocal chords so heavily."

Adolf nodded, and tried again to sing as the Friar instructed. He thought he understood what the Friar had meant when he said to use his diaphragm, but he could see from the Friar's face that he was still doing something wrong.

"Your diaphragm, Adolf. You sing with your gut, not with your chest. Here." The Friar took Adolf's hand, and placed it on his stomach over his brown robes. Friar Roald then sang, and revealed a sonorous voice that Adolf would never have believed could belong to the slender man. He felt the man's muscle moving beneath his robes as his voice climbed and descended a scale.

Adolf believed that he understood and tried again to sing as Friar Roald had, but the Friar was again shaking his head in the negative.

"Closer, but still not right. Here."

The Friar put his own hand on Adolf's belly. The Friar's other hand came to rest on the boy's buttocks. He pressed gently then on Adolf's stomach. "Sing," said the Friar, very softly.

Adolf tried to sing, but never liked being touched, and the Friar's proximity made him nervous. His voice, strained by his discomfort, sounded far worse than before. Still, he did become aware of what Friar Roald was explaining as he felt his diaphragm move when he climbed an octave in the scale of e flat.

Adolf felt very uncomfortable. The Friar's hand had moved bellow his belly button, and now pressed itself against his abdomen. The hand on his buttocks had firmed its grasp ever so gently, now cupping one cheek through his twill trousers. The Friar had bent slightly to position his hands in this manner, which put the Friar's lips rather close to Adolf's ear. The man spoke softer than he had in his previous instructions.

"You are far too tense, Adolf. You must relax yourself to sing properly. Relax. Would you like more wine?"

"No, Friar. I will . . ." Adolf swallowed in an effort to dispel his discomfort. "I will relax. I am not used to anyone being so close to me."

"Relax and sing, Adolf. I am only here to help you. You may come to enjoy my closeness. There is nothing to fear, just relax and focus on your notes."

Adolf could smell the wine in the Friar's words. The man was so close that Adolf could feel warm breath on the nape of his neck. He closed his eyes and again tried to sing, but as he came to the highest note of his falsetto measures, the Friar's hand fell further and pressed what his mother had told him was a very private place. The boy's voice cracked, and he jerked himself instinctively away from the Friar's hands.

"Adolf, you were doing so well. What happened?" The Friar spoke in the most innocent and normal of tones.

Adolf was not sure himself. One moment he was singing like an angel, and the next he was being fondled. Except, he was not sure that was what happened. The Friar seemed so matter-of-fact about this lesson that Adolf could not help but feel guilty and embarrassed by both his discomfort and his reaction. He was standing just a few paces from where he had moments before, but he felt as if he were looking across miles at his teacher.

The Friar recognized the scared and confused look the boy was giving him, but did nothing to credit or validate it. Instead he continued speaking calmly and naturally. "I cannot properly instruct you if you are standing over there. Perhaps you are too tired to continue this exercise. It is okay to be uncomfortable. Many people experience apprehension when trying a new thing. We can try this exercise again some other time, and we will see if you do not feel better about it then."

Adolf was silent, staring at the Friar while he regained the breath that surprise and shame had stolen from him. Had he been rude to have jerked away like that? The Friar only wanted to help him, and he had been very kind to him all these months now. He should trust the man, and yet he knew he should not. He could still smell the man's breathe and feel it on his crawling skin.

At last he said, "I—I think I am just tired, Friar. I am . . . I am sorry."

The Friar only nodded. He then moved back to the chair behind his desk and sat. "It is all right, Adolf. Learning to be so great as you could be takes time. Time and trust. You do trust me, do you not, Adolf?"

Adolf did not speak, but nodded.

"Good. Go through your breathing exercises one last time, and then we can be done for the day."

Adolf nodded again, glad that he only had to breathe and not sing again before he left. He still felt very strange inside, and the giddy feeling the wine had imparted was now soured into a sickly feeling. Perhaps most confusing of all, while he was certain he did not like being touched, especially how the Friar touched him, he was not sure that he disliked the feelings that touch had stirred in him. Somewhere beyond the surprise and past the embarrassment, guilt and shame, there was the smallest hint of enjoyment.

Friar Roald had no idea what Adolf had thought or felt about the entire experience, but that briefest moment of contact, even through the fabric of school uniform trousers, had been enough to excite the Friar in a way he had not known since he had taught his last prodigy a few years before. Once the boy left, he would open another bottle of wine, and his excitement would turn to ecstasy and, ultimately, satisfaction when these memories combined with his own imagination. Surely a lifetime of serving the Lord, living here in the Abbey, would redeem his soul of being guilty of such sin.

Adolf went through his breathing exercises, which calmed him further as he progressed from counts of four to ten. He did not even notice the glint in the Friar's eyes, which were fixated on his mouth. At last the exercise was done, and the wine's effects were diminishing into a drowsiness that would couple with Adolf's emotional exhaustion. He doubted he would even eat dinner once he reached home. He had lost his appetite and wanted little else besides the solitude of his room.

"Keep practicing, Adolf. You did well today. Very well. I will see you in rehearsal tomorrow, and I look forward to our meeting again next week." The Friar rose and moved to the door, where he paused, his hand on the doorknob. "And remember, Adolf. You have promised not to mention anything that we do here to anyone. I have your word, and the Lord has it also. Say hello to your parents for me, Adolf."

Adolf did not cringe when the Friar patted him on his head before the door opened. He just nodded and began the long walk through the Monastery's cold halls. He was very slow in his walk from the Abbey up the long hill to his home. Too many thoughts and feelings filled his young mind, and if it were not for the cold weather that day, his mother would surely have questioned why he returned home with his cheeks so red.

Adolf's trials should have been over for that day. With the cold wind chapping his lips and lacing through the grogginess that lingered from the Friar's *reward*, he walked with dour purpose toward his home. His demeanor was sullen; his cloudy appearance would not provoke a courteous exchange of conversational pleasantries from any of the hardy folk that walked the cold streets. He could not have been more startled by the stranger's voice calling out to him from a storefront doorway.

"You there, be a good lad, and take a small job for a modest wage?"

The elderly gentleman was holding a short leash on a handsome Shepard pup. His attire was common to any member of Lambach's affluent upper class: A long, brown trench coat covered a tweed suit that doubtlessly fended off the brisk air better than Adolf's own attire. He really should have listened to his mother that morning, when she had told him to wear his heavier woolen coat.

"You like dogs, don't you?" the gentleman continued. "This shopkeeper won't let me take Kaiser into the store with me. Even leashed! Against store policy, he says!" The gentleman sounded absolutely incredulous of the store's draconian laws.

"Of course you like dogs," the man continued. "What is a boy without a dog? Here, take Kaiser's leash, and simply hold him until I conclude my business within this uncompromising establishment. There will be a coin in it for you, and two if you can keep him from barking at the fine ladies who might happen by. He is a real dog when it comes to the ladies, if you understand me." The man winked.

Adolf did not. He did, however, understand that this was a good opportunity to make a little extra money.

"Very well. Will your dog obey me?" asked Adolf at last.

"Certainly!" exclaimed the gentleman, holding out the dog's leash for Adolf to seize. "Thank you so much for your help. I will not be more than a moment. Just a short minute, dear boy!" And without any further instructions, the man left Adolf standing with Kaiser's leash gripped tightly in his hand.

The Shepard pup was content to rest on his haunches and wait with a playful sort of patience. The pup's tail wagged vigorously from side to side, and a mischievous glint was in his eyes. After a few moments, Kaiser pushed his moist black nose closer to Adolf, giving him a tentative sniff before backing off again.

The pup was old enough for Adolf to feel cautious. Shepards

were powerful dogs when grown, and while Kaiser was not yet in the prime of his puppy-hood, he would still be a challenge to keep under control if the animal decided to bolt after a stray cat. What the owner had said about his pet's behavior when encountering the fairer sex must have been an exaggeration for comedy's sake. Adolf saw no sign of it.

"You be a good dog, and you will be rewarded, the same as I am being rewarded for holding your leash." He did not feel quite so groggy now that he had been charged with a responsibility, especially because his task was appointed and carried out in public. His mind moved pendulously between the furry charge at his feet and the soured, lingering taste of the Friar's tainted port. The wind still whipped outside the storefront's embrasure, and it was only becoming colder as the day moved closer to night.

"Here, boy, let's find you a stick." Perhaps he could entertain the dog until his owner finished his purchases within. Adolf had not even bothered to notice what it was the shop sold. He was still in shock since waking from his final lesson with Friar Roald.

"This one. This one here." Adolf bent and retrieved the small stick that lay in the street just out front of the shop. "Can you fetch? Fetch."

The stick did not travel far. Adolf had no desire to be suddenly yanked by the pup, so he had taken careful aim to land the stick within the leash's limits. It was a very small stick, almost a twig, and certainly no thicker than his finger. Playing with the pup was better than thinking about school or breathing exercises.

Kaiser dutifully bounded after the short toss. The dog's eyes had not left Adolf's hand since the boy bent and took up the stick.

"Good boy." Adolf did not cheer the dog or speak with a tone of praise. The compliment was as much an affirming command. "Now come."

Holding the stick in his mouth, Kaiser looked toward Adolf. The pup's ears perked toward Adolf, but Kaiser did not return to him. Instead, the dog sat in the street, entirely unbothered by the cold wind whipping past the storefront. Now the dog pinned one end of the stick with one paw, holding it levered over the other paw, and gnawed contentedly at its elevated end.

"I said, *come*." Adolf enforced his command this time with a firm pull of the leash.

The dog was hesitant at first, but Adolf continued to call and pull Kaiser closer. At last, Adolf could reach out to take hold of the stick in the dog's mouth. "Drop it."

Instead, the young Shepard bit down harder on the wood and began to back away. Adolf tightened his own grip, again commanding the dog to release the stick. "Come on boy, drop it. Give it to me, I said!" But the harder he pulled, the harder the dog pulled back. Kaiser started to growl and tossed his head in an effort to wrench the stick from Adolf's grasp.

Surprised by the aggressive sound of growling, Adolf's other hand grabbed the pup by his throat. He squeezed tightly and still pulled at the stick. The Shepard's growl became strangled yelps of pain, and at last Adolf let go. With the dog's throat still in his grip, Adolf used the stick to discipline the pup. He hit the dog on his snout repeatedly, until the twig snapped in Adolf's hand.

Without thinking, Adolf rose and gave the dog a swift kick in his ribs. "Stupid dog!" He dropped the half of the stick he still held and left it in the street, covered in drool that would soon freeze in the cold air. "Useless mongrel. No wonder you are not allowed in the store. You probably do not listen to your owner any better. Next time, obey your master!"

The pup whimpered and continued to back away from Adolf. Now free of Adolf's grip, the dog tried to back away from Adolf as far as he could, but whenever he began to pull against the leash, Adolf would pull back much harder.

"*Come*." Adolf commanded, expecting the dog to have learned his lesson. Unfortunately, the dog had, and was staying away from the ill-tempered boy. Adolf would not abide being ignored. He would not be disobeyed by a stranger's dog. "I said, *come*!" But the step he took toward the pup only frightened him more, and because it could no longer back away, Kaiser simply lay against a stone wall and whimpered with his head down and tail tucked tightly between his legs.

Adolf no longer had any patience for the animal. Whether or not he was someone's pet, Adolf wanted nothing more to do with him. "Stupid dog." Adolf repeated, just before aiming one last kick at the animal. Kaiser had only wanted to play, and his whimpers did nothing to soothe Adolf's outburst of rage. Cringing had never slowed the strike of his father's hand, either.

The dog dodged away from that second kick and cowered against the shop's front door. Adolf was breathing hard, surprised by how easily the dog had made him lose his temper. He looked around the street, to see if anyone had seen his interaction with the dog. So close to the dinner hour, the street was all but empty, and the stranger who owned the dog still bartered within the ... wine shop? Looking in through the shop's door window, Adolf finally noticed why the dog was not allowed inside.

At last, the dog's owner emerged with a large brown bag tucked into the crook of his left arm. Kaiser darted away from the door as it pushed open, and Adolf gave the animal a final sharp tug of his leash to bring him to heel. The owner hardly seemed to notice the pup's yelp.

"Thank you, young man. I am sorry that took so long. That store's proprietor is a thief as well as a tyrant! But his is the only shop that stocks my favorite vintage of French wine. Anyway, you managed to keep Kaiser quiet enough. I hardly heard a sound over the wind out here. I am sure you are anxious to be on your way home again. Sorry to have troubled you, but I hope this at least makes it worth your while."

Adolf accepted the two silver marks the man pressed into his palm, speaking with an arrogant tone the stranger found odd in one of Lambach's youth. "Your dog is ill-mannered and ought to be taught to properly respect the holder of his leash. Don't worry though, I showed him who is master."

The gentleman raised an eyebrow as he took his dog's leash back from Adolf. "Indeed . . . well, thank you once again."

Adolf gave the young Shepard a quick pat on his head, even as the dog was recoiling from his touch. "Good boy," spoke Adolf, before dropping the silver pieces of his payment into his coat pocket and continuing on to his home.

By the following Thursday, Adolf had largely forgotten the discomfort of his last meeting with Friar Roald. He had performed that Sunday and attended both rehearsals on Monday and Wednesday, during which the Friar was as kind and natural with Adolf as he was with the rest of the choir.

Friar Roald was again sitting at his desk when Adolf entered his office. He set down the quill he preferred using instead of a pen and smiled at the boy. "Hello Adolf. You did very well in rehearsal. I expect we will make a great deal of progress today."

Adolf quietly closed the door behind him and approached the Friar's desk. "Thank you, I have been practicing at home, too."

Again Friar Roald had a bottle on his desk, but this time the two glasses were already filled. He lifted one glass, and then motioned for Adolf to take the other. "I am glad to hear that. Cheers."

Adolf watched as the Friar drank first, and then drank as well. Even before he tasted the glass's contents, his nose felt the gentle burn of stronger alcohol. The liquid was very sweet, tasting of a blend between fig and plum. It was smooth, and easy to drink, but the burning that chased the sweetness was much stronger than the wine had been before.

Friar Roald smiled and set his glass down. "I thought you might enjoy a port more than last week's wine. It will coat your throat and relax it even more." He did not mention it was nearly twice as strong. He simply watched Adolf, waiting to see if the port's sweetness was strong enough to disguise the bitterness of his own medicative ingredient.

The boy only smiled and continued drinking until the glass was empty. "I do like it, Friar Roald. It tastes almost like candy."

The Friar smiled. "Indeed. I hope it was not too strong for you, but you are very mature for your age, so I am sure you can handle it."

Adolf took confidence from the Friar's words and ignored the warmth that was spreading rapidly throughout his body. It was different from the effects of last week's wine, but with that experience in mind, he allowed himself to enjoy the feeling.

"Now, let us have you begin with your breathing. Try and count to twelve this time. Each week, we will expand your lung capacity. Remove your shirt so I can watch your diaphragm. I want to be sure you are doing it properly."

Adolf removed his sweater, and then his undershirt. He was glad the Friar could discern whether or not he was breathing properly simply by watching him, instead of having to endure the man's hands on him again. Friar Roald watched closely, standing once Adolf was breathing in for a count of seven. He moved around his desk and came to stand closer to Adolf as the boy passed counts of eight and nine.

By the time Adolf was breathing out his count of ten, he felt very strange. He was light-headed, as he had been the week before, but he also felt drowsy and paused to yawn before he began his count to eleven. He was about to apologize, but Friar Roald only shook his head,

"It is all right, continue." The Friar did not even bother to disguise the underlying and unsettling anxiousness in his encouragement. Was he coaching Adolf or coaxing him?

Adolf nodded and breathed in while silently counting, but before he could reach the number nine in his count for eleven, he felt a wave of warmth overcome him. The last thing he would remember was the Friar's arm catching him as he lost consciousness and drifted into velveteen blackness.

By the time he woke, the sun was very low and bright, lighting the room with prismatic color from the light streaming in through the stained-glass windows.

Adolf's head felt heavy, and tongue was thick and dry in his mouth, which tasted strangely of salt. He found himself lying on Friar Roald's cot, still shirtless. The bright, colored light hurt his eyes, but he squinted and willed himself to sit upright. It was then that he noticed that his entire body felt sore.

Friar Roald had been sitting at his desk; when he saw Adolf sit up, he set down his quill and smiled at the boy. "Oh, thank the good Lord. I was just penning a note for your parents. I was afraid you would sleep through the entire day and into the night. I would have had to share a room with Brother Dominic."

Adolf's eyes blinked first at their blurred dryness, but were soon blinking back tears of fear—or perhaps guilt.

Friar Roald smiled his deceptively kind smile, "It is all right, Adolf. It is not your fault. I did not think the port would be too strong for you, but it seems you had some sort of reaction to the libation. Are you allergic to figs or plums by chance?"

As Adolf listened to the Friar's words, he felt as if his ears were stuffed with cotton. He was very confused and frightened.

"No matter. I am sure it is something you will grow out of some day. Just avoid ports. I blame myself, of course. I should not have given you wine again, but I thought you would enjoy the port's sweetness. I meant it to be a reward for how well you sung this past Sunday."

"Friar?" Adolf spoke, his voice raspy and hoarse in a throat that was also sore. "I would like to put my shirt back on. I would—I would like to go home."

Friar Roald nodded, "Of course, so long as you are well enough. I will send someone to walk with you. I would not want you to faint again and find yourself alone in the street."

Adolf stood slowly, finding both his balance and just how sore he was. His trousers, and even his underpants, were twisted awkwardly, and he found that his pant's buttons had been undone.

Friar Roald offered Adolf his shirt. "When you fainted, I called for Brother Dominic. He could have been a doctor if he had not chosen to serve the Lord instead. He undressed you to make sure whatever reaction you had did not cause swelling in your glands, but I am afraid it did. You may be sore for the next few days."

Adolf took his shirt and sweater and pulled both garments over his head. Something was very wrong, but he did not know what it was. The Friar's explanations made perfect sense, but they did not feel right. There was a glint in the Friar's eyes that had not been there before, a certain tightness around his eyes that was normally absent from the kind-spirited man.

"Brother Dominic left for the evening prayers. He did not think there was much else to do for you until you woke, but if you would like, you can speak to him before you go home. Just remember, you made a promise to both me and the Lord that you will not tell anyone of what we do in these private lessons. I do not think your parents would be happy to know I gave you port. That was supposed to be a reward for you. I am very sorry it made you sick."

The Friar then walked back to his desk and dipped his quill in a blue ink pot. He scribbled swiftly on the heavy paper used for official letters, and then looked back to Adolf. "Would you like me to send for Brother Dominic?"

Adolf did not want to talk Brother Dominic or anyone else. He shook his head vacantly at Friar Roald, and began walking toward the door.

Friar Roald reached the door first and kept the handle in his hand. "Your word, Adolf. It is very important that you do not break your word." The Friar handed Adolf the letter he had just written. "Go home now, and take this to your parents. It is mostly filled with praises, but also provides the excuse that our lessons ran late today. They will be very proud of you when you perform your solo. Let us hope our next meeting goes better than this one. I am looking forward to it already."

Adolf took the Friar's letter and nodded. "Thank you, Friar Roald." But the words sounded hollow, and he looked to the door, instead of the man in front of him. Adolf still felt strange, and his head was fuzzy, but he noticed that Friar Roald did not send for anyone to walk him home, as he said he would. That was just as well, since Adolf wanted nothing more than to be alone.

The Friar smiled at the boy's heartless thanks, not his warm, kind smile, but a smile of sin. A smile of satisfaction. The heavy oak door opened at last with a soft squeaking of its hinges, and without looking back to the Friar, Adolf began the long walk home.

Once he was outside the Abbey, he spat, trying to rid his mouth of the salty taste, feeling that uncomfortable and primitively wrong soreness.

He knew nothing, other than that he would not visit Friar Roald ever again.

Chapter 4

ADOLF DID NOT go to school the next day. He convinced his mother that he was too sick to attend classes and instead remained in his bed. He was still very sore, and worse, he continued to feel as if something had happened that he did not understand.

The boy who had inherited his father's desire for control had never felt so emotionally powerless. It was different from feeling physically powerless, as he did when his father had beaten Al. That had made him angry and sad. This, though, this feeling was closer to despair.

He did not sing in the choir the following Sunday, either. By Monday, Klara wanted to call the doctor. Instead, Alois came into his room and felt for a temperature. He found none and demanded that Adolf return to school that day.

The soreness was gone by then, but the feeling of wrongness was as pervasive as it had been since he had awoken on the Friar's cot. Adolf presented a note from his mother to Brother Dominic, explaining why Adolf had not attended classes on Friday, but the teacher did not seem concerned. Brother Dominic just took the note and placed it in the drawer of his desk without reading it. Adolf thought he noticed a similar tightness around his teacher's eyes as had been around Friar Roald's. He knew something, but was not saying it.

It was difficult to focus on assignments. Unable to pay attention, Adolf's mind wandered during lectures. Strangely, Brother Dominic never called on him to answer a question, as he did with other boys who were guilty of daydreaming. It was the sort of oddity that only increased Adolf's suspicion that something was different from what it had been before he had tried Friar Roald's port.

As the week went by, Adolf hurried from his classes to home, always worried that he might run into Friar Roald in the hallways.

He did not attend any of the choir rehearsals, and he skipped his private meeting with the Friar that Thursday. By Friday, Adolf had failed his first exam, and had barely passed two other quizzes. Just as he was leaving class, Brother Dominic stopped him and handed him a note to take to his parents.

As soon as Adolf handed the note to him, Alois knew his son had done something wrong. He had been so quiet all week—what else could trouble him besides guilt? Now, perhaps, this note would explain the boy's silence.

Adolf could see the anger building in his father as his eyes scanned Brother Dominic's note. His eyes drew tighter, his jaw clenching against deeper breaths. His veins were already beginning to throb at his temples.

"You failed a Latin exam? And almost failed quizzes in history and German? History is one of your favorite courses!" Alois clenched the letter in his hand, ruining the paper as Adolf's young pride felt similarly crushed. That was only the beginning of Alois's reproach. "What do you have to say for yourself? What have you been doing in your room all day? You have not been to rehearsals, and it says you missed your private instruction, as well!" Alois threw what remained of the crumpled letter at Adolf, utterly disgusted with disappointment.

Adolf was taken off guard by the mention of his absence from choir rehearsals and private time with Friar Roald. He had meant to apologize to his father, and was not going to offer any sort of excuses. He flinched from the harmless paper ball, unable to say anything at all.

"Well? Are you going to explain yourself? Speak boy, unless you would rather save us both the time, and I will just punish you now. Well?"

Adolf just could not speak. He did not know what to say. Tears formed in his dark eyes, and before his father's hand ever rose, Adolf was crying.

Alois, thinking the tears were, at best, an admission of guilt and, at worst, fear of what was to come, decided he would give the child a definite reason to cry.

The old man's hand was hard and calloused. The arm that swung it had lost none of its strength or vigor over the years. Nor had Alois learned that corporal punishment was not always the best form of discipline. His hand struck Adolf's cheek with a crack that staggered the boy and immediately left red fingerprints in his pale skin.

Alois did not hesitate, but advanced directly on the boy even as he staggered. The man's hand roughly gripped Adolf's shoulder, and Alois dragged his son to a chair, where he sat and pulled the boy onto his lap. "Still do not want to tell me anything, eh?" Alois's hand fell across the boy's buttocks, which stung even through the fabric of his trousers. It was a pain that was very different from the soreness he felt last week, but it only reminded Adolf of that pained area all the same.

He was wailing and choking with pain within minutes. All the stresses that had been building since the last time Alois punished his eldest son were now coming to a head. Alois struck his new eldest son on his buttocks and the back of his thighs time and again, releasing his own frustrations without understanding that his punishment had nothing to do with discipline at all.

As the blows fell, Adolf cried and sobbed, allowing the physical and emotional stresses that had been building within himself to find release in a sadomasochistic form of therapy. He cried, and cried, and cried, until he could not breathe, until he could not cry any more.

Alois slapped his eldest boy over his knees until his own hand was stinging painfully, his arm too tired to deliver another blow. He slapped Adolf and wondered what would have happened if he had punished Alois Jr. in this manner, instead of using the branch. Perhaps the boy would still be here with the family. He wondered if slapping Adolf like this now would prevent the need to ever take a branch to him in the future. Neither had noticed Klara's cries for Alois to stop the punishment or Edmund's frightened tears.

At last Adolf felt his father relax his grip, and so he rolled off the man's lap. His rear was by then too numb to feel the short fall to the floor.

"I never want to see another note like that again. Are we clear, Adolf?"

Adolf looked up from the floor and started to nod, but then stopped, and instead stood.

"Well? Or do I need to hit you with my other hand? The Lord was kind enough to provide two." Alois narrowed his eyes at the boy who now looked at him so coldly. "You have not said a damned word since you gave me that note. Do you not have anything to say for yourself?"

Adolf continued to stare at his father, silent, until the older man blinked. He then spared a glance to his mother, clearing his throat. "I cannot go back to that school."

His voice was so clear, so calm after all his crying, that Alois and Klara were both taken aback by the statement. Klara moved to stand next to Alois. "Why Adi? What happened?"

Adolf was quiet for another moment, but as he sensed that his father was about to begin demanding answers again, he started from the beginning, breaking his word to Friar Roald and the Lord.

When he was finished speaking, his mother hugged him very tightly. His father stood slowly, watching his son all but collapse in his mother's arms. He knew the boy was not lying. What child could imagine such an evil lie? He did something he never did: He reached out and put his hand on Adolf's shoulder. It was the strongest gesture of comfort the man would ever offer.

There was nothing either parent could do about what had happened. Adolf himself was not sure what had occurred, but his parents had very strong suspicions. They might speak to the Abbot, but even then it would be Adolf's word against Friar Roald's—and perhaps even Brother Dominic's.

"Adolf, go play with Ange and Ed," Alois gave the boy a squeeze that was nothing like the forceful grip he had just used to punish him only moments before.

The boy stepped back from his mother, out of his father's touch.

"Yes, Papa." He left for Angela's room. Once the door was closed, Alois ran a hand over his moustache and sighed. His wife had tears brimming in her eyes, and the stoic man was surprised to notice that there was a sting at the corners of his eyes, too.

"We cannot stay here, Alois. He cannot go back there!" The hand that had settled on his son's shoulder now reached out to his wife. He hugged her as she had been hugging Adolf. "Calm, Klara. You must be calm. He is too young to know what happened. He may even forget." But the words sounded as hollow in the air as they had in his mind.

"He is not going back there." Klara repeated again. She stepped back from her husband and looked him in his reddened eyes.

To surprise, he agreed. "No, he is not. I should never have let him go there to begin with. A monastery is no place for a civil official to receive his education. He needs a city, not a backward market town."

Hearing the anger returning to her husband's voice, Klara nodded. She agreed. "You always enjoyed working in Linz. We will find a house close to the city, something better than living on top of a hill. I am tired of walking up and down it just to get to the market."

Alois was indeed becoming angry. He began tugging at his white chin hair. His jaw clenched against the pulls and his own conscience. He was as angry with himself as it was at the man who had wronged his family. He should not have spanked Adolf, but his impatience had snapped his temper. Now he owed the boy an apology he knew he could never bring himself to give. He began to wonder if God were repaying him for breaking his first marriage vows—or for taking Klara as his third wife, even though she was his niece in the eyes of the church.

"It will be all right, Alois. You are probably right. He is young, and he will forget."

Alois sat down. "Yes, yes he will. The sooner we leave here, the better, I think. I will begin looking tomorrow."

Klara nodded. As she turned to look at the door behind which her children were at play, she could not help but wonder if this was yet another punishment from the Lord for falling in love with her uncle.

Adolf knew even less of his parent's sins than he did of the Friar's. While they were making the decision to leave Lambach, he sat in his stepsister's room and watched Ange brushing little Ed's hair. His own arms were occupied with the task of cradling his baby sister.

Paula was already very different from her siblings. Angela had inherited her mother's raven dark hair; Adolf had dark hair as well, but it was a boy's black. Edmund's hair was just a shade lighter than Adolf 's. Paula, by contrast, had blond hair that could almost be called flaxen. She was a happy baby, quick to smile and giggle at the silly faces Adolf made to amuse her. Just as Angela had done with Edmund, so did Adolf turn his adoration to Paula. He rocked his baby sister gently; the soothing motion helped calm him as much as it soothed his sister.

"You should not invite Papa's anger, Adi." They were the first words Angela had spoken since Adolf had come into the room. His shouts had been heard throughout the house, sounds from which Angela had distracted Edmund and Paula.

By then, his tears had long since dried. "I did not know that I had." Adolf said quietly. "I was afraid he would not believe me. I was afraid he would not understand."

"Well, he must have. At least he did not cut a new branch . . ."

Adolf 's eyes flickered up to meet his stepsister's. His eyes were as dark as his hair, but now they were not only dark, but hard as coal. "That is not funny."

Angela blinked, blushing at the reproach. "You are right—it was not." The words were sincere, but they did not soften the look Adolf continued to give her. Angela realized it was the same hard gaze that her father often gave just before his temper snapped. It frightened her to see that intensity in her little brother, so she let her eyes fall on innocent Edmund instead. Even in his terrible twos, he was still her little cherub.

Adolf continued to stare at his stepsister. He could not help the renewed pang of jealousy he felt seeing Edmund in her lap. It had been so long since she had held him that way. But he was too big for that now. It was a rare occasion that he was allowed to sit in his mother's lap, either. This was the first time he had realized that. He was growing up.

The door opened, and Klara looked in on her children. Finding Edmund with Angela and Paula with Adolf, she smiled, silently apologizing to God for thinking she was being punished. With such beautiful children, she must surely be blessed. Losing young Ida and Otto to diphtheria had been punishment enough. It had to be. What had happened to Adolf was horrific, and she could not understand how the good Lord could allow one of his children to endure such an experience. She could not understand how one of the Lord's servants could commit such sin, but it had nothing to do with her own sins. It could not.

"Is dinner ready, Mother?" Angela had never grown out of using the formal address, even with Al absent and unable to continually remind her that Klara was not their real mother.

"Yes, Ange. Help Ed wash his hands and come to the table." Klara then looked to Adolf. "Can you carry Paula to her crib, or would you like me to take her? She ate earlier, and will not be hungry for a few more hours."

Adolf felt his muscles protest as he uncrossed his legs and first got to his knees, and then, when he tried to stand, he gritted his teeth as the soreness of his father's spanking returned. "I can take her," he answered, not bothering to hide the tightness the discomfort gave his voice.

Klara just watched as Adolf walked stiffly out of the room, carrying his baby sister in a cradling embrace.

Dinner was a simple stew of sausages and bratwursts. The family ate in relative silence, broken only by occasional requests for more bread or to pass the water pitcher. It was a somber dinner, because, Angela assumed, of whatever had caused Adolf's punishment.

At last Alois finished his second portion and sat back in his chair. "At least Linz has better sausages."

Klara looked up from what remained in her own bowl and smiled.

Seeing her mother smile, Angela looked to her father. "Linz, Papa?"

Alois nodded. "Yes, your mother and I have decided that we are moving back to Linz. Lambach is . . ." He could not help but spare a glance to Adolf, and then looked back to Angela. "It is not right for us here. Linz will be much better for you children. There is culture in Linz. You will like it."

Angela had been moving all her life. She was only six when the family began its odyssey in Braunau Am Inn, and now the family would move for the fourth time. Her brow furrowed, and she turned her attention back to the stew, deciding it did not truly matter. She was nearly fifteen, and soon she would find a husband. Her prospects would certainly be better in a city.

Hearing his father's words, Adolf was sure he had never loved his father more. The sooner they left Lambach, the better. He still believed the Abbey was an incredible structure, and he held the Abbot as an ideal man. It was the Abbot's monks and friars of whom he never wanted again to think. The farther he was from Friar Roald, and even Brother Dominic, the better.

After less than a week searching for a suitable home, Alois decided on Cape-style house in Leonding. On a large plot of land, the house had two floors and ample attic space. Linz was only three miles east. Klara would come to call it the "garden house," simply because the soil was so rich. She spent days working the earth around the house, planting flowers and bushes about their lush acre. Adolf helped his mother dig deeper holes for the shrubs and small flowering trees that would benefit Alois's bee-hives at the rear of the yard. His father had never lost interest in keeping the industrious insects.

Although it had taken far more hardship than he had ever anticipated, Alois finally had his retirement dream home.

For almost the first year in Leonding, life went very well for the Hitler clan. Adolf attended his last year of grammar school and was again doing very well in his classes. He dropped his study of music, but worked on his drawings more than ever. He was also quieter than he had been and no longer sought Angela's attention. He still adored baby Paula, but he gave little attention to young Edmund.

Adolf would come to regret his familial negligence greatly just before the family's first anniversary at the garden house. Nothing, it seemed, was ever easy for the Hitler family, and tragedy again struck their household when Edmund contracted measles.

Alois and Klara both did all they could for their youngest boy. Alois hired three different doctors from Linz, but the virus was too aggressive for the child's system, and Edmund passed away on February 2, 1900.

Alois faced this latest act of God with a stoic detachment, sometimes believing he was no longer being punished for his sins, but rather, that he and all his line were simply cursed. It was a thought that had occurred often in the younger years of his life. He had believed hard work had changed his luck, but ever since his retirement, it felt as if life had nothing but cruelty left for him.

Klara took Edmund's death much harder than Alois. She had largely isolated herself with the child on the second floor, while Angela, Adolf and Paula were quarantined on the first floor, in an effort to keep them safe from the sickness. Klara had brought all Edmund's meals to him, staying with her blotch-spotted boy almost day and night, leaving Angela to prepare dinners for the family. After Edmund's death, Klara refocused all her maternal energies on her three surviving children, but perhaps on Adolf most of all. She knew her boy was different, and thought that only love might help him recover from his traumatic experiences.

Adolf felt definite guilt when Edmund passed. He had given so much of his affection to Paula that he often had no time for his little brother. How could Adolf have known that it was Edmund who was so short of time?

Grief and its resulting guilt would gnaw at Adolf the way his memories of Friar Roald often filled him with guilt and shame. Suddenly, without warning, he would feel *wrong*, a feeling he could not dispel, but upon which he dwelled until the emotional pain felt ... good.

The only surviving Hitler boy—Alois Jr. was still as good as dead to the family—Adolf drew back from his father in the weeks to come. He distanced himself from Angela, as well, but tried to give Paula what attention he could. He always had time for his mother. His days consisted of attending school, where, after Edmund's death, his grades once again suffered.

The following September, Adolf and Angela attended high school in Linz, walking six miles round trip each day, which guaranteed them an abundance of fresh air and exercise. Adolf's physical health seemed to be returning to what he had enjoyed in Hafeld's high airs. His grades, however, did not show similar improvement.

High school was a hard adjustment for Adolf. The school was much larger, and there were different floors and wings in which sat hundreds more young people than at the monastery, where the average class size had been much smaller. This new school did not have the rigid structure of prayer time, nor did church bells strike each hour to keep the children and the teachers on pace. But it was not only the lack of structure that caused Adolf's troubles; the Friar had robbed him of his self-confidence that day in his office.

On Adolf's first day at the new school, he found himself lost from the start. Unable to find the room assigned to him, he wandered the school's halls for the better part of a half hour before a janitor noticed him walking past for the third time.

"Lost, eh? Where are you supposed to be, lad?" The Janitor was friendly enough fellow, in his gray overalls with his bristling mustache and balding head that shined brighter than the school's floors. He looked as though he had just finished trying to clean his face of some dark dust, or soot. He had not managed a very good job of that, either.

Adolf's lost confidence had been replaced with a wary shyness. He was also embarrassed. His voice high and shaky, he answered the older man, whose moustache held more bristles than the broom he carried. "Room 309-B, sir. I see no numbers on the rooms down here in the basement, though."

The janitor could only chuckle softly as he leaned his broom into a vacant corner. "'B' does not stand for "basement." It means the other half of room 309, which is on the third floor with the rest of the 300-numbered classrooms. Come, I will take you up in the service lift. You will be late enough to your class without having to climb all those stairs."

Adolf could not believe the stupidity of his mistake. He was so nervous about meeting new classmates and his new teacher that he had allowed himself to become fixated on his first presumption—that "B" would stand for "basement." He had seen other children on this level, but, as the janitor explained, that had probably been because the gymnasium was also on this floor. Adolf had seen lockers and assumed that his was among them. Now he found out his locker would be with his classroom, on the school's third floor.

The service lift shook horribly as its steam-powered engine raised the janitor and Adolf to the third floor. Electric elevators were still a fairly new invention, and the school could not afford such technology. The school was very proud indeed to have any sort of lift; not all schools did.

Adolf felt awkward having to stand so close to the man in the small lift. He stared straight ahead during the slow ascent. When the lift came to a stop with a sudden jolt that staggered Adolf into the man, his face turned redder than even his father's ever would in his most terrific moments of rage. The janitor put a hand on Adolf's shoulder to steady himself, and then opened the sliding door of the metal cage that protected passengers from a nasty fall into the shaft's depths.

Adolf was very happy to be out of the lift and back on the solid hallway floor. "Your classroom is the last on your left," the man pointed. "Tell your teacher your small fingers were helping me fix something, and you will not be penalized for tardiness—this time."

"Thank you, thank you very much, sir." Adolf's nervousness and discomfort made the words sound rudely hollow.

The janitor only nodded, and then closed the gate, descending back into the school's depths.

Now came the harder task: facing his teacher and his new classmates. He could not help but visualize his entrance: the door opening, all eyes suddenly turning from the teacher's lecture to Adolf and his tardiness. Even armed with the janitor's excuse, he could not help his anxiety about what lay on the other side of the large wooden door. Without the janitor's kindness, he would never have had the courage to open that door at all.

A deep breath, and his sweating hand grasped the large brass knob. He tried to enter quietly, as inconspicuously as possible, but the knob and the door's hinges squealed as he moved the door, so Adolf's face was already flushed red by the time his foot passed over the classroom's threshold.

The teacher, occupied with writing the classroom rules on the grey chalkboard, paused and turned her sharp blue eyes, narrowed at Adolf's intrusion. "May I help you, young sir?"

Adolf had never seen so massive a woman. His own mother, almost as tall as his father and much heavier, was large by feminine standards, but this woman must have at least doubled his mother's weight. Her gray-streaked hair was pulled into a horribly tight bun that seemed intent on stretching the wrinkles from her brow.

Adolf, taken off guard, did not answer directly. "I . . . I was . . ." He paused, trying to regain his composure, but his mouth felt dry and his tongue cloven. "I mean, yes ma'am. I believe this is my classroom."

The woman set down her piece of chalk, dusted her hands in a vigorous clap, and then settled those hands on the enormous bulge of her hips. "You must be Mr. Hitler, as you are the only child not present for this morning's roll. You may call me Frau Spinnen. What kept you from my web, Mr. Hitler?"

Adolf's stomach was turning on itself. As if the domineering presence of this ogre of a teacher was not enough, he could hear children at the back of the classroom already giggling at him. He had not dared to look at that sea of faces just yet. "I was helping the janitor, ma'am. He told me to explain that he needed my small fingers—"

"And decided to keep you from your first day of classes? His need must have been great, indeed. I will speak to Mr. Gustolf during the lunch period. As you will see from the board, my first rule is about tardiness and my second about interrupting my classroom. You have broken both rules. You are excused from punishment this time, but do not allow this behavior to become a habit, Mr. Hitler."

"I will not, Frau Spinnen. Thank you, Frau Spinnen." Relief was evident in his genuine gratitude.

The teacher narrowed her eyes. "You should thank Mr. Gustolf, I suspect. You may hang your coat on the rack in the rear of the classroom, and then find yourself an empty desk in the back row. Consider it a reminder that responsibilities begin here in the classroom. If you can fulfill those responsibilities, perhaps you will work your way forward."

"I would not take that bet," sniggered a boy from the middle of the classroom, quiet enough for the teacher to ignore him, though she likely heard every word. She turned her impressive girth back to the chalkboard and continued writing the rules of the class.

Adolf found a desk next to a window at the rear of the classroom. Aside from meeting Mr. Gustolf, a window seat was the best luck he had had since leaving Hafeld. Nothing in Lambach could be considered lucky, anymore. He did not know who had spoken, but if that were the worst taunt he received that day, he judged himself to be well enough off.

Frau Spinnen at last finished her list of rules and went over each in detail while the children wrote them on the first page of their fresh notebooks.

Rule 1. Tardiness is not to be tolerated and will be punished with the classroom's yardstick.
Rule 2. Interrupting the teacher or other classmates will not be tolerated and will be punished with the same yardstick.
Rule 3. No copying, passing of notes or other forms of cheating will be tolerated, and will be punished

not only by the yardstick, but also by a trip to the Principal's office. You will be suspended or expelled.

The rules were short, but simple. Plenty went unsaid; Frau Spinnen's demeanor made it clear that she would allow no foolery. Adolf, finding the rules no different from those he knew from his school in Lambach or Hafeld, did not worry about crossing Frau Spinnen again. He was a fly as surely caught in her web as were the other children, but he had escaped from the center of her attention to the web's outer edge.

Frau Spinnen spent the rest of the class outlining what would be taught in the next week. Adolf was not the only child to spend more time furtively glancing at his fellow classmates than paying attention to those plans. Most of the children were dressed as he was, and all had the same crew-cut hair. The boy seated to his right seemed slightly better dressed than the other children—there was a definite elegance to the cut of his clothing.

More than once that day, Adolf could have sworn he heard the boy whistling to himself. Soft and airy, the sound would never carry to the front of the room, but Adolf could hear it clearly enough. The sound was distracting, but Adolf did not mind. The notes were pleasing. The boy clearly possessed no small degree of musical aptitude. Sensing this boy was an artist like himself, Adolf decided to introduce himself formally to the boy after class.

Adolf approached the boy after class was dismissed, his curiosity greater than the shyness he would normally feel. At this new school, he would need friends. Holding out his hand in greeting, he said, "Hello, my name is Adolf, Adolf Hitler."

The boy seemed surprised by the introduction, and at first only blinked at Adolf. Then he spoke, in an almost lilting tone of High German that must have been accentuated by the boy's musical proclivity. He was very formal in his response. "Greetings, Mr. Hitler. I am Ludwig Wittgenstein. You may call me Mr. Wittgenstein."

Adolf was put off by the boy's insistence of using such formal titles. Perhaps he was a noble? Adolf, having recently moved to

Leonding, did not recognize the name Wittgenstein any more than he would Spinnen or Gustolf, but that hardly mattered at the moment. Adolf decided to indulge the boy's eccentrics. "Well, Mr. Wittgenstein. It seems we are going to be classroom neighbors. I heard you whistling today. You are very good at music, yes?"

The boy smiled at the compliment and nodded. "My family is well known for our musical talents. I had a brother who was going to be a great composer, but I think the stress of his own criticism was too much. He passed away, last year."

Adolf was sorry to raise a sore subject. "I am sorry for your loss. I have had siblings pass away, also. Though I doubt any would have grown to be a composer or anything so great."

Ludwig only shrugged. At last he said, "It was a pleasure meeting you, Mr. Hitler. I will look forward to your company in the classroom. I am afraid I must be heading home now though. Our studies are light enough this first day, but I cannot be late for my clarinet lessons."

"Of course, I am sorry to keep you. I will see you tomorrow." The fact that the boy could afford a Clarinet, never mind Clarinet lessons was impressive to Adolf. Here, perhaps, was a boy of some quality. Ludwig would certainly be a peer worth forging a friendship with.

The next day, Adolf was already seated when Ludwig walked in. Adolf offered the boy a nod of greeting, but he received none in return. Instead, Ludwig hung his coat on his peg and moved to his chair as if he had not seen Adolf at all. Then another boy greeted Ludwig, and his High German was perfectly civil with a short, but courteous greeting.

Rebuked, Adolf clenched his teeth and turned his head forward. He had never been slighted in that way before, and he decided that it was fine if Wittgenstein did not want to be a friend, but if he would not be civil, then they were at the least rivals. The longer Adolf sat and dwelled on the matter, the more he thought "enemies" might be the better term.

The classroom continued to fill, but there was no sign of Frau

Spinnen. The teacher would break her own rule of tardiness, it seemed. When the boy sitting ahead of Adolf turned in his chair, Adolf did not bother looking up from his desk. He was too absorbed in the umbrage Ludwig had incited.

"You are new to this school, just like him." The boy looked to Ludwig, and then back to Adolf. "Do you like it here?"

Adolf looked up. His eyes were obsidian in his pale face, and for an uncomfortable moment, he stared at the boy in front of him.

"Forgive me, how rude. My name is Byron, Byron Silverstein. Pleased to make your acquaintance, Mr ?"

"Hitler. Adolf Hitler." Adolf's tone was hard, even less social than Ludwig had been with him. This Byron was a tall boy, but lanky. His sunken cheeks made the deep sockets of his eyes seem nearly hollow. The precipice of his long nose jutted precariously over an upturned lip, which, when he spoke, revealed that his left eyetooth was gold.

Adolf recognized the boy as another classroom outcast, and he had no desire to ally himself with the weak, the slow or the ugly. Better to keep himself isolated, to associate with no one at all. He had learned more by saying nothing than he had by trying to extend his own friendship. It was interesting to know that Ludwig was new to the school as well.

Byron was nonplussed by Adolf's cold response. He ignored Adolf's reluctance to engage in conversation, determined to carry it himself. "Since you are new, I assume you do not know Frau Spinnen's reputation. She is a difficult teacher who cares only for students who excel. If you fall behind in your studies, she will not wait for you to catch up. You will simply be left behind. Osmond there is repeating this grade. So are Wilhelm and Sigmund." He pointed to each boy in turn.

Adolf's patience was beginning to run thin. Each boy Byron named looked to Adolf, for they could easily hear Byron's loud voice. Other eyes in the classroom began to turn toward his seat in the rear. Adolf wanted no part of this attention.

"Perhaps they will study harder, then," said Adolf, low, but confident, just loud enough for Osmond and the other two failures to hear. "Perhaps you should study harder yourself, Mr. Silverstein. Your people are not exactly known for their intelligence."

Byron's mouth fell open, revealing two other fillings, silver instead of gold. "'My people'?"

Adolf sat straight back in his chair. He was not sure himself what he had meant, but he could not back down now. His temper was heating his words, his tone becoming more aggressive as the more students turned to watch.

"You Jewish Gypsies are defiling these Christian lands. You are all thieves and liars, murderers and parasites that sicken the lives of good Austrians. Is that clear enough?   I have heard how your people covet gold. How you make others repay your loans. Your people murdered our Christ. Now turn around. Do not speak to me."

Byron blinked, rendered speechless and mute. He turned around quickly to hide tears of embarrassment. There must have been other Jewish boys in the classroom, but none said a word. No one defended Byron.

No one spoke to him for the rest of the day. Frau Spinnen arrived and class began. The work was challenging, but Adolf did not fear Byron's warning. He began sketching in his notebook pictures of landscapes or architectures, giving little attention to Frau Spinnen's teachings.

As a treat for Adolf's twelfth birthday, Alois purchased tickets to a performance of *Lohengrin* at the Linz Opera

House. Paula was left in the care of Aunt Johanna, who was still living with the family. Klara and Angela wore their finest dresses and frocks, while Alois and Adolf donned their best Sunday suits.

From the exterior, the opera house was not particularly impressive. It was large, and had many windows, but it was rather plain. By contrast, once inside, Adolf found himself immersed in a world of red-velvet wall coverings and gold-leafed woodwork. The vaulted ceilings were coffered in copper that had long since oxidized to a distinguished green patina. The building was unlike any Adolf had ever seen.

He felt awed by the place's majesty in a way that was very different from the feeling of his first look at Lambach Abbey. This was no place of worship. Its columns were decorated by busts of bare-chested women, heads of lions and eagles. The opera house was a place of fantasy, and its décor sent a thrill through Adolf before they even reached their distant balcony seats.

As the houselights dimmed and the pit orchestra began its resounding music, Adolf realized he had never felt so grateful in all his life.

On the stage was a set depicting a field of battle. Alois knew his boy had been reading books about various wars for some time, ever since the lad had discovered the volumes concerning the Franco-German War. He thought the boy's love of art, music and battle, all of which he would find in *Lohengrin*, would make this a perfect birthday present.

But the opera proved to mean much more for young Adolf. *Lohengrin* was the story of a princess and the knight who protects her honor, an ideal that was as appealing to Adolf as it would be to most boys his age. He already had a fantasy-love for battle. Seeing a hero arrive magically on the back of a swan to save a princess and win her hand in marriage was precisely the sort of inspiration that awoke adolescent desires to find and protect the honor of his own princess.

Until now, the only girls he had seen were his sisters. He had not yet reached that state of maturity in which he would begin to notice the other gender or excite emotions of attraction. He did not yet dream by day of romances or by night of passions. But he was about to change.

His eyes were wide and sparkling, miniature stars in the firmament of the opera house balcony. He had never known such emotional stimulation; the opera restored his love for music, which had been lost since leaving the choir. Delighting in the music, Adolf again thought that artists should be as respected as any civil servant. They were serving society as just well, if not better. If anything they should receive even more respect for their talent.

Alois did not see the opera from that perspective. For him, the opera was a moment of escape from normal life, an exercise in culture and, ultimately, an indication of his social status. That status, however, had been earned through his profession as a Customs Official, and without people such as himself, there would be no society for whom this opera could perform.

That would have been his argument, at least, had he known his son's thoughts. But all he saw were the boy's shining eyes, and he knew that he had done something good for the boy of whom he was so proud. He even squeezed his wife's hand when she caught him looking at the boy.

Just a few weeks after the family's attendance of *Lohengrin*, Alois became very ill. Normally so strong and vigorous in his manners, he was instead reduced to a man unable to rise from his bed.

The doctors treated the sixty-four-year-old man for influenza symptoms. For nearly three weeks, he was debilitated by infirmity. He retched almost daily and suffered from fevers. His temperature fluctuated, but refused to spike or break. Perhaps most troubling, however, was the color and thickness of the mucous he violently spewed. It was at first a brown so dark that the doctor feared there must be blood in it, but as the weeks went by, the color lightened to something more akin to a rusted yellow, and yet the doctors were hesitant to declare his health was improving.

Then, by the third week's end, the old man made a sudden and miraculous recovery. His fever broke without ever spiking, and his stomach calmed and accepted again foods of any weight and consistency. His coughing never stopped completely, but what mucous it did produce was light and relatively normal in color.

It would not be until the summer of the following year that Alois again found himself in bed with a doctor holding a stethoscope to his chest.

The rest of the family enjoyed a healthy and prosperous year. Adolf's grades did not match the excellence he had enjoyed in grammar school, but they were adequate enough to avoid his father's wrath. But escaping his father's fury was no longer a problem: The man could hardly raise his hand, never mind hit someone with it.

The head of the Hitler household had been filling a basement coal bin for the approaching autumn months, when he suddenly collapsed. It was not until Adolf returned home from school, and his mother sent him to call his father up for dinner, that the boy discovered his father lying against the coal bin. His cigar had fallen and burnt itself out on Alois's work shirt.

When the doctor at last removed his stethoscope, he looked to Klara, sitting at her husband's bedside. "Your husband, I think, has suffered a minor hemorrhage in his left lung. The shock must have startled him, causing him to fall, as it is this lump on his head that explains why he was unconscious for so long. He must have hit his head on something in a panicked collapse. Poor fellow probably felt as if his lung had exploded."

Klara listened with open-mouthed horror at the grisly picture the doctor had painted.

"Oh do not worry, Mrs. Hitler. The hemorrhage was mild, I think. Otherwise I would have heard more fluid in his lungs. There is a rattle, but it is nothing with which I would concern myself. No, if he had not taken that knock to his head, it is possible he might have recovered and never known about the hemorrhage at all.

"It is actually quite fortunate that he did hit his head. Had you not called me, I would not have known to tell you that he must stop smoking his cigars. He should stop handling coal, as well. The smoke from the former and the dust from the latter will only put him at risk for larger hemorrhages in the future."

Klara was not sure if she should slap the physician for scaring her or hug him for bringing her such good news. Alois would recover. She elected to offer a simple nod of understanding. "I see. I will be sure to destroy whatever cigars he has left. I suppose Adolf is old enough now to move the rest of the coal."

The doctor rose. "Very good. Your husband is a man of advancing years, and he should not have to perform such chores at his age. Alois will wake soon enough. Keep him in bed for the next day or two, but he should recover swiftly. Do not hesitate to call if his condition does not improve, but I am all but certain it will."

With that, the doctor let himself out. The bill, of course, would be in the mail.

The Hitler household enjoyed a few months of peace while Alois recovered. It was not until Adolf's first report card came home that Alois summoned the strength to return to his duties of administering corporal punishment.

His approach to solving the problem of Adolf's dismal grades was the same as ever. His belt proved an even better instrument than the tree branch. The belt, at least, would never break.

As he whipped the boy, he proclaimed, "You will never pass the service exam if you do not apply yourself, Adolf. You earned excellent marks in the past. You are not stupid. You can do well again. Stop daydreaming, and apply yourself!"

Adolf tried to hold back his tears, but failed. His back was surely striped by the first five lashes his father administered, one for each of his failing marks, but by the time the fifteenth blow landed on him, he almost anticipated it with welcome. It was strange. He did not cry from the pain any more. No, the source of his tears was solely from the frustration of not being able to strike back.

"I do not want to pass the service exam."

Alois gaped, feeling shock that would surely be replaced by irate anger once it wore off. "Do not want to . . ." He shook his head, mouth still open in disbelief. At last he asked, "And what exactly is it that you *do* want to do?"

Adolf knew he had gone too far, that he had chosen a poor time to make his stand. Only a few weeks earlier, he had been rummaging through his father's library and found a collection of books that contained accounts and illustrations from the Franco-German War of 1870. His love for history aside, the boy had found refuge from his depressive thoughts in the heroic war stories the volumes recounted.

Perhaps it was that inner sense of heroics that gave him the nerve to tell his father he did not want to be a Customs Official. But the longer his father allowed him to answer, the stronger his conviction became. At last he spoke with cold seriousness. "I want to become a painter. I want to be an artist."

Alois continued to stare at his son, no longer in shock, but in utter disbelief. The boy was mad. Entirely mad to even consider that painting could be a career. "Boy, you have lost what little sense I had hoped was left in you. What sort of living do you expect to make as a painter? You may as well dream your life away!"

Adolf said nothing as he withstood the berating and debasing of his life aspirations. He knew another beating was about to begin, but he had chosen this ground to make his stand, and even if it were tactically a poor position, he would not withdraw now, lest he see his dreams defeated.

Seeing the defiance in the boy's eyes, Alois realized it was the same gaze Al had met him with the day he announced he wanted to live on his own. He saw the same stubbornness that would become a juggernaut if allowed to gain any sort of momentum. Beating the boy had done nothing, and so Alois decided to try something his temper generally did not allow him. He was not sure how he had not flown into a rage at the boy yet, but he would make a concerted effort to first reason with the boy.

In a voice much calmer than it had been with the disowned son, he said, "I will tell you what I told Al." Taking a deep breath, Alois said with reservation, rather than true calmness, "I have given you a home. I have given you food. I have given you clothes. And I have given you an education. But more important than any of those things, I have given you a name. You are a Hitler, and no Hitler will degrade himself to become a painter. I worked harder than you will ever know to gain my positions. All you have to do is pass the service exam, and thanks to the people I know, you could begin your career as a Customs Official where I had to end mine. Do you understand how great a gift that is?"

Alois waited for any sort of recognition in his boy's eyes. Finding none, he said "No, of course you do not."

Adolf listened carefully to his father's words, and spoken as they were, without specks of spittle flying from a belligerent mouth, they did make a great deal of sense. He started to respond, but his father held up his hand and went on.

"No, how could you understand? You have not had to work for anything but good grades in your young life. Now that those do not come easily, you want to give up and draw pretty pictures for people instead." Alois shook his head. "Artists are crazy people. Their contribution to society is not recognized until after they die, and that is if they are ever credited at all. I do not think you know what sort of life you are striving for if being a painter is truly your goal, and not some adolescent fantasy."

Had Alois stopped at the end of his first speech, Adolf might have taken his words to heart. His talk of artists being crazy, however, hit far too close to Adolf's own feelings as of late. Nothing had been the same since leaving Hafeld, and his bouts of depression were often only alleviated by drawing. He might already be crazy, for all he knew. That was not what bothered him most, though. No, it was his father's final two words. "Adolescent" . . . "Fantasy" . . . they tore at what very little pride Adolf possessed. Fearing he would lose that precious pride utterly if he now let his father's words stand, he gathered what resolve he could muster, and just shook his head.

"You are wrong, Papa. I have a great amount of talent, and with formal instruction, I could be a great painter. I do not know what sort of life it will be, but it will be *my* life. You have lived yours, and I could not be any more grateful for what you have given me. All I ask is that you now give me the one thing I have always lacked from you—love. I also want you to trust that I will do you proud."

Alois listened to his son's words and knew they were true. Having never known his own father's love, he had never been sure how to truly express that sentiment to his children. He demanded they do him proud because he was so proud himself. He had every right to be proud, for he had worked to earn that pride. He did not have the right to then demand his children make him proud in his context. They had to work themselves, and earn their own pride as he had.

"Adolf, I do love you, very much. I loved your brothers, also, just as I love everyone in our family. I know you are very good at drawing. I have at times thumbed through your notebooks, and you certainly have skill, but . . ." Alois looked out the window and pointed to the beehives. "I am a very good beekeeper, but that does not mean my profession should be making honey. It is a hobby. You can be very good at drawing or painting, but let it be your hobby. You have too much potential. Do not throw that away."

Adolf considered his father's words. He could hardly believe the man had not begun beating him again, and that fact alone forced him to closely deliberate what he should do next. He had made his stand, and he had already gained some degree of respect, or else he would be feeling his father's belt again. His father was trying very hard to treat him as an adult, and he did not want to do anything to disvalue his father's effort.

"I will study harder, Papa." Adolf said at last. He saw his father's face soften and was glad he had chosen those words first. "I will study harder, but I will still draw. When the time comes, I will take both the service exam and entrance exam to art school. If you are not convinced in my ability to draw or paint by then, and Mama agrees with you, I will be a civil servant like you."

Alois listened to his son's words and was disappointed when the boy insisted on still taking the art exam. However, the boy was being reasonable, and Alois found that dealing with his son this way was much like dealing with a merchant on the train platform. Calm reasoning could often be as effective as subtle threats. In this instance, talking to his son had at least provided better results than only beating the boy. He had no headache from his blood pressure climbing. His arm was not tired, and his voice was not hoarse. But perhaps best of all, Adolf was looking at him with respect, not fear or hatred.

For his part, Adolf was proud of himself. He had chosen his ground, had stood that ground and now came away with a marginal victory when otherwise he would have endured a brutal defeat. His back was still very sore from the fifteen belt lashes, but he deserved those. He expected to be bleeding after he had told his father he wanted to be a painter, but instead they had forged a different sort of relationship.

This was not just a turning point in Adolf's life, but began a climatic shift in the entire Hitler household. Alois was not cured of his abusive tendencies, but he repressed them with greater frequency than he ever had before. Klara even began to wear shorter sleeves again, since the bruises on her arms from Alois grabbing her had had time to heal.

Adolf held up his end of the bargain with his father, and his grades improved. For an entire year, the Hitler household could forget about curses or punishments from God. Paula grew into a beautiful toddling girl, and Angela grew into a beautiful young woman.

It was easily the most peaceful period in the family's history.

Chapter 5

A JANUARY WIND blew down Leonding's main street, swinging shop signs and forcing flags to flap and snap in the frigid air. The street was barren. The outdoor vendors who would normally brave the cold to sell their wares to weekend customers did not open their carts or stalls. Meat, vegetables and poultry would freeze in this climate. Vendors who sold newspapers or magazines would freeze as well. Even the boys with their boxes for penny-cent shoe-shines were nowhere to be found.

Bundled from his bald head to the well-shined boots, Alois made his way from the Garden House across town to see a friend who normally sold fruit here on Main Street. Alois, a man who had always put work before all else, shook his head at the vendor's failure to fulfill what Alois deemed a societal duty. Now, instead of the man doing his job and enduring the cold, Alois had to walk twice as far to see the man in his home.

Why Alois was out on this foolish mission to acquire apples was a mystery. He was developing either a softer heart or a softer head. Oh, he liked Klara's apple pies and apple crisps and apple scones and everything else apple the woman baked into desserts that were bigger and better than any the town's bakery had ever produced, but that was hardly a valid cause for this fool-headed mission of braving the elements and returning with frozen, over-ripened and out-of-season apples that would join sugar, cinnamon and nutmeg to create indulgent desserts. He had perhaps overindulged in such sweets this holiday season—as he passed the town hall, he was beginning to feel out of breath.

The wind was incessant, seemingly its only purpose to sweep the street of any human presence, but Alois was a stubborn man. Klara had told him to wait for the weather to warm before he went for the apples, but who could say when that would be? It was Saturday morning, and if there were to be pies for Sunday dinner, then he might as well go out for the fruit now.

Since the episode of his hemorrhage nearly five months ago, Klara had been more like his mother than his wife. He had made a full recovery as the doctor supposed he would, but Klara no longer allowed him to smoke his cigars. Oh, he had beaten her the first time she suggested he stop smoking. He drew blood from his wife's lip when she was so bold as to forbid him from doing so, but when she then broke his cigars and threw them into the fireplace, he at last gave in to the guilt with which she charged him for endangering the health of the family by endangering himself.

Yes, he was softer in the head after all. In his younger years, he would never have allowed such behavior. Now he was reduced to smoking his cigar through the folds of his woolen scarf as he made his way into the bitter wind's teeth. He had undertaken this expedition as much to get away from his house as to get apples for pie. The cigar's heat helped warm his lungs. The rough coughing that seized him at times was surely from the cold air, not the hot smoke.

He was not so frail as his wife believed. His eyes, his only flesh exposed, burned from the air's bite, but the sun was up, and the sky was clear of all but the faintest clouds. The wind-chill was well below zero, but the absence of people gave him a surreal and pristine feeling as he avoided patches of ice and piles of snow.

Leonding's only tavern was now within sight, and Alois wondered if it was too early to pause there for a warming cordial. He was well known in the tavern, as he was throughout the small town, so even if the tavern was not yet open, Alois was fairly confident that the owner would do him the favor of serving him, even at this early hour. It was his last thought before he felt a sudden twinge in the back of his skull. His steps then faltered, and Alois Hitler collapsed in the center of the cobbled street.

When sensation returned and he had regained his faculties, he found himself lying on one of two long, wooden tables he had come to know so well. His coat had been removed and now served as a pillow. His thoughts were jumbled, and when he attempted to sit up, he found he was entirely unable to move so much as his hand.

"Easy, Mr. Hitler. Be still, the doctor has been sent for."

The man's voice sounded very strange to Alois, who could only shift his blurred eyes. But even with his vision failing, he recognized it was the town's locksmith who had apparently helped him off the street and into the tavern. He tried to speak so as to thank the man, but his mouth made the words all wrong, and instead he managed only to mumble something entirely unintelligible.

"Wine. I think a glass of wine might help revive him," said the Good Samaritan. It was a lucky thing that Alois had been found by the locksmith. The man had used his talents to open the tavern door, much to the surprise of the barkeep who was busy hauling new kegs of ale and wine from the tavern's cellar for the weekend crowd. Seeing one of his more affluent customers stretched out on his table, looking so pale and drawn, had added a certain alacrity to the owner's actions.

Their efforts would go unrewarded. Alois Hitler endured one last spasm before passing from the world in which he had worked so hard to succeed. Neither the wine nor the doctor could reach him in time. He died that Saturday morning, January 3, 1903.

The stain of the cigar's tar was still on Alois's bloodless lips when Klara arrived at the doctor's office later that day. "I am very sorry for your loss, Mrs. Hitler. If it is any consolation, the hemorrhage was in his brain this time. I believe he died a painless death. Had it been in his lungs again, the poor man might have drowned in his own fluids."

Klara stared at the doctor through reddened and puffy eyes. If she had not felt so numb at that moment, she might have slapped the fool man. Was thinking about what might otherwise have happened supposed to console her? Her beloved husband was dead.

She was a strong woman. She had had to be strong to endure her husband's abuse and the deaths of four children. Alois had been a hard man, but he also deserved the authority and respect he had always demanded. Knowing that had always given Klara the strength to endure his beatings. It was not an admission that those beatings were justified—no, she merely accepted the circumstances of her love. Alois had always provided for the family. He had worked extra shifts to buy almost anything for which Klara asked. He loved his children, perhaps too much in some cases, and it was for those qualities that she would remember him and miss him deeply.

When Klara had been summoned into the doctor's office, Adolf had been charged with the task of caring for his little sister, Paula. Angela was in Linz with her boyfriend, who was taking her to the Opera House, and Adolf was jealous of his sister's opportunity.

"Mine!" said Paula, snatching one of Adolf's toy soldiers with which he had not yet outgrown playing. His recent discovery of the works of Karl May had excited his imagination, and when he was not studying or reading May's books, he pretended his toy soldiers were savage American Indians. His favorite toy soldier was one of May's heroes, Old Shatterhand.

Reaching for the toy, he said, "No, Paula, that is not yours. Play with your dolly."

The girl was now seven, more than old enough to understand the concept of possession. She simply enjoyed teasing her brother. "You play with Dolly. I like this!" She triumphantly raised the toy soldier in her small hand.

"Boys do not play with dolls, Paula. Give me back Shatterhand before I take him!"

Paula pretended to consider her next move, no doubt hoping to aggravate her brother further. Had she truly considered her actions, she might have understood just how thin Adolf's patience was growing.

"I said, give him now!" With that, the older and faster Adolf snatched the toy from his sister's hand, striking her with his larger hand as he ripped the toy from her small grasp.

Paula began to cry.

"Stop that," Adolf shouted. "Stop crying!"

But Paula was frightened and hurt by her brother's sudden force.

He was always so gentle with her. He had far more patience for her than anyone else in the family. This new behavior was terrifying, and she could not stop her crying.

"Here, play with your doll." Adolf held the doll tightly in his hand, waving it in front of her. When Paula still did not stop crying, he lost his temper and threw the doll at her. A large doll—its face painted porcelain—was a very expensive toy, passed down to Paula from Angela. It struck the girl with an audible thump, and then fell to the floor, face first. A crack appeared on its cheek like some horrible scar.

Seeing the damage to Dolly, Paula cried louder than ever.

Adolf did not know what to do. All he wanted was to finish his mock-battle, but Paula would not stop crying. Before he understood what he was doing, he had pulled his sister to a chair, where he proceeded to sit and force her over his knees. "Stop crying right now!" he said, even as he hand began spanking the girl.

"Mamaaaa! Mmaaamaa!" Paula began to wail, but Klara was by then far from home.

Adolf continued to spank his sister until he felt a hand on his shoulder. Startled, he paused mid-slap and turned to find Aunt Johanna hunched behind him. The disfigured woman rarely left her room on the second floor, her disabilities so prevalent that Klara had not even considered leaving Paula with her instead of with Adolf.

For his part, Adolf feared his aunt. He believed she was either sick or cursed and wanted nothing to do with her either way.

Now she sounded stern. "That is quite enough, Adolf. Let her up."

Adolf's eyes narrowed at the command. He was the man of the house. He always listened to his beloved mother's wishes, but he had no tolerance for orders from his disabled aunt. His hand hung suspended in the air fell a final time, with emphasis that could not be mistaken. Only then did he let the sobbing girl off his lap.

"What happened?" Aunt Johanna's own patience was thin, as standing for too long hurt the hump in her back.

Adolf remained seated, though he turned somewhat to face the woman better. He would not give her the equality of standing to address her. "She took one of my soldiers and refused to give him back. I told her to play with her doll, and she refused that as well. I took my soldier from her, and she began this crying you hear now. I told her to stop, but she refused."

Aunt Johanna looked to Paula, whose cries had subsided into snivels. "Is that the right of it, child?"

Paula bent and picked up her doll. "He hurt Dolly! He broke her!"

"*You* broke her, you mean," Adolf interjected. "If you were not so clumsy, you would not have dropped her."

Paula could not believe how cruel her brother was being. She began to cry again, without explaining what she had meant by, "He broke her." It was as if she had been the one to break the doll.

Aunt Johanna moved over to Paula with shambling steps and took the doll from the girl. "Oh, this crack is small enough. Nothing your mother's makeup could not hide." Johanna had no use for cosmetics, but that did not mean she had not played with them as all girls do. "Paula, shall we leave Adolf to his soldiers so you can help me fix Dolly?"

Paula was frightened of her aunt's appearance as much as anyone. The woman's reclusive life made her into some monster that happened to live behind the door at the top of the stairs. Because of the recent Christmas and New Year's celebrations, the family had seen more of the woman these past few weeks, but she was still a mystery to the Hitler children. They did not understand why she looked the way she did, and Klara's explanation of God's plan did not seem remotely adequate for what they saw when they looked at their deformed aunt.

Just the same, when faced between the choice of her brother's newly violent and terrifying company and the chance to play with makeup, she decided she could keep her eyes on Dolly and not so much her aunt. "Okay, Auntie."

"Very good. Come with me." Johanna looked back to where

Adolf still sat in his father's chair. "You should go and play in your room. Your father would be angry to find you sitting in his chair when he gets home, I think."

Adolf knew his aunt was right, but she was the last person he would allow to order him into doing anything. With an elevated chin, he said, "I must tend the fire, and then I intend to play with my soldiers in front of that fire."

Johanna pursed her lips, and then clicked her tongue before slowly turning to direct her shambling steps back up the long staircase.

Paula looked at Adolf, her brow furrowed as she tried to hold back the tears she felt returning. Adolf returned her stare with a gaze that was hard and lacking any of the warm adoration she usually found within. With a renewed case of snivels, the girl cradled her doll and followed Aunt Johanna up the stairs.

As he heard the door to his aunt's room close, Adolf could still feel his blood pumping. Why had she disobeyed him? If the girl had only handed the toy back to him, he would never have had to spank her. Her childish behavior was at fault; his own actions were impeachable. If his little sister would not listen to him, who would? He was not about to let a seven-year-old girl—or a crippled aunt, for that matter—order him or disobey him. Since Al Jr. had run away, Adolf had been treated as Alois's successor.

He had only been doing what his father would have done.

Adolf had only been to one other funeral in his young life, the short ceremony for dear Edmund. His baby brother had not been old enough to experience much of life, and as such, there was little of it to celebrate at his funeral. Grief had been abundant, but beyond tears, sobs and prayers for his innocent soul's mercy, the funeral had been brief.

The funeral for Alois Hitler was a vastly different affair. There was still an abundance of grief—even Adolf could not hold back the tears that came as he prayed before his father's casket—but there was also laughter within the funeral parlor.

Alois had lived to the dignified age of sixty-five. He had what the town considered to be a lovely family and had worked an honest (from what his peers knew) and admirable career as a civil servant. It seemed that the entire town had come to pay their respects, as did distant relatives from Spital and former colleagues from the customs offices—even a handful of representatives from the other civil service departments.

Klara, Johanna, Angela, Adolf and Paula were somber throughout the wake that began Sunday evening and ended the following Monday afternoon. Those hours were more for the town's benefit, so that everyone in the community could offer their respect to the well-regarded man.

For Adolf, those hours of standing in line, just a few feet from his father's casketed corpse, watching strangers parade by, one after another, felt as if they were a part of some opera. The minor characters had their entrances and their exits, but he was one of the main characters. No, he was *the* main character, tragic and miserable, just as he now was the man of the Hitler household.

Many of his father's friends told him how good a man his father had been, that the apple did not fall far from the tree. The men shook his hand with appraising eyes, judging him, despite their encouraging words. The women took him into smothering hugs that smelled of cheap perfume and mothballs. Adolf, who never invited any physical contact, endured these sympathetic gestures with a cold fire in his dark eyes that hid the sick twist in his stomach and began to wish he could trade places with his father.

Worst, perhaps, was the volume of voices within the room. Whether it was a woman crying or an outburst of raucous laughter from Alois's friends, when they had remembered a particularly humorous anecdote, Adolf could not help but liken the wake to a carnival. Instead of being dressed in costumes, the participants were all garbed in black. Formality was merely a formality, it seemed, and Adolf hated that so many people could be laughing while he felt only an expanding emptiness inside.

He had loved his father, as most boys do. Despite the man's

authoritarian nature and vicious temper, Adolf had been provided with an education, a home and, perhaps most importantly, a name. No matter how savagely he had dealt with instances of disobedience, his father had loved his family.

The numb feeling with which grief had infected him lasted throughout the wake, staying with him until the funeral. His mother, aunt and sisters still cried at the funeral, but by then Adolf had grown a thick and calloused scab over his wounds. He sat, stoic, in the front pew of Leonding's church, listening to Catholic prayers and hymns far too uplifting to be appropriate for what should have been a solemn and mournful ceremony.

Adolf tried not to think about the choir. He tried not to think about anything, letting his eyes wander the church's interior until one of his father's friends, the Mayor of Leonding, began to give his father's eulogy. For the first time since stepping into the church, Adolf's full attention was captured as the Mayor began addressing the surviving family members.

"Angela, you have grown into a young woman whose intelligence was the fodder for your father's barroom bragging, as often as he spoke of your beauty. He loved you very dearly."

Angela cried all the harder at those words, and Adolf could not help but swallow hard against the lump that was growing in his own throat. The Mayor then turned his attention to Adolf, the next oldest surviving child, making no mention at all of Alois Jr.

"And you, Master Adolf. You are growing into an admirable young man of whom your father was so very proud. He always boasted about your intelligence and character. He was quite convinced that you would rise even higher in society's ranks than he could. He could think of no better son to carry on his legacy of civil service. You have a very bright future ahead of you, lad. Remember your father's examples, and you will be a successful and respected man, too."

Even in death, his father had managed to have the final word about Adolf's career.

He should have felt some measure of pride that his father had shared his aspirations for his son with his friends. Knowing Alois had praised him to others, it must be truly how his father felt—his proud words to Adolf were not merely words spoken to mold him into such a man. But Adolf was not proud. He was frustrated. His father would be resting in his grave soon, and yet reached out from beyond life to counter Adolf's desires to become a painter. If nothing else, the Mayor's words only reinforced Adolf's resolution to defy his father's plans.

It was still bitterly cold when Alois Hitler Sr. was lowered into the earth. It had taken the gravedigger almost twice as long to scratch and chip away the first few inches of frosted soil as it had to dig the rest of the grave, but after the priest spoke the final prayers, Adolf laid a single rose on his father's casket, and then walked away from Alois's dreams for him.

His father's obituary portrayed a man that could have been a stranger to his family. To say that he was always cheerful in company was almost comical. The following sentence attempted to excuse the "harsh words that sometimes fell from his lips," but would have been far more accurate if the sentence did not to make mention of a "warm heart." Adolf would have said that his father was a man of great extremes, and that hot or cold could be accurate, given the circumstances, but warm was simply not a part of the man's existence. A statement that Alois "could always be counted on to pronounce authoritatively on any subject" was entirely true, though that was more than likely due to his authoritative personality than it was his actual knowledge of the subject. After all, his insufficient education had restricted his promotion to higher ranks.

What Adolf learned from his father's death was that much of life depended greatly on others perceived you. He was all-too aware of his father's shortcomings, but he had lived with the man. To his peers, Alois had been a model citizen, recognized as such when he received the title of *Honoratioren*—

No, perception was the foundation for any such accolades. If Adolf manipulated people's perceptions of himself, he would be just as respected as his father had been, without ever needing to endure a life in service. Society would service *him*.

The weeks following his father's death brought a marked change in Adolf. He had always been shy and selective with friendships, but now he went from simple detachment in the classroom to unmasked elitism that separated him from his peers. He wasted no opportunity to display his superiority to classmates who did not pass his rising standard of physical appearance, social manner or intellectual ability.

Perhaps it was his own ego that absorbed what attention he received from his teacher and classmates. Perhaps he felt the attention of snide remarks as vented jealousy, and modest agreements as great victories for his particular opinion. He thought himself well-regarded and felt empowered by the occasional mirth his wit might produce. Indeed, many of his peers admired his ability to command confident language when he chose to answer a question posed to the class or corrected a student who had misspoken. Others thought him arrogant, but they were of course below Adolf's attention to begin with.

Even his nature at home began to alter as his belief in his own righteous prowess grew. Paula suffered most from this shift in Adolf's attitude, as she was his easiest target. Throwing her dolly at the girl had only been the beginning, and Adolf's treatment of his baby sister was soon little different than had been his father's treatment of him, Alois Jr. and his mother.

At first, Klara believed that he was merely venting the stress of his father's death. Adolf's treatment of Paula was surely only sibling rivalry or the natural fighting between brothers and sisters. Though she did not condone his actions, and reprimanded him harshly whenever Paula came running to her in tears, she continued to believe her boy was only in a phase, and he would soon be the quiet and studious boy she knew him to be.

It was not until Paula came to her mother with a bloody nose that Klara understood Adolf was actually striking the girl. Withholding dinner as punishment was no longer adequate, but Klara was not sure what else she could do. She did not want to strike the boy. She could never bring herself to harm her own children.

There seemed only one solution: Adolf was sent to live at a home in Linz, where a handful of other boys boarded while in school. Adolf no longer had to walk to his classes, which Klara believed might also help to improve his grades, which had continued to decline since Alois's death.

Five other boys were living at Frau Sekira's boarding house. The eldest boy in residence was turning seventeen in two months. Adolf soon discovered he was the youngest boy, but his demeanor commanded an authority that proved that while the other boys were older, they were not necessarily more mature.

His father's pension provided Adolf with the financial comfort to rent his own room. The space was smaller than his room at the Garden House, but Adolf did not mind the smaller space. He was on his own. He kept his quarters immaculate, and for his first few months of freedom, his grades improved. He spent his hours of new-found freedom drawing sketches or reading fantasies of savage Indians in distant lands, wearing feathers and wielding tomahawks. These books would remain with him all his life.

As was usual for him, he remained the most solitary of the boys that boarded at Frau Sekira's house, cold and distant at best. Because Adolf boarded alone, several of the older boys, those who had to double up in rooms, resented that younger, smaller, frailer and more arrogant Adolf could afford his own room. Four of the other five boys staying at Frau Sekira's home were Jewish, their parents frugal enough to arrange lower fees for their sons sharing rooms.

This situation created tensions for which Adolf was hardly prepared. He found himself thinking of the man often. He wanted to command the authority and respect his father had possessed, but he had no desire to gain those rewards through civil service. Instead he affected a manner that resembled his father's public self-important bearing. He was not nearly as boisterous as his father had been, but when he spoke, it was with definitive statements that presented an air of superiority.

"No, Handel, you could not be more wrong. Wagner was not attempting to spread Pagan beliefs" Adolf's hands cut sharply through the air before him, as if he were cutting down Handel's opinion, "but rather was converting Nordic and Germanic myths to Christianity. Oh there are plenty of fanciful creatures and strange ceremonies and pacts, but there is also an abundance of purely Christian elements.

"Consider the role of marriage in *The Rings of the Nibelungs* as compared to its function in *Lohengrin*. The rings might well be considered Pagan, but the Prince's inability to reveal his true name, lest he lose the powers the grail has granted him, is a device of the romantic plot more than it is a central theme of the plot.

"Siegfried's use of the magic cloak to convince Brunhilde to marry him, on the other hand, is not so much a device of the plot, but a main theme that contains more Pagan elements than *Lohengrin*, and yet its marriage scene portrays Christian beliefs in a far greater capacity than the marriage in *Lohengrin*. Furthermore, Wagner combined the story of the Swan Prince with that of the Holy Grail, and I can hardly think of anything more Christian than the Grail."

Since attending *Lohengrin* at the Linz Opera House, Adolf had taken almost as strong an interest in the works of Wagner as he had in Karl May. Johan, the oldest boy in Frau Sekira's boarding house, was the only person with whom Adolf deemed worthy of carrying a civil conversation. He addressed everyone else—including Handel—as if they were children, and he the professor. These boys were no different an audience than those he instructed when he gave an answer in class. His words would assert his importance, and these fellows were at first willing and eager to listen.

Johan liked the newest addition to the boarding house. Adolf was quiet and formal, and yet self-possessed; the other boys admired, envied or even hated that confidence. For his part, Johan chose admiration. He enjoyed employing his own wit to test Adolf in a way similar to how Adolf was testing Handel. So far, Adolf had proven far better suited to the task of disguising what he did not know.

Johan was three years Adolf's senior, in the final year of his education. He, too, was an enthusiast of opera and was surprised to find such cultured knowledge in a boy Adolf's age.

As Adolf delivered his lecture to Handel, Johan only nodded with quiet appreciation of Adolf's argument as he watched the lost and simply out-matched expression settling on poor Handel's face.

The eldest of the four Jewish boys, Handel was less than a year younger than Johan. He considered himself to be cultured and was always anxious to denounce Christianity's influence on the arts. He listened carefully to Adolf's argument, but although he knew the Nibelung saga well, he was unfamiliar with *Lohengrin*, so he was not able to present a sufficient response. "And so a wedding is supposed to offset the greed and lust so prevalent in these works?" Unwilling to admit he was not familiar with *Lohengrin*, Handel hoped both sins were present in both opera.

Adolf smiled wolfishly. "Lust? The Prince arrives to save the Princess of a realm without a king. If not for the Prince's offer to defend her honor, she would have been charged with the murder of her brother. The Prince and Princess marry just after that. What instance of lust were you citing, exactly?"

Handel swallowed and glanced furtively toward Johan, hoping the other boy might interject some comment that would allow Handel to backtrack. Johan only smiled in his silence. He knew this argument was already won.

"Well?" asked Adolf, a confident and wolfish smile still at the corners of his lips.

At last Handel sighed and put up his hands. "You have me . . . lust was a poor example. Wagner may indeed have Christianized these myths, but they still are founded on Pagan beliefs."

Johan put a hand on Handel's shoulder. "Most of the world is founded on such stories. Neither the Christian God nor the Jewish God was worshipped before Zeus or Odin. So far as I am concerned, it is the teachings that are important, not the teacher."

Handel was about to argue against that statement, but Johan's hand closed on Handel's shoulder as the lad was opening his mouth. "I know, I know," Johan said. "Your God is great, and I am damned. I do not want to hear about it now. If you will excuse me, I would like a word with Adolf before Frau Sekira calls us to dinner."

Handel closed his mouth and gave Adolf one last look before offering a curt nod to both boys.

Adolf broadened his triumphant grin.

Once Handel had closed the door to his room, Johan opened the door to his own and invited Adolf inside. Johan's room was larger than Adolf's and much better able to accommodate company; Johan had not only a desk chair, but also a sitting chair.

"You know a lot about opera for someone your age. Handel has been to many, but I think you have read more. Reading them usually helps you remember them better."

Adolf settled into the sitting chair. It could certainly use reupholstering; the fabric on its arms was worn almost to the wood. "I remember my first opera quite distinctly, but I think you are right just the same."

Johan sat in his desk chair, and then leaned it back until it reclined against the wall. "You obviously enjoy the arts. What are your feelings on sports?"

"I have never played any—not seriously, at least." Adolf did not like to admit there was anything about which he did he had no knowledge, but it seemed best to be honest with Johan.

"That is fine," Johan said. "You do not need to play them to enjoy them. I always enjoy playing more than watching, but watching is good, too. Listen, I am going to a soccer game tomorrow after classes. Some friends are going to meet me there. Would you like to come along?"

Although Adolf's social arrogance precluded him from displaying any emotion akin to excitement, Adolf was pleased by the invitation. Rarely were new acquaintances worth the time it took to learn their names. However, Johan was an interesting enough fellow.

Surely his friends also would be of some quality. At last in a tone in which he might have thanked Johan for passing salt during dinner, Adolf answered.

"Very kind of you to offer. I accept."

"Excellent. I will meet you in the street once classes let out. The field is only a few blocks from the school."

The ring of Frau Sekira's dinner bell then sounded throughout the three floors of her boarding house, and her six tenants soon reported to their dinner stations. The meal of pot roast, potatoes and carrots was hearty, even though Frau Sekira had gone a bit overboard with her usage of rosemary and basil. Adolf ate the meal and cleaned his dishes before retiring to his room for the night.

If he was going to watch a game tomorrow, there was a lot of work he should do tonight. Yet as he sat with his history book open in front of him, he could not focus his mind. He kept daydreaming what the soccer match would be like and who Johan's other friends could be. He liked Johan well enough; he respected, perhaps even admired, the older boy. What of his friends though? What sort of people would they be? The more Adolf thought about it, the more nervous he became.

That nervousness persisted throughout the next school day. He prepared himself for the dismissal bell almost five minutes early, just so he could be certain he was among the first children to escape the classroom. He did not want Johan to forget and leave without him.

Adolf did not consider what it would feel like to instead be the one waiting. His excitement contested with his mounting anxieties, and he must have looked somewhat ridiculous standing statuesque in the center of the street while he waited to catch sight of Johan.

Minutes passed, as did his fellow schoolmates. Some of his lesser acquaintances stopped to ask for whom he was waiting or why he was standing there at all, but his nervousness made his answers sharp, cold, and so he was left to stand alone against the waning tide of students. Still there was no sign of Johan. As he was beginning to wonder if Johan had played a cruel joke on him, he felt a hand on his shoulder.

"Been waiting long?" asked Johan.

Never one for being touched, Adolf gave a startled shout before turning to recognize Johan. "How did you get past . . . ?"

Johan smiled roguishly. "Cannot come out of a school that you did not go into, can you? I was busy preparing a surprise for one of the friends you will meet. Let us go—the match is starting soon."

The older boy did not wait for agreement, but marched toward the field; Adolf, with his smaller frame, had to hurry to keep up. Johan was a native to Linz and knew its side streets and alleyways as well as did the city's rats. Adolf was still learning the city, but he always enjoyed exploring new places. The alley might not be the deep forests of the wild Americas, but all the same, it was new, foreign and exciting.

By the time they reached the field, Adolf had expended most his anxiety in his effort to keep up with his friend. Johan was very fit and did not think twice of climbing fences or jumping rails. Adolf followed, albeit at a slower and slightly clumsier pace. Having reached the field, Johan then lead them into a small section of wooden stands.

Adolf followed, wondering where amongst the assembled crowd Johan would choose to sit. His anxiety returned to its previous volatile state when Johan made a turn down a row of benches upon which two very pretty girls sat. One was shorter, perhaps Adolf's height, but entirely opposite from him in all other comparisons. Her hair was gold spun into curls that ended just beyond her slender shoulders. Her eyes were the most startling shade of blue, sparkling like ice in the afternoon light. Her smile was large and confident when she saw Johan approaching, and she stood to offer her hand, before lightly kissing each of his cheeks, one after the other.

The girl sitting beside her was also very pretty, although tall— prettier than the shorter girl, thought Adolf as he shyly appraised her. While the other girl's height was somewhat intimidating to the younger, smaller Adolf, her dark hair was long and neatly braided. Her eyes were also dark, resembling his mother's in their shape and color. He realized she was appraising him just as closely as he was summing up her.

Johan then hugged the second girl, while Adolf was left to stand awkwardly behind the embracing pair. At last Johan began introductions. "Helga, Elise, I would like you to meet Mr. Adolf Hitler. He is one of my boarding fellows, a man whose somehow established maturity long before his age could catch up."

The girls smiled kindly at Adolf, who fought back a flush of embarrassment as he smiled timidly. He may have achieved maturity beyond his years when it came to such things as the opera, but so far as girls were concerned, he was a virgin in the purest and most fundamental sense. If any conversation were to arise, it would be the first he had held with members of the opposite sex who were not his relatives.

"And these fine young ladies, my dear Adolf, are Miss Helga and Miss Elise Faveshra. They claim to be twins, and while I would never dare to call their honor into question, you can imagine why so many people have!"

Helga, the blond twin, slapped Johan swiftly on his knee. "Called into question, indeed!"

Elise leaned her longer frame forward, so as to look down the row at Adolf, "Very nice to meet you, Adolf. My sister may be offended, but Johan is welcome to put *my* honor to the test whenever he pleases."

Helga made a girlish yelp of indignant reproach before slapping her sister's knee. Johan laughed and smiled his roguish smile. Saying anything more would likely have earned a slap from Helga, and he was far more interested in her than he was in anything Elise so boldly offered.

Adolf did not understand any of the innuendos, and so only smiled at the twins. "It is very nice to meet the both of you."

Johan turned to Adolf, speaking quietly. "Helga is my age. Elise I think is closer to your age, whatever their claim of being twins might be. Convenient for us, is it not? As much as I normally would be more than happy to put Miss Elise's honor to that test of which she speaks, my attention is on the lovely Miss Helga. I hope you do not mind playing second fiddle, as it were, but Helga would not come without her sister, and Elise would not come unless I brought a friend, so here we are."

Adolf listened and nodded while he watched the girls hold a similar conversation. Adolf could only wonder what was being said.

In a low voice, he said, "You could have told me we were coming to meet girls. You told me we were meeting your friends. If I had known, I would have gone home to change first."

Johan shrugged. "There was no time for you to change. That is partly the reason I did not go to school today. As for telling you they were girls, well, dear Adolf, you will learn that telling your version of the truth is oftentimes better than telling the full truth. You might not have agreed to come if you had known you would be with older girls. I remember being your age. I would have been very nervous all day. This way, I have spared you of that.

Adolf was incredulous. He *had* been nervous all day. He might proceed straight to panic if this Elise expected him to do anything besides sit and watch the game. Adolf had no idea what teams were playing, but he decided that rooting for the red team was as useful an occupation for his attention as anything else. Anything that did not lead him to direct eye contact with either of the girls would be useful for the moment.

They were maybe ten minutes into the match when Elise rose from her seat. Helga and Johan had been conversing with each other more than watching the game, and Elise seemed anxious to partake in the same social intercourse. Her efforts to intrude on her sister and Johan's conversation failed, but Elise was not a girl to be ignored.

Turning her attention to Adolf, she said, "Adolf, would it be too much of an imposition to request the pleasure of your company? It would seem that my view here is obstructed by my sister's incessant twittering in poor Johan's ear."

Adolf, surprised to be addressed, never mind asked to keep

a girl company, blinked a few times and began explaining that it would be no imposition at all. Before he finished speaking, Elise was already making her way past Helga and Johan, moving her lithe form between the narrow space past other knees. She was not so graceful to avoid stumbling at least once in her journey, although she caught herself with her hands pressed to Johan's broad chest before she recovered, and then slipped into the seat next to Adolf.

Helga narrowed her eyes at her sister, whose eyes had locked on Johan's the moment she had pressed his muscles with her clumsiness. Johan, for his part, stared back for a moment, before blinking and offering a hand to steady Elise. Her smile was certainly not from embarrassment, as the mischievous glint in her eye forced Johan to wonder if it had really been an accident at all.

"It is a lovely day, is it not?" Elise said. "I am so glad the snow has melted."

Adolf could not bring himself to look at Elise. She was the prettiest girl he had seen since his night at the opera, beauty that was intimidating. "Oh yes, it is a fine day." His response was timid, after which there was an awkward silence.

Elise continued to watch him, observing the angles of his face. He was so very formal, so polite, and yet self-possessed, with tensile posturing. He was trying so hard to hide his nervousness that he was making it even more obvious. It was cute, and mildly endearing. She would enjoy teasing him.

She did not allow that silence to last long.

"You have very distinguished eyes, did you know that?" She could not see his eyes at all the way the daylight fell on them, but she had to compliment something just to end their boring silence.

His cheeks had not yet lost their baby fat, and his chin lacked the chiseled strength of Johan's. His eyes though, his eyes contained a sharpness that suggested intelligence. There was fire in his eyes, even if the rest of his body language showed him to be shy.

"Thank you." He said formally, though could not help the color from filling his cheeks.

Elise pressed her lips into a thin line. She hoped for more than two words of response. Was he just timid? Or uninterested in her? No, that was impossible. She would simply have to try harder. She had flirted often enough to know that sometimes boys Johan's age took a great deal of effort to relax so that they would just be themselves. She would simply keep talking, and he would eventually say something at least mildly interesting. He had to, even if it were just a matter of dumb luck.

"So, Adolf. Have you lived in Linz very long?"

Adolf, still afraid to meet Elise's eyes, continued to look between the girl and the game as he answered. "No, not very long at all. My father passed away recently. I have been staying at Frau Sekira's since then."

At last he managed to string together entire sentences. She was making progress, even if it were aggravatingly slow. She would not give up. Just the sound of Johan and Helga laughing together made her try all the harder to dispel Adolf's insecurity. She hated when Helga was enjoying herself with a handsome fellow, and she was not.

"I see," she said. "I am sorry for your loss. You must be happy to be living here in Linz, at least. This city is the most Austrian of cities. I would rather be here than, say, Vienna, any day. Let them have their royalty. We have our sports, our arts!"

At last Adolf smiled at Elise's enthusiasm. "You enjoy the arts?" Still nervous, but glad to find a mutual interest, he spoke with a concerted effort to keep his voice even.

Elise smiled mischievously, "I enjoy many things, especially something as romantic and passionate as art. You are passionate, aren't you?"

Adolf only felt the wind of that innuendo as it sailed over his head. "Oh yes, I'm very passionate about the arts." Adolf missed the open invitation to flirt, and instead decided to carry the conversation and impress Elise with his goals. "I draw in my spare time and attend whatever opera I can manage. I am going to be a great painter, some day." Adolf's own conviction in that statement almost surprised him. Elise was the first person outside his family to whom he had admitted his life's dreams, and it had felt so natural, so right, for him to announce his passion to someone new.

Elise let her mischievous smile relax into something more genuine. "Such confidence! Would I be too forward if I asked to see your drawings some time? I also like to draw and sing. And dance! I love to dance. Do you dance, Adolf? You must! You must dance very well, I think."

Adolf was beginning to feel that he must dance very well indeed, despite never having tried a single step. Elise's faith in his ability gave him a very fuzzy, muddled sort of feeling. He made no answer, not knowing what he could say.

Elise did not allow the younger boy's silence to deter her. "We must meet again, and you will bring drawings. We can share our work. We can critique each other, like the famous artists do!" Her hand then fell on Adolf's thigh, "We will become very close friends, I think. That is, if you would like to share your work. Some artists are very picky about letting people see their work, but I do not think you are silly like that. What is the point of creating something if no one is allowed to see it?"

With that, Adolf could not agree more. Her words almost distracted him from the girl's hand on his thigh. He hated to be touched, but his flesh had never felt more alive through the fabric of his trousers. "Of course you may see my drawings."

Helga leaned forward to peer around Johan, "Be careful, Adolf. My sister has a habit of talking people into doing the strangest things. Be sure you do what you want, and not only what she wants."

Elise wrinkled her nose and briefly stuck out her tongue in a very unladylike gesture.

Johan laughed. "Aye, she might see your drawings, say they are quite good, and then later decide she wants her taste back."

Adolf took the jibe in stride, "If the work confuses her tastes, there is hope, I think. Even finding some small merit before the faults appear means there is something good and talented in the piece, even if it is not perfect, yet."

Elise gave his thigh another gentle squeeze, and then a pat that succinctly terminated the contact. "Well said, Mr. Adolf. Very well said. I am looking forward to seeing your art."

Adolf was looking forward to it too, but he was more interested in seeing her again. His dark eyes no longer fled back to the field when they met Elise's. Her complexion was flawless, rosy in her cheeks with dimples that showed her mischievous manner when she smiled. Her eyes were bright, and her nose small, as were her ears, which hid in her dark braided hair. She was very pretty, indeed. Did she know how pretty? Did she know he thought she was? What did she think of him? Was he handsome? Homely? He must be handsome, or she would not have spoken to him or wanted to see his drawings. She was so pretty.

The four of them ended up talking more than they watched the match. They were still laughing and smiling over some poor joke or quick wit while the game ended and the other attendees exited the rickety wooden stands. Before long, the sun was just above the trees, and the girls were pulling their frocks tighter to themselves against the oncoming chilly air.

"We will miss dinner if we do not leave, and Papa will be upset." Helga always worried about her father's interests.

Elise was more selfish, and would have stayed out until the late hours if her sister did not bring her home.

Johan nodded, "And we will miss our dinner as well. Shall we do this again next week? Or should we meet somewhere else, so that Adolf and Elise can share their pretty pictures with one another?" Johan grinned. "Unless, of course, they have made plans of their own?"

"They had better not have," said Helga abruptly. "She knows she is not allowed to go anywhere without my company. The same as I cannot be without hers."

Elise made another of her faces at Helga, adding to Johan's theory that she was, in fact, the younger of the two, even if she were taller. They were certainly not twins, no matter that they claimed to be.

"I could bring my drawings here. I keep most of them in a notebook." Adolf did not notice Elise narrow her eyes. "Here is as good as anywhere."

"Well," Elise began. "My drawings are mostly done with charcoal crayons on very large leafs of paper. They are not so transportable. However, I would love to see your drawings, Adolf. If we prove to have similar tastes, then perhaps you will be so kind as to visit my home after, where I can show my own work."

Adolf was curious to know what sort of talent Elise had, but it was certainly not a prerequisite for sharing his own work. He was very happy just to have any sort of audience at all.

Johan grinned and put his hand on Adolf's shoulder. "I am sure Adolf would be happy to attend. Of course, he only goes where I go."

Helga elbowed Johan in the ribs, but Elise smiled coyly at Johan. "I was rather counting on such." But when Helga shot her sister a harsh look, Elise went on. "Who else will keep poor little Helga entertained and away from us artists? We need our privacy, after all."

Adolf swallowed hard at that thought, but then smiled as wide as had Johan.

"Then it is settled," Johan said. However, I am afraid that we cannot meet you here again next week if we do not leave you here first. Hurry, lest you excite your father's displeasure. Then neither Adolf nor I will be welcomed anywhere next week."

Helga smiled, and then offered her hand for Johan, who took it and formally kissed it farewell. Elise did the same with Adolf, although her eyes lifted to Johan, to whom she was obviously more attracted. Adolf's own were lowered.

""Til next week," she said.

"Farewell," Adolf said, managing to raise his gaze at last.

"Farewell!" And with that excitement, the girls left the boys in high spirits.

"Well, Adolf, you performed admirably. I knew you were just the fellow to entertain Elise. You may be the youngest of Frau Sekira's tenants, but your demeanor exudes maturity. Handel's tongue would have been tripping over his teeth. What is more, I think Elise truly likes you!"

Adolf was not so mature as to avoid the color that came to his cheeks. "She is a very pretty girl. I am just lucky she enjoys art, I suppose."

Johan shook his head after jumping a low wooden fence. "No, no her eyes suggested luck had nothing to do with her interest. Your art certainly helps, but I think Elise is more concerned with a lad's physical appearance than she is ability."

Adolf hurdled over the fence and smiled, "You really think so, do you?"

Johan slapped Adolf on his shoulder, "I do not really need to think about it at all. I know the look. She is given it to me plenty of times, but I have always liked blonds better. Not to say Elise is not attractive. She is beautiful by any standard, but she is not my type. But she is *your* type, is she not?"

Adolf did not particularly like to know Elise had been interested in Johan, as well. He was very glad, however, to know Johan was conversant enough with the opposite sex to confirm Adolf's suspicions. She had told him that it was all very romantic, and her dark eyes had said even more.

"Thank you, Johan," Adolf said. "I must thank you again for taking me with you. I am not sure I have ever been so happy or excited in all my life." And indeed, Adolf's words were spoken through a smile, with a wild light to his own dark eyes.

He knew how Adolf felt and laughed at the boy's thanks. Johan was still young enough to remember the first girl who had taken an interest in him. "Thank me now, before you learn how much of a headache girls can be."

They were making their way down the last alley before the boarding house, dodging puddles and stray animals as they went. The sun had long since fallen over the western hills, and what had been an invigorating chill earlier was now a nipping cold, but Adolf felt flushed and heated in his excitement.

The two boys ended up being late for their own dinner after all, but Frau Sekira was kind enough to save their plates atop the wood-burning stove. When one of the other boys, David, asked where they had been, Johan spoke of the soccer match, but never mentioned either of the girls. Sebastian, the youngest of the Jewish boys and the only boy among the four Jews to whom Adolf even considered offering his friendship, asked Adolf later that evening, curious about why the normally stoic Adolf was smiling so much. Adolf, though, supplied the same answer Johan had and, in doing so, gained more of the oldest boy's respect and trust.

For the next six days, Adolf all but ignored his studies. What time he did not spend talking to Johan, whom he was beginning to regard as an idol, even as much as Adolf thought him a good friend, he spent working on his drawings.

For the first two or three days, he reworked old sketches and drawings from his days in Hafeld and Lambach, pastoral works full of panoramic depictions of the countryside and mountain ranges. His efforts at revising the pieces resulted in drawings with rural sentimentality and rustic elements that married well to his natural talent for depicting proportions, whether they were the architectural structures, apple orchards or riverbanks. He was very proud of these edited versions and was sure Elise would notice and appreciate his devotion to the small, but intricately beautiful, details of his subjects, such as wildflowers blooming or the shadows lengthened by the setting sun.

He thought of Elise quite often while he worked, as he did during his classes and when he lay in bed at night, trying in vain to sleep. By the fourth night, he had gone over the few hours he had spent in the soccer stands a thousand times. He had considered what altering words or gestures might have done to make her like him even more; he wanted to say the right thing when next they met.

The more he thought about Elise, the more perfect for each

other he convinced himself they were. She enjoyed the arts! She was knowledgeable and intelligent, and very, very pretty. She had only met him once, but once was enough to convince the adolescent Adolf he was in love for the first time. By that fourth night since he met her, that love for the arts and the fact that he was obviously such a talented artist was enough to convince him that she loved him back.

By the fifth night, he had finished working on old drawings and decided it was time to create something entirely new. He was in Linz, a city full of Austrian beauty and wonder. Although there were fewer trees here, and no mountains to recreate in ink, there were an abundance of buildings whose architecture was inspiring. Adolf began wandering the city after school, learning its alleys as Johan had. By the sixth night, he had drawings of the Opera House, not only as it was, but also how Adolf would have made it, with formal fluted columns forming a receiving pavilion before the opera house doors, and the vaulting dome of a roof that would offer both aesthetic beauty and more expansive and encompassing acoustics within the opera house itself. Or at least, so he believed.

His pride in his work had never been firmer, nor had his confidence in himself ever been greater. Kept so low by his father's abuses over the years, and by the incident with Friar Roald, Elise's attention had bolstered his confidence, and he had never been happier.

He also had never been more arrogant. Without his father's hand to humble him, Adolf's growing ego only made him even more authoritative. He no longer gave any attention at all to Handel, Sebastian or any of the Jewish boys. He never offered a civil hello in passing, nor answered any such salutation they offered. The more he considered Johan's words about Handel tripping over his own tongue if he had been introduced to Elise, the more Adolf saw other flaws in the older Jewish boy. His nose, for instance, was ridiculously large, as were his ears. His oily, black, tightly curled hair looked like it belonged on a sheep. Handel believed Wagner supported pagan beliefs! No, Elise would never have seen anything in Handel.

Johan noticed the change in Adolf's personality and liked it. He had taken Adolf under his wing and thought of him more as a little brother than he did as a true friend, but Adolf's own ego did not allow any understanding of the difference. Indeed, Adolf would not learn the difference until it was too late.

By that sixth night, the eve of his second date with Elise—it was a date, was it not?—Adolf began to believe his love was in fact so strong, and so mutual, that he could express his feelings simply by *thinking* them to Elise. As he lay in darkness, waiting for his body heat to warm his cold sheets, he thought very hard—so hard that surely their love would permit the transcendence of physical barriers of distance. She was miles away on the opposite end of Linz, or that was what he imagined, at least; he had no idea where she lived. Just the same, his feelings of love would be more than enough to arrest her subconscious attention. He would use telepathy to profess his love.

On the seventh day, Johan decided it was probably a good idea to give Adolf further advice about girls in general. As they walked to the soccer field, Johan put his hand on Adolf's shoulder. "You probably do not have a lot of experience with women yet, correct? Do not be embarrassed. Everyone starts somewhere, and I think you are going to start somewhere today. Your drawings are going to impress her. You need the same confidence you had the last time—more even. Sit close to her while you show your pictures. Go through them slowly. If she compliments them, touch her when you thank her. Take her hand, lean your shoulder into hers and press your leg against hers, but be sure to make contact. The more she feels such innocent contact, the more used to you she will become."

Adolf nodded. "I understand," he said, before breaking into another of his wide smiles. "What else?"

Johan grinned. "Well, if you find her looking at you strangely, in a vacant, dreamy sort of way, she probably wants you to kiss her. If you do, make sure you do not hesitate. Kiss her, and depending on her reaction, either kiss her deeper, and perhaps put your arm around her, or break off the kiss yourself. Whatever you do, do not let her pull away first. You want to leave her wanting more, not the other way around. Understand?"

This task sounded more difficult than simply holding the girl's hand. How was he supposed to know when she was going to pull away? If he did not know that, how could he know when to back off himself?

Johan saw Adolf's uncertainty. "It is not easy, I know. All I can say is to trust your intuition. Whatever you do, do not worry about a kiss. Chances are she will be nervous, too." But Johan was not entirely convinced of that. Elise was different from most girls, with confidence that was rare in anyone her age. Adolf was mature for his age; Elise was just as mature.

Helga displayed a similar strength, which made the claim that they were twin sisters more plausible, even if he still greatly doubted it. Helga was more reserved; she would never eye him in public as mischievously as had Elise. The more Johan thought about the difference between the sisters, the more he hoped Adolf could keep Elise entertained.

"Thank you yet again, Johan. I will try not to disappoint you or Elise." With his sketchbook under his left arm, and his continued attempts at employing telepathy, he was certain the day would go very well. It could hardly get any worse—he had received grades on three exams earlier that day, failing two of them. If he planned to pass his courses, his studies would need to come before his drawings next week.

It was warmer that day, being later in the spring. Adolf's birthday was only a few weeks away, although his mother had made no mention of it to him, yet. She was likely far too busy making arrangements for his half-sister Angela's wedding in the fall.

This time, it was the boys who arrived at the match first. Johan led Adolf high into the stands, marching straight to the uppermost row, although there were at least three rows empty beneath them. "It is not always bad for a girl to have to work a bit for your company," Johan said, explaining his choice of seats. Besides, we will have more privacy up here."

Adolf agreed, feeling again like a young apprentice learning from his master, a strange relationship for Adolf, used to being the ringleader.

The stands continued to fill with fans for both teams. This week, some yellow-shirted team with green shorts played the red-shirted team. Adolf had still not learned what the teams' actual names were. Never being particularly athletic in his frame or constitution, the allure of sports might have been entirely lost on Adolf, except it excited in him a competitive spirit of which he had otherwise been ignorant.

The match started, and less than two minutes had passed before a referee issued the first yellow card to a member of the red team. Adolf was not sure what the card meant, but the red team's fans were booing and cursing the referee. Adolf decided he liked the color red more than he liked yellow, so he booed too. He was about to holler an acidic obscenity when Johan's restraining hand redirected his attention to the arrival of the twins.

Helga wore her golden hair in braids, and Elise's was loose enough to show that while her hair did not have Helga's curl, it was very wavy and longer than Adolf had imagined. Adolf was surprised to find the look very attractive. The girls still wore their black frocks, covering their school uniforms. "Hello boys," Elise said when the girls at last reached

the stand's top row.

Helga then made a show of looking over the wooden railing, evaluating the distance to the ground. "Sitting in the clouds today, are we?"

Johan grinned. "We were among the first ones here and thought the crowd would fill in below us. Rather than having people climb past us, we thought to sit here, where we would remain unmolested. If you had not been so late, we might have had closer seats." He winked to soften his words.

Helga narrowed her eyes at the reproach, but did not say anything. Elise made one of her faces at Johan, and then moved past him to sit next to Adolf. "Do you not have a hello for me?"

Adolf smiled, hoping it would stop his cheeks from blushing. "Of course! It is good to see you again. I missed you. I brought my drawings."

Elise just raised one of her beautifully shaped eyebrows. "Missed me? How sweet. I suppose I missed you, too. You are far more interesting than Johan's last friend, and I have looked forward to seeing your artwork."

Adolf was not sure what to say. *Johan's last friend?* Why had he not considered that before? If Helga only went out with her sister, and Johan had obviously met the two before, it could only mean that previously Johan had brought another boy to keep Elise's attention. He wondered who it had been. For a moment, Handel's face came to mind, and fierce jealousy darkened Adolf's mood. Had Johan given the Jewish boy similar advice? He tried not to think about it and instead opened his sketchbook. Handel was not sitting next to the beautiful Elise.

Adolf slid on the wooden bleacher until his hip was pressed to hers. "I spent most of the week redrawing my older pieces. If you would like to see the original version in comparison and my new renditions, it may help to illustrate just how much my art has improved since moving to Linz." "Fascinating, I am sure," said Elise. She then turned away from Adolf as he offered her the sketchbook. Instead, she leaned across Johan's lap to interrupt his conversation with Helga. "Excuse my intrusion, but I was just wondering if either of you are hungry? Perhaps it was the walk up all

those extra steps, but I am positively famished."

Helga did not appreciate her sister's interruption any more than her current proximity to Johan. "No, I am not hungry. Perhaps you should ask Adolf."

Adolf had been listening, but remained quiet. Elise narrowed her eyes at Helga, and then turned back to Adolf. "How rude of me," she said with evident sincerity. "Forgive me, but I am so used to thinking of my sister first. Are you at all hungry?"

Despite Johan's advice not to be nervous, anxiety over the upcoming date had ruined Adolf's appetite at lunch, and he had a feeling it would be a long time until returned. "No, no, I would hate to spoil my dinner. Frau Sekira is making a pork roast with her cinnamon-honey glaze."

Johan laughed. "Aye, which is far too sweet for my taste. I would love to eat something now, actually. Wait here, and I will bring something back for you."

But Elise shook her head. "No, no, it is not fair to make you walk there alone. I will go with you. Helga would enjoy seeing Adolf's drawings as much as I would, and I will have plenty of time to view them once we return."

Helga shot her sister a particular look, but the taller girl was already stepping down into the next row, which had remained unoccupied, pulling Johan's pant leg just below his knee as she went. With a shrug, Johan rose and followed her, leaving Helga and Adolf alone.

Helga smiled, making the best of the situation. "You will have to forgive Elise. She is headstrong and used to getting what she wants. She has always been Papa's favorite, and he spoils her dreadfully."

Adolf smiled and slid closer to Helga on the smooth wooden bench. "That is all right—I am sure they will be back soon enough. If you would like, I will show you my drawings until they return."

Helga returned his smile and nodded. "I think I would like that more than I would enjoy watching the match. Sports do not hold my attention very long. Elise has more talent when it comes to creating art, but I have always enjoyed critiquing it. I'd much rather be looking at a gallery than this field . . ."

If Adolf had not been so confident in his work, he might have become even more nervous at the prospect of showing her his art. Instead, he opened his sketchbook and, after Helga had a few moments to look his drawings, began describing the stories behind each sketch. He had no interest in the match either, and Helga's attention to his efforts made him feel even more excitement than

Elise's cold interest had the week before.

She liked his work, complimenting him many times and offering hints of constructive criticism as he turned the pages. If Helga were Elise, Adolf would have had ample opportunities to take the girl's hand in his. Instead, he let the sketchbook rest on the bench between them.

They were perhaps halfway through his sketchbook before Helga began to wonder why Elise and Johan had had been gone so long. It should not have taken them that much time to get a sausage sandwiches and return. Adolf had been so absorbed by the opportunity to show his work, had lost track of the time. Seeing Helga's eyes searching for her sister, Adolf at last began to wonder as well.

Helga's gasp came only a moment before Adolf followed her eyes to see Elise and Johan sitting on a bench near the sausage vendor. Even at this distance, there was no mistaking the fact that the two were kissing, not only publicly, but from what Adolf could tell, rather passionately.

"That bitch," said Helga, her voice strained by the tears filling her blue eyes.

Adolf did not know what to say or do. His thoughts of love had meant nothing. His feelings had meant nothing. Elise did not love him as he loved her. She had no interest in his artwork—or in him. Perhaps she had only been trying to raise some jealous sentiment in Johan.

Helga looked away and reached out to take Adolf's arm, directing his attention away from the scene. "My own blood would betray me for . . . for him! He would betray me for . . . for her!" Her tears were wetting her cheeks, and she was surprised to find Adolf's were also wet.

"You poor boy," she said, her voice filled with compassion, "this must be even harder for you, young as you are. You are not like Johan, just as I am not like Elise."

But Adolf did not want Helga's sympathy, especially when it

sounded so much like pity. He had just begun to think he knew what love was, when already his heart had been broken, not once, but twice in one instance. He had thought he loved Elise, but worse, he had trusted Johan.

Looking at Helga was too much; he stood and began turning away. But Helga reached out and grabbed his arm. "Please do not leave me, Adolf. Do not make me wait here alone for them to return. I cannot go home to Papa
without Elise. Please?"

Adolf did not want to stay. He wanted nothing more than to return to his room and never again emerge. "I am sorry" he said, his throat tight. "You are a beautiful girl, and if you do not want Johan, there are plenty of other boys next to whom you can sit at soccer matches. I would guess that Johan still likes you more than he does Elise. You could him if you decided to forgive him. Me, though? Well, I think it is obvious that Elise never liked me at all." He almost said "loved," but caught himself in time.

Helga stood, and before Adolf knew what was happening, she kissed him quickly on his lips.

"You are a very handsome boy, Adolf, and talented. There will be many other girls with whom you can watch soccer matches, too. But for now, please, stay and sit with me. I do not want to be here alone."

Adolf wanted nothing more than to be alone. He was reeling, no longer from Johan's betrayal, but from his first kiss, about which he did not know how to feel. His heart was still fixed on Elise, and so Helga's kiss had felt wrong. Perhaps Johan and Elise could betray their friends, but Adolf could not. He did not want Helga; he wanted Elise.

"I am sorry, Helga."

Adolf gathered his sketchbook and walked away.

Chapter 6

LENGTHENING HIS STRIDE, the blood throbbing in his temples stronger than the anger forming within him, Adolf fought the tears brimming in his eyes. How could he have allowed himself to believe so many lies? Elise did not love him. She had never been interested in him at all. And Johan? Johan had been the older brother Adolf had lost when Alois had run away. Johan's betrayal was even harder to accept.

The women walking home with the evening's groceries gave Adolf a wide berth as he marched down the streets, back to the boarding house. He was in no mood to use the shortcuts Johan had taught him, even those Adolf had found on his own; he would not hide in alleyway shadows. He wanted everyone in Linz to know his condition. He wanted the world to see his jaw clenched as tightly as his fists, to see the fires that must surely be burning beneath his tears. His reddened eyes challenged anyone who dared look at him. Unlike his normal desire for privacy, he wanted all of Linz to know his hurt and fury.

Few did. Most saw the purpose in his gait and smartly decided not to cross his path. They knew nothing of his heart, was broken not once, but twice in the same day. If he were older, sitting in a tavern with that look, many there would recognize it for what it was: heartbreak.

He had hidden his anger from Helga. She had all but begged him to stay in the stands with her, but he simply could not do it. He was doing a very poor job at controlling his emotions, and he had not wanted her to see him cry. He did not want to cry at all—only his strained pace kept the tears from falling. Why had he allowed himself to believe Elise was so perfect for him? How had he ever convinced himself that she loved him? He had been so naive . . .

By the time he reached the boarding house, he had all but blinked away the tears that had never fallen. His features were still strained, but he had a tighter rein on his emotions. As he turned his heavy house key in the lock, the left side of the double-door opened, almost pushing Adolf off the landing. The boarding house must have been a school at one time, considering the size of its front doors, an architectural curiosity that Adolf had never considered before. It was yet another source of irritation, even if incredibly minor compared to the larger sources of Elise and Johan, and now of course his surprised embarrassment of nearly being knocked from the front stairs.

It was Handel, of course. "Oh, Adolf, excuse me."

Adolf recovered his balance before retrieving his key from the lock. "Oaf. Next time be more careful. The door has a window for a reason." Although he spoke with the alto of youth, his voice was rough, almost guttural, muting its intended severity.

Handel saw that Adolf was in a bad temper. The younger boy's eyes were fierce red. But Handel had grown tired of Adolf's condescending manner. "Yes, the door *does* have a window. Perhaps you will be kind enough to grow so that I will be able to see you from it."

Adolf was a good four inches shorter than Handel, and he was no fighter, but even the smallest stature can often be strengthened by intensity, which Adolf had been accruing his entire walk home. He punched Handel in the stomach, the heavy house key wrapped in his palm.

The older boy doubled over, clutching his gut, his face pale.

"Can you see me now, Handel?" Adolf leaned over, whispering into the injured boy's ear. "Am I on your level?" When the boy remained silent, Adolf stood up, saying, "I am never at your level, Handel. I always stand above you. Remember that."

Handel tried to answer, standing upright, but Adolf had driven the wind from him with that punch. Adolf, accustomed to being the victim or the abuser of those weaker than him, had never been in a real fight with a peer. He had not intended to hurt Handel so greatly, but it was lucky that he did, or else the other boy might have returned the favor. "Never again use a glib remark or stand in my way. Next

time I will do worse."

Adolf walked past Handel, who allowed the smaller boy to push him aside, gasping as he struggled with his breath. Inside the house, David, the youngest of the Jewish boys, had witnessed the entire exchange from just inside the front hall. He did not say anything to Adolf, just watched

him walk into his room.

It was the smartest thing anyone had done all day, thought Adolf.

Behind the privacy of his latched door, Adolf at last relaxed his grip on his sketchbook, setting it on his small desktop with resignation that quickly gave way to a dark and smoldering mood. The fire of his emotions had left him once he reached the relative private confines of his room. He had no desire to look at the drawings of which he had been so proud just a few short hours ago. Now he wanted no part of anything he had drawn with Elise in mind. He would destroy the sketch of the two of them sitting in the soccer stands. Maybe he would destroy every piece he had reworked in the past week. But first, he needed to lie down. He was light-headed from the wild emotion and unrelenting thoughts of hurtful betrayal.

Less than a half hour passed before Frau Sekira's dinner chime roused the boarders from their rooms. Adolf's stomach was still twisted with a range of emotions, from furious anger to heartsick despair. Food was the furthest thing from his mind, although he had eaten very little that day. He had skipped breakfast that morning and eaten only a meager lunch of an apple and a pear. With his slight frame, he did not, as a rule, have a particularly large appetite, but in times of nervousness or stress, he often did not eat at all.

In the works of Karl May, he had read about an old trapper who insisted that hunger sharpened a person's senses. Adolf had found this to be true: his own mind was sharper when he felt pangs of hunger, but he did not understand that sharpness also made him more irritable and further shortened his already short temper. Now that he was sitting alone in his room, the adrenaline from his long walk wearing off, he felt utterly drained and wanted nothing more than to bury his face into one of his mother's hugs.

A knock sounded at his door, a short, polite rapping. It would not be his mother, and in her absence, he had buried his face into his pillow. He did not want to speak to anyone. Had Johan returned? The older boy would certainly want to talk to him. Could it be Handel? The taller boy would have recovered his breath by now. Would he come seeking retribution? At least a minute passed, and Adolf thought that whoever it was must have gone away. But the knock came again, this time with a more staccato—and thus insistent—sound.

"Mr. Hitler? Mr. Hitler?" Frau Sekira's tone would never be mistaken as motherly. Matronly, perhaps, but despite her inclination toward inquiry, the woman's voice always maintained an inflection of authority. "Mr. Hitler, please answer your door so I might have a word with you."

Adolf gritted his teeth and gripped the corners of the pillow even harder, burying his face deeper into it. He was in no mood to answer the woman. He did not care at that moment that she was the owner of his residence. She could have been a maid for all he cared about her just then.

Again Frau Sekira's voice sounded. "Mr. Hitler!"

At last Adolf let forth an aggravated groan that was muffled and muted by fabric and feathers. He rose and answered the door with rude abruptness, wrenching the knob and almost pulling the door from its hinges. "What?" Frau Sekira was a stern woman. She had to be, given her occupation as owner of a boarding house for boys. "'What'?

What indeed, Mr. Hitler. What kept you from answering my first knocks for your attention?"

In no mood for the woman's reproachful tone, Adolf looked up at Frau Sekira. "Nothing, beyond my refusal to jump in my own quarters and rush to welcome an intrusion on my privacy."

Frau Sekira had run her boarding house for over a decade now.

Never had she been answered in such a manner. "Well then, Mr. Hitler. Allow me to apologize for so rudely interrupting whatever you were doing to remind you that dinner is served. Also, I was told that you had an altercation with one of the other residents. It was alleged that you actually struck him."

Color rose in Adolf's normally pale cheeks. David, or perhaps Handel himself, had tattled to Frau Sekira about the incident at the door. He thought a moment, and then said, "That is true." There was no sense in lying about the confrontation, but Adolf could at least make Handel look like the aggressor. "I was at the door, having just inserted my house key, when Handel rudely threw the door open, nearly knocking me from the landing. I told him he should be more careful in the future. He then made a remark that suggested my stature was to blame for the accident, as I was not tall enough for him to see through the windowpane."

"So you struck him in his belly?" she asked with an arched eyebrow.

He nodded. "I doubled him over, actually, which I had not meant to do. Really, if Jews had any sort of manners, he might have apologized sincerely, instead of offhandedly. Then there never would have been any violence. But he did not, and I simply will not stand idly while a larger fellow tries to bully me with his size."

David had mentioned none of those facts in his report of the altercation, and now, after hearing Adolf's side of the story, there was little else Frau Sekira could do, unless Handel himself came with a complaint to her with yet another version of the events, which would compel her to investigate further. Unwilling to be bothered by this matter, she decided that boys would be boys, and she need do no more.

"Well, Mr. Hitler, if you would like, I can make it very plain at dinner that such rudeness will not be tolerated in my boarding house. However, you must also understand that violence will not be tolerated either. I expect you to offer an apology, regardless of who began the altercation.

Now come, the roasted chicken will be cold by the time we sit. I rang the dinner bell minutes ago."

Adolf still had no appetite, but a painful twist of his stomach reminded him that he should eat something whether or not he had a taste for food. As for an apology, the woman could expect whatever she liked from him; what she got, however, might be disappointing.

Sebastian, David and Morris were all seated and waiting respectfully for Frau Sekira. Neither Handel nor Johan was present. Adolf's eyes fell on the boys already filling their plates, his gaze lingering perhaps a moment longer on David than the others. He then noticed a new boy at the table—and in Adolf's chair, no less!

"Excuse me," Adolf said, approaching the new boy. "That is my chair."

The boy, busy salting his meal, did not respond.

Adolf could hardly believe this boy's lack of manners. Raising his voice, he repeated himself. "I said excuse me, but that is my chair you are sitting on."

The other boy shrugged. "You are too late. I got here first."

Adolf's barely contained fury began to rise again. "You little rodent . . . I will give you five seconds to get out of that chair."

The boy did not respond.

"All right, what is your name?" Adolf's tone had become aggressive. He spread his feet shoulder-width apart, opening his stance while setting it. His shoulders hunched forward somewhat, making the muscles in his shoulders appear larger as he loomed over the new boy.

But the new boy paid no attention to Adolf's escalating tone. After what had occurred with Handel earlier, and Adolf's regular reputation at the home, the other boys chose to keep out of Adolf 's business, for now. The new boy of course knew little at all about Adolf, and simply answered, in a mocking manner of pleasantry, "Why my name is Samuel—Samuel Eisenberg. What is yours?"

"Adolf Hitler," he said proudly. He eyed Samuel's tightly curled black hair and bushy eyebrows and could not help himself. "You are one of *them*, are you not?"

"Excuse me?" The question was genuine, evident in the surprised confusion in the corners of Samuel's eyes.

"You self-indulgent louse! I bet you have never dirtied your hands a day in your life, have you?" Adolf pointed an accusing finger at Samuel. "You think the world owes you a favor, do you not, you lazy, good-for-nothing swine!"

Samuel had no idea what this Adolf fellow was talking about or why he was speaking to him in such a vehement manner, but he chose to answer with his usual off-handed cynicism.

"Boy, your parents certainly taught you well."

Adolf lost what control he had held over his temper. The veins in his neck strained as his father's often had in such times of fury. "How dare you insult my parents, you filthy Jew! They worked hard for a living, which is more than I can say of yours."

"What do you know of my parents, anyway?" Samuel withstood the undeserved attack with a mature patience. His tone did not invite any escalation of the conflict. His question was sincere and without any measure of the hostility in Adolf's assault.

Adolf snorted. "I know they must be inferior, just like you. You deserve a good whipping. That would teach you to stay away from my place at this table. Get out of that chair, or I will force you out. You can sit on the floor where you belong."

He suddenly realized that the new boy had not just sat in his seat, but stolen it, which fanned his anger even more hotly. "How dare you come to this table and usurp my chair? I paid good money for that seat. It is just like your kind to try and steal it."

Samuel slid the chair back and away from Adolf. His manner was still calm and civil. "Really, this is just a mistake. I arrived here first and saw no names on the chairs. There was no flag proclaiming this space as yours. If you were not so rude, I would have given you the chair gladly." And at last, a certain look came into Samuel's eye, a change in his demeanor so subtle, but so complete, that it made his next words sound gravely serious. "Now perhaps I think I will stay here on principle."

"Principle?" shouted Adolf. At last, he felt provoked. "What do you gypsies know of principles? Thievery and insolence are not principles. Where I come from, liars and cheats are not given a chair at the table. They certainly do not take the chair of honest, Christian Austrians."

Adolf moved behind Samuel, gripping the back of his chair. "I will give you one last opportunity to rise of your own volition. Then I will push you from this seat like the cur you are."

The boy, reluctant to get into a fight with an apparent lunatic, finally began to rise from his chair, muttering, "I pity you."

Adolf caught what Samuel had said and could not restrain himself from getting the last word.

"Funny, no one will pity you, Jew. Not when I am through with you. Now get out of my chair!" Adolf wrenched the chair out from under Samuel. Although he did not fall, he stumbled awkwardly before he regained his balance. He was about the same size as Adolf, but he had no interest in confronting the boy physically. Word had already spread about Adolf's earlier encounter with Handel.

Smiling smugly, Adolf took his seat.

What would Frau Sekira have said about all this? She was lingering in the kitchen much longer than usual; it had been close to a quarter hour since she had rung the dinner bell. But Frau Sekira had heard every word of the exchange, and while she may not agree with Adolf's attitude toward the Jews, she did agree that Adolf had paid for his chair—or at least paid more than had Samuel's parents—so Adolf had the right to it.

The boys were utterly quiet in the other room. Perhaps the rudeness of the entire exchange had shocked them into silence. Or perhaps David had already told the others what Adolf had done to Handel. Either way, instead of defending Samuel—or summoning Frau Sekira so she could witness Adolf's intolerable behavior—none of the boys had spoken or moved since Adolf had entered the room.

Sebastian decided to act as though nothing out of the ordinary had happened, filing away the scene in his head, in case he could use some part of it to later take revenge on Adolf. "Good evening, Adolf. How very kind of you to join us."

Adolf took his portion of chicken, potatoes and carrots from the communal dishes on the long table. He also took Sebastian's bait. He simply could not resist putting in a superior remark. Little did he realize that allowing others to goad him thus was not a mark of intelligence or superiority.

"It was kind of you to wait," Adolf responded, "although I will not go so far as to thank you for something that was not necessary. After all, we are not waiting for Handel or Johan."

"Handel is probably seeing a doctor."

David had avoided eye contact with Adolf this whole time. His eyes remained on his plate, hoping Adolf would not be able to discern whose voice had spoken.

Frau Sekira at last was ready to sit at the head of the table. She stood, waiting as Morris pulled out her chair. The other boys had enough manners to stand until the lady took her seat.

"Thank you, Morris." Frau Sekira waited for the boys to seat themselves again before bowing her head in prayer. "Gentlemen, may God bless this evening's meal and bless you with health and wealth alike. May he bless this house, that shelters all of us from the spring's storms, and let us remember that this place is indeed a refuge for us all." She might have glanced at Adolf. "Finally, we also pray for the boys who are not present. May their absence be short and their company enjoyed at our next meal. Amen."

Adolf often wondered which god Frau Sekira addressed. With so many Jews lodging in her house, it would not surprise Adolf to learn that Frau Sekira had Jewish blood herself, even if she did attend Catholic masses.

His mother and the priests had often insisted that there was only one God, but Adolf refused to believe that the Jewish God and the Christian God could be one and the same. The Jews believed they were a chosen people, and Adolf's God would never choose Jews.

He began eating his chicken—picking at it, really, since his appetite was still weak. The empty chairs left by Handel and Johan bothered Adolf, but not as much as either boy's presence would have. He did not truly care where Handel had gone, but wondered where Johan was. Could he possibly still be with the girls? Was he still with Elise, kissing her on the bench? At that thought, the embers of his anger stirred again.

His fork scraped his plate rudely with the force with which he pinned his meat. If he pressed any harder, he might dull the edge of his dinner knife on the heavy porcelain dinner plate.

Adolf, absorbed by his thoughts of Johan and Elise, had not noticed the sound at all. It was only when Sebastian asked that he use finesse instead of brute force when cutting his food that Adolf noticed he was pressing hard enough to bend his fork.

Frau Sekira forestalled Adolf from responding with his acidic wit. "Would you care for some mulled wine, Mr. Hitler? We have all had stressful days, and I usually find that a bit of spice for your sips can be quite relaxing."

There was always wine on the table for the boys. Frau Sekira watched the contents of each boy's glasses like an eagle, but it seemed to sedate the boys better than ales; for the younger boys, like Adolf and David, the wine could be cut with water. To be offered mulled wine, however, something Frau Sekira normally reserved for her own pleasure, was a rare treat.

The other boys looked far more excited by the offer than Adolf felt. He could not help but wonder why Frau Sekira would offer him the drink. Was this her way of apologizing for intruding on his privacy earlier? No, she had every right to demand he speak with her on her terms. She owned his room, after all. He merely rented it from her. Perhaps she was genuinely concerned for his attitude. He was self-conscious enough to know that he was very tense.

"That is very kind of you to offer, Frau Sekira. I graciously accept with thanks."

Frau Sekira smiled, and then rose and went to the stove, where she was keeping a carafe warm.

In her absence, Sebastian continued to pick at Adolf's manners. "A true gentleman would have retrieved the libation himself and poured first for the lady. Perhaps Johan has not taught you well enough, after all."

Adolf stopped chewing and stared malevolently at Sebastian. He set down his fork and swallowed the chicken he had been eating. Still holding his dinner knife, he pointed it at Sebastian. "You are just frothing with advice for me, are you not, Sebastian? Let me be very clear. Whatever Johan has taught me is no business of yours. Nor do I appreciate your commentary on my every action—or lack thereof. Unless you would like me to begin needling you over trivial matters of courtesy, such as your tendency to gulp your beverages or your proclivity for allowing bits of food to become stuck between your teeth, I suggest you finish your meal in silence."

Sebastian snorted. "Will you sucker punch me, as well? If having a scrap stuck between my teeth is my worst affront to etiquette, then I am still a courtesan—and you the most boorish of commoners. I understand that your father was a very well-respected man. It is a shame you are so eager to spoil his good name, is it not?"

Frau Sekira returned from the kitchen, steam rising from the carafe of mulled wine she carried. She had not heard the boys' conversation—she had been busy putting plates of food for Handel and Johan's on the woodstove's warmer—but she caught Sebastian's last remark and responded.

"A name such as Mr. Hitler's is something to grow into, Mr. Henkel. You should concern yourself less with his name and more with your own, lest you risk providing your peers with reason to believe you are jealous of Mr. Hitler."

The smell of cinnamon, nutmeg and, perhaps, ginger, wafted from Frau Sekira's carafe, opening the nasal passages of everyone present. After filling Adolf's cup, she filled her own, and then returned the carafe to the kitchen, making no offer to the other boys. She would enjoy its contents when the night's drafts began chilling her old bones.

A slow sip was all Adolf's tender palate could endure, both for the wine's heat and the strength of its spices. It was very good though, very good indeed. Its steam drifted up his nostrils, tingling, opening the vessels in his chest so that he seemed able to breathe better. The tightness that had gripped him since he had seen Elise and Johan kissing began to relax.

But the wine did not have a similar effect on Adolf's words.

Looking again at Sebastian, Adolf said, "You will learn, Sebastian, just as has every other person who has had the insolent gall to compare me to my father, that we are nothing alike at all. He earned his reputation by serving society's fools, like you. I will earn my reputation with my talents, my intelligence and my will." There was no arrogance or bravado in Adolf's words. They were measured, deliberate and brutally certain. "Three concepts about which I think you know positively nothing. If it were not for your family's generations of thievery, hoarding and miserly ways, you would not be in this boarding house at all. Now stop talking to me, or else I will do far worse to you than I did to Handel. You certainly deserve no less."

Frau Sekira spoke up, preventing Sebastian from retorting. "I trust the wine was not too strong for you, Mr. Hitler. I would hate for you to say something you might later regret because I erred in judgment. I know my mulled wine is particularly pungent to the nose, but it is also known for loosening tongues. I trust your capacity for the drink is such that you will remember to keep your speech civil."

Adolf ignored the wine's pungency and its nearly scalding temperature and took a long draught, a stubborn challenge to Frau Sekira's words, and then said, "My capacity is enough to recognize such proximity to inebriation and to stop myself short of that irresponsible mark. My words only matter if I mean every one I use. Be sure that I do."

Sebastian silently glowered at Adolf, not the least intimidated by the other boy's carbon-dark eyes staring back at him over the brim of his raised glass. Why was Frau Sekira protecting the boy tonight? Was it because Adolf's rent was higher than everyone else's except Johan's? Surely it was not because the other boys were Jewish? Whatever the case, he had tired of aggravating the boy for one night. He would remain silent for now.

Frau Sekira ate her dinner, occasionally hiding smirks of amusement behind her glass. It was true that she liked the Hitler child more than her Jewish residents, and it was just as true that she liked his higher rent. Adolf's mother had been willing to pay whatever she asked; she had experienced a very different negotiation with the Jewish boys' parents. She protected Adolf, currently the better investment.

Morris had hardly spoken a sentence throughout the entire meal. As he rose from his seat, shortly after David's departure, he looked at Adolf and said, "Just remember, Mr. Hitler, that although a surprise attack might gain you what you desire in the short term, violence is never the answer. God will forgive you for this incident, but I will pray that in the future you will find another way to settle your disputes" Nodding at each of them, he said, "Good night, Mr. Hitler, Mr. Henkel and, of course, good night to you, Frau Sekira."

Morris brought his plate to the kitchen, where he washed it and his allotment of pots and pans.

Adolf nursed what remained of his mulled wine. Its literal and figurative warmth had spread through him, relaxing him as Frau Sekira had promised.

He had developed a distaste for receiving advice from anyone, be they priest, teacher or Frau Sekira herself. His mother was perhaps the only person he still obeyed as dutifully as the distance between them allowed. Still, he paid heed to Morris's words, if only because he knew the boy chose them with even greater care than he did.

Sebastian was the last of the Jewish boys to leave the table. He bid Frau Sekira a cursory goodnight, and then left to do his own share of dishes. The woman nodded to the boy, and then sat sipping the dregs of her glass, while Adolf continued to pick at what remained of his meal.

The Frau spoke. "You made more than one enemy tonight, and

of the two, I think Mr. Henkel is the more dangerous. I am almost sorry I forced you to answer the dinner bell, Mr. Hitler."

Adolf dropped his fork and knife and pushed his plate away from him. He sat back in his chair, one arm draped over the chair's backing, the other bringing his glass to his lips. The mulled wine had cooled significantly by then, and although its initial warming effects had diminished, the spices were enjoyable. He savored the last taste and was glad when it continued to linger on his palate.

"Yes, I suppose I have made another enemy," he said, in no way concerned. Indeed, he made a rare joke. "And to think, Johan has not even arrived home yet."

Then his manner lost any trace of levity. "I must warn you, Frau Sekira. I have managed to keep my temper so far. With Johan, however, I will not be so inclined to restrain myself."

"And just what did Mr. Rainmayr do to deserve such hostile intentions?" Frau Sekira was curious, not only because she enjoyed her vicarious knowledge of the boys' lives, but also because Johan's rent was the only amount greater than Adolf's own. Just as she had protected her investment in Adolf, so she did the same with Johan.

Adolf said quite simply, "He betrayed my trust."

Frau Sekira had been renting Johan his apartment for almost four years. His parents had been killed in some tragic accident while on vacation, and his father's pension had since provided the funds for his residence in the boarding house. The old woman had seen the boy grow into a young man, and she well knew of his various relationships. She did not need to be told specifically what had happened, but she could guess. Woman's intuition, perhaps.

"That is a dire transgression," she said in a serious tone. "The worst, maybe. I am sorry to hear that, not just for your friendship, but also for the peace of my home." She gave him a meaningful look. "Do remember, Mr. Hitler, that this is *my* home, and I do not like when children squabble over grudges. I expect better manners from Handel, Sebastian and you. If you do not mind, I will speak to Mr. Rainmayr when he comes in. I would guess that I will find him slinking into the kitchen in an hour or two's time. Perhaps if I tell him how much his betrayal upset you, he will be more inclined to offer you an apology. I will not waste the effort though, unless I know you will be mature enough to accept such an apology."

Adolf set his glass on the table and rose from his chair. "Maturity will have very little to do with my decision of whether or not to accept his apology. Its manner and scope will decide me. But what issues I have with Johan I will settle myself. Thank you for the wine, Frau Sekira. Good night."

Without waiting for a response, Adolf took his dish to the kitchen, where the other boys had already finished their share of cleaning. Adolf was relieved that they had retired to their rooms already. Before Johan came slinking back—how very appropriate a term Frau Sekira had chosen—Adolf was back in the privacy of his own room.

He was still angry. He was still hurt and disappointed. Nothing had gone as it should have. The entire day was marred by betrayal, and it felt as if he had spent the previous week in absolute futility. He had ignored his studies to prepare his sketchbook for Elise's appraising eyes. Now it sat on the corner of his desk, sheets of paper protruding from its binding where he had torn old sketches out and replaced them with his revised pieces.

The more Adolf thought about the day's events, the more he decided Morris was wrong. Violence might be the only answer. He would never have been offered the mulled wine without his act of violence. He would probably still be sulking, close to finally spilling tears over his tragedy. Yes, Johan might as well have been Judas, and that was a true tragedy.

Tears again began to sting the corners of his eyes, but he took steadying breaths, still refusing to cry. Perhaps he had not seen things as they were? At that distance, how could he really know whether Elise and Johan were kissing? Perhaps they merely had been whispering secrets to each other. What if it had meant nothing at all and he had made a fool of himself by storming off? Perhaps Johan had not betrayed him at all.

But what of Helga's reaction? It was her words that had accused and condemned the pair. Had he simply overreacted to her overreaction? Life had become so infinitely complicated now that girls were involved.

Inasmuch as it pained him, his feelings for Elise were now stronger than ever, surely stronger than those he had known earlier in the week. She did like him, he was sure of it. She was interested in his work, but she had been ravenously hungry when she arrived at the game. It had been his fault for remaining in the stands with Helga instead of escorting Elise to the sausage stand. Had he done so, it might have been him kissing sweet Elise.

His door abruptly swung open, startling him from where he daydreamed on his bed. He had forgotten to throw his latch after returning from dinner, and now Johan's frame filled the open space of his doorway.

"You had better be as sick as you look, Adolf."

Adolf did not rise or move at all. He let his gaze leave Johan in the doorway, fixing instead on the ceiling over his head. His doubts had eroded the foundation of his anger, and he was caught wondering if Johan had indeed betrayed him, or if Adolf had been wrong all along.

"I am talking to you, Adolf. Look at me." When the other boy's eyes were once again affixed to his, he continued. "What were you thinking? How could you leave Helga alone in the stands like that? I trusted you to keep her company, and you left her there alone."

Adolf took a deep and steadying breath. He sat up and swung his legs off the side of his bed. "I did not know what else to do. Was she right? Were you kissing Elise?"

Johan closed the door behind him and threw the latch shut. "You do not even know? You left, and you do not even know whether I kissed that girl or not. Well, I did. Rather, she kissed me, but I certainly allowed it. The chances of either of you looking at just that moment were astronomically slim. Why were not you showing Helga your drawings? She appreciates such things more than Elise, anyway."

"You were kissing the only girl I have ever loved, and I am supposed to explain why we caught you?" Adolf's alto voice sounded whiney compared to Johan's tenor, but his words were heated.

Johan covered his face and laughed openly. He could not help himself. The only girl Adolf had ever loved? Adolf clearly was not as mature as Johan had believed him to be.

"Stop that," Adolf cried. "Stop laughing at me! You liked Helga. Why would you betray her? Why did you betray me? Stop laughing, and answer me!"

But Johan could not help himself. He laughed until tears glistened on his face. "Oh, oh, Adolf. Really now." He tried to wipe his eyes and suppress his laughter at the same time. "I am sorry, I should not laugh. You are just so very serious. Love! You met the girl once. You knew her for only a week, and you are ready to profess your love for her? Johan's mirth had finally calmed. "You do not love Elise, Adolf. You do not even know what love is yet. Oh, I am sure you lusted for her. What man would not? Why do you think I kissed her? Not because I love her or even particularly like her much. She is far too ... predatory. No, no, I like Helga—a great deal, actually—but I do not love her. Which is good, I suppose. I doubt she will ever speak to me again." He shook his head regretfully. "Why in God's name did you leave her alone?"

Adolf's heart was pounding in his chest. His fists tightened and gripped his comforter. He gritted his teeth, and his nostrils flared as he struggled to keep a reign on his emotions. He was being laughed at. His love for Elise was being laughed at, but what was worse, was that he deserved no less. Oh he had been a fool, all right.

"You should never have left her," Johan continued. "I trusted you to provide her with company. Elise trusted you, and Helga trusted you, too. You left her all alone, and it was not until she came down from the stands and joined Elise and I, eating our sausages, that we had any idea you had left. She would not talk to me, of course, but she told Elise what had happened. If you think my laughing is bad, then it is good you did not hear hers. I can only imagine what she would have said if you ever admitted your . . ." he could not help another snigger, "*feelings* for her."

Adolf's alto tone was now strained by the tremendous lump in his throat, and it made for a hoarse, rasping voice. "You dare speak of trust. You knew I liked Elise. You told me what to do if she kissed me! Did you pull away before she did, Johan? Did you leave her wanting more? Damn you! Get out."

Johan shook his head. "I told you, *she* kissed *me*. She was the first to pull away, and although I wanted her kiss as much as would any red blooded Austrian, I was not interested in her beyond that. I have said it before—Helga was my prize. Now there is no bloody hope of that at all!"

"Get out. Leave. Now!"

Johan shook his head again. "You have no idea how much you disappoint me, how much you disappointed your 'love,' how much—"

Adolf interrupted him, all but exploding upward from the bed. "Stop it. Just stop it, damn you. I do not want to talk about it. I do not want to talk to *you*. Just leave!"

Whether Adolf was on the verge of tears or violence, Johan was not sure. There was a definite possibility that both would occur, and, with the wisdom an extra three years of dealing with girls and life in general had given him, he understood that despite his intelligence or demeanor, Adolf was still very much a child. He would not listen to reason, nor accept responsibility for any action. The younger boy had grossly overreacted to the entire situation and responded badly, but there was nothing to do about it now. Helga was surely gone.

"If nothing else," he said, "I hope this proves to be another good lesson for you. You cannot fall in love with a girl you have only seen twice and known for a week. Remember that."

Adolf did not answer, only continued his relentless, tearing stare.

Johan sighed, chuckled again softly and let himself out, closing the door behind him.

The school year came to a disappointing end for Adolf. He never regained the motivation to pursue his studies and did poorly with his final marks. Even drawing had become a chore.

Elise still occupied his thoughts. Regret for what might have been ached in his heart and mind, regardless of what Johan or anyone else thought. He no longer spoke to Johan or any of the other boys at Frau Sekira's. He was alone. He had thought that the loss of Elise was what troubled him, but his loneliness was more profound than that which the loss of a weeklong infatuation should have caused.

His mother had been understandably disappointed when she learned that he had failed so many of his subjects. She had traveled from Leonding to Linz so that she could meet with Adolf's teachers. They all explained that although Adolf was certainly intelligent and talented, he was also arrogant and difficult to teach. He could be very moody, often seeming withdrawn into his own thoughts or activities. It was not as though he were simply daydreaming, for he always produced something from his apparent inattention to the class lessons. He answered well what questions piqued his interests, articulate, and even insightful, in his responses.

At last it was decided that if Adolf retook his French examination, he would be allowed to proceed to the next grade. The catch was that he would not be allowed to continue at this school. He would be transferred to the town of Steyr, approximately twenty-five miles east of Linz, putting him even further from his mother, who lived west of Linz.

"You must not squander this opportunity, Adolf. I do not like that you will be even further from my attention, but I trust you have learned your lesson." Klara knew she must be sterner with her boy than she had been in the past. Even sitting in her rocking chair, the methodic creaking of its runners on the floor warned Adolf that his mother's words were measured and deliberate.

"Promise me you will work very hard at your studies in Steyr, Adolf."

Seldom did his mother ask that he promise her anything.

His intolerance for authority had been growing, but especially toward women, understandable given the condition of his heart. Frau Sekira had tried speaking with him more than once since the night she had offered him the mulled wine, but each time Adolf had dismissed her out of hand. She could think him rude, if she wished, so long as she left him alone.

He had missed his mother. He also missed Angela and Paula, but Angela had married a man with whom Adolf got along poorly. A tax collector, he was constantly lecturing Adolf on the merits of civil service. Even with his father dead and buried, Adolf still could not escape the man's wishes.

"Promise me, Adolf," his mother said. "You must do better in your studies. Otherwise you must return home with me, and I will begin looking for someone to take you on as an apprentice."

That would be the end of his freedom for certain. Apprentices often worked more than ten hours a day learning the skills of their trade. He would have no time for drawing or opera or reading his savage Indian stories. "I promise, Mama. I will not waste this opportunity. I will not disappoint you." He resolved that these words would not be lies.

Klara smiled and hugged her son. She could hardly believe what the teachers had said about Adolf. Around her, he was almost always such a sweet and mild-mannered boy. Oh, he had a temper—he had his father's hot blood in him—but it was hardly any fault of his. He tried hard to keep his temper under control.

Thinking of how Adolf had beaten Paula at times, Karla shuddered. But those times had been rare, and Adolf had been much provoked.

Her Adolf was a good boy, and she loved him very much.

Once Adolf was settled in his new situation in Steyr, his mother returned to Leonding. Their goodbye was especially difficult for Adolf, as he was left alone again, but now it was even worse: The distance between them had more than doubled. Living so much farther from his mother, he would see her even less frequently.

In Steyr, he did not stay in a boarding house like Frau Sekira's.

He lodged at the home of Petronella Cichini and her husband, who was at least twice her age, rarely, if ever, left his bedroom. Another boy attending the Steyr Realscule lodged there, but Adolf avoided him. He had no desire to make friends—what had transpired at Frau Sekira's was still fresh in his mind—and if he were going to study as dutifully as he had promised, it was best he kept to himself.

During his first weeks in Steyr, his grades improved. Although he had never been the most athletic boy in school, his passions for winning and achieving superiority over his classmates drove him to earn very high marks in gymnastics. He soon led the class with his efforts and drew to himself a small following of boys who admired his leadership in games like tetherball or soccer. Although Adolf did not enjoy soccer—it reminded him of Elise—it seemed that he was good at it.

He led the class in freehand drawing, which came as no surprise. All his other courses he passed with adequate or satisfactory marks, except for one subject: handwriting, the only course he failed at the Steyr Realscule. He had excellent motor skills, as his competency with drawing and sports indicated, and yet he could not write a legible sentence. His teacher believed that improvement was a matter of discipline and effort, but Adolf knew the truth: His mind thought faster than his hand could write.

All things considered, Steyr was a great improvement over Linz—and yet he often missed Linz. Knowing his grades were adequate enough to no longer be a true concern, he decided that he could forego a weekend of study, that he had earned himself a trip to the opera. Now 15 years old, he was independent enough to travel to Linz and attend the event on his own. He did not particularly care what was playing. All that mattered was that he would be there.

When he arrived at the Linz Opera House, he was initially disappointed by the playbill: Gustave Charpentier's *Louise* was opening that night, a fairly new French play. Only its worldwide popularity had brought it to Linz so soon after its premiere four years ago, on February 2, 1900. The playbill described the opera as a love story between a young artist and a seamstress living with her parents in Paris. Since failing his French courses in Linz, he had only attained adequate marks in the subject at Steyr, but as soon as he discovered that the story revolved around a young artist, he decided he was very lucky to have chosen this weekend to attend the opera.

On a student's budget, he could not afford the sort of seats his father had purchased. He could pay for a place in the standing room section. But his location was of no concern. Just being inside the opera house filled him with excitement. He experienced an unexpected twinge of sentimentality thinking about the time his father had taken the family to see *Lohengrin*. It had been only a little more than a year ago, and yet everything was so very different.

Arriving alone, Adolf did not dally in the concourse outside the theatre. Among the first to claim his viewing space, his artist's eye considered the various vantage points available in area. He decided that the best viewpoint was next to a fluted column to his right, against which he might lean if his legs should grow weary of standing.

He arrived at his intended spot just as another boy his age approached with the same intent. Adolf, unwilling to relinquish the territory, lengthened his stride to cut off the slighter taller boy off before he could reach the column himself.

"Well played, young sir," said the boy with a wry, good-natured tone.

Adolf grinned, wolfish in his victory. "It is kind of you to acknowledge such, although I think I was perhaps only lucky enough to have been a mere moment's thought ahead of you."

The boy laughed and nodded. "Aye, if you have seen enough opera from here, you know which places are choicest. Congratulations, Mr ?"

"Hitler. Adolf Hitler."

The boy stuck out his hand. "My pleasure to meet you, Mr. Hitler. My name is August Kubizek." He held no ill-will for the other boy for beating him to his favorite vantage point, for all was fair in the standing section when it came to claiming one's place. More than once, shoving matches had begun over a patron's desire to claim and keep their place. Proud to possess a more civilized demeanor, August had yielded the spot as soon as he had seen Adolf's strides lengthen.

Adolf took the offered hand and shook it as firmly as his smaller hand allowed. "Well, Mr. Kubizek, it sounds as though you view the opera from this section rather frequently. Tell me, do you know much about tonight's performance?" August had indeed seen many performances from this area, but thought it somewhat rude of Adolf to point it out, suggesting such admission was all he could afford. Then

again, perhaps the boy was only making conversation.

August shook his head. "I am generally not interested in the French performances. I find their plots to be as pretentious as the rest of their much-flaunted culture. What about your? I do not think I have seen you here before, and given my frequency here," he winked, "I think I would have marked a young man such as yourself. I would hazard to guess that this is your first opera"

Adolf laughed softly. "No, not my first, but you are right in that this is my first time viewing a performance from here." He gestured around him.

Nodding, August said, "Well, you were smart to find something on which to lean. If you will excuse me, I believe

I am going to claim that column there"—he pointed to an area to the right of the column Adolf claimed—"while I still can. It might be off-center of the stage, but it will be better than standing in the throng."

"The throng?" asked Adolf, somewhat incredulous.

There was hardly anyone else around them.

August smiled. "Many people are in the concourse outside the theatre, waiting to meet people, or perhaps indulging in libations at the theatre's bar."

"Ah," replied Adolf. "Well, hopefully it will not become too crowded."

August was content to offer a last nod, and then let the

conversation falter.

Silence was more than acceptable to Adolf. His eyes were soon drifting about him, lingering on the rich, red velvet that hung on the walls to improve the acoustics and the gold-leafed busts of rams, bulls, horses and eagles that overlooked the crowd from pillars on either side of the audience. He was just taking note of the copper-coffered ceiling when he noticed a familiar face in the incoming crowd.

He blinked once, and then stood fully upright, turning away from the column so he have a clear view of the girl. Having already noticed him, she was making her way toward him. Adolf could not have felt any more nervous or surprised.

"Hello, Adolf," Helga said.

Adolf bowed ever so slightly. "Hello, Ms. Faveshra." He thought to make some comment about how pleasant a coincidence it was to meet her again, but his mouth had gone quite dry, as if all the moisture there had been diverted to his palms.

He could hardly believe his misfortune. Of all the weekends to attend the opera, and of all the places to stand . . .

Helga smiled warmly, remembering Adolf was the nervous sort, so very formal, and aside from leaving her in the soccer stands, so very polite. She had long since forgiven him for that transgression, guessing that he had been far more hurt by Elise than she had been by Johan. "What a strange coincidence this is. Although . . ." she paused to consider for a moment, a dimple appearing in one corner of her cheek, as if her face sought to explain her pause. "I understand that this opera is about a young artist, so perhaps it is not much of a coincidence after all, being a young artist yourself, that is."

Adolf could hardly believe the girl would still speak to him. That she remembered he was an artist was even more to her credit. After all, it had been weeks since they had last seen each other. She looked even prettier now than she had then, although it was still a very different beauty than Elise's. Elise was striking and mischievous, while Helga possessed a more subdued, simpler beauty. For the first time, Adolf understood what Johan had been trying to explain about the difference between the two girls.

"Are you here alone, Adolf?" Her voice was excited, perhaps tinged with nerves, as she came closer. Happy would be the best description for her tone, and that made Adolf more nervous himself.

"I . . . well, yes. I am."

Her cheeks flushed with embarrassment, Helga regretted asking such a rude question. It was no business of hers whether or not he was here on a date—not after the incident at the soccer field. "I am sorry—," she began.

When she saw his eyes narrow in response, she quickly continued, "I am sorry to have asked, that is. It is, of course, no business of mine if you are unaccompanied. How very brave and independent of you, though."

The compliment eased Adolf's mounting tension. He even managed a small smile of his own. "I enjoy the opera, and there was no one else to ask, so . . .".He flinched inwardly. How pathetic that must have sounded to her! He shrugged. "So here I am. What about you? Should there not be a young gentleman escorting you? What of your sister?" Afraid she would appear as if conjured, he could not bring himself to say Elise's name. "I thought you could not be anywhere without her."

Helga gestured toward the theatre door. "Oh, she is still fluttering about the concourse, I think. Her escort is late, and she is probably convincing some other gentleman to buy her a glass while she waits. I came ahead to find our seats—and found you instead! It is all rather serendipitous, really. That is, assuming I am not imposing on you at the moment?"

Momentarily distracted by her mention of Elise approaching other men, he shook his head. "No, no you are not imposing at all."

She reached out and patted his shoulder. "Thank you, Adolf. You are a very sweet boy."

Adolf flinched almost imperceptibly at her touch, but bristled inwardly at being called a "boy." Alone as he was in public, attending an opera by himself, he did not feel much like a boy at all, but a young adult. Just the same, Helga had meant well, and he was happy to be called sweet.

"It is kind of you to say so, Ms. Faveshra." A thought occurred to him. "You had said that . . ." he paused for a brief moment before saying the name, "Elise's date is late. Is your date then tardy as well?"

One rude question deserved another, thought Helga. Of course, Adolf did not realize the question was rude, perhaps because Helga had asked him first. Regardless, Helga laughed softly, "I had best hope he is not late, as I have no date at all."

Adolf lifted his brow in question.

She continued, "After what happened with Johan and you, I decided that boys were more trouble than they were worth. No offense, Adolf—I somehow doubt you are much like most other boys. Anyway, my sister is . . . well, she is my sister. Just because I want no part of a relationship right now, it does not mean I should deny her of the chance to do the same."

But he had all but stopped hearing her at her first words. "Wait, do you mean to say that you are also alone here tonight?"

Helga smiled. "Well at the moment, I am enjoying your company. In about five minutes, when they begin seating everyone else, I will be enduring the company of my sister and her date." She sighed in frustration. "I very much want to see this play, and it will be difficult to enjoy it fully with my sister carrying on next to me. Did you know the opera is set in Paris? Paris!" Her cheeks were flushed and her eyes large with excitement.

Aside from Vienna, he could think of no other city than Paris that would better accommodate an artist's bohemian lifestyle, the very life he had imagined for himself since he had first told his father about their conflicting plans for his future.

Helga smiled. "I must admit that when I learned it was about a girl seeking her freedom who falls in love with a young artist, well, I thought of you."

Stunned that she had thought of him for any reason, Adolf blinked.

"You are the only artist I know," she said. "So you see, it is really not a coincidence at all that I find you here. it is serendipity, I think."

After considering the opera's plot, Adolf could not help but agree. "Yes, I think you are correct."

Before their conversation could continue, people began filing in through the broad double doors. Serendipity only brought you so far, it seemed.

Helga sighed at the interruption of their conversation. "Well, I should find Elise. I hope her date has arrived. I would hate to miss the first act because my sister has to wait, and I could not possibly leave her alone once the opera begins."

Adolf cringed imperceptibly, wondering if she realized her words had special meaning for him given their last encounter. No, he should never have left Helga alone after all. Perhaps tonight he would be able to make amends.

"Perhaps we could meet again during the intermission?"

Absorbed as he was in his regrets, her request surprised him. "Yes, I would like that."

Helga smiled, a far more genuine and beautiful expression than any Elise had ever given him. "Wonderful! Since I already know where you are seat—" She blushed again. "I mean, *situated*, I will come to you."

That plan suited Adolf well. He had no desire to see Elise with her date. "I will be here," he said with a smile. Her slip did not offend him. In fact, it was kind of her to correct herself mid-word. He was not particularly embarrassed to be found in the standing-room section, but he would have become uncomfortable had she made an issue of it.

He watched her turn and move against the flow of people entering the theatre, looking like a beautiful fish struggling to swim upstream. What had prompted her to climb so high to the theatre's rear to begin with was anyone's guess, unless she had made the ascension purely for the view? It was impressive, if not exactly comfortable for the duration of an entire performance. It did not occur to him that she may have seen him and made her way up to where he was standing.

He felt a mixture of incredulity and pleasure. What were the odds they would meet again? His heart was beating with adrenaline and anxiety. Helga was so different from Elise. If only the roles had been reversed, and Johan had liked Elise, everything would be so very different . . . but there was no use fantasizing about what might have been.

In the short months since that day in the soccer stands, Adolf's perspective about love was far more mature than it had been since he had allowed Elise to break his heart. He would not recklessly devote his heart to Helga. He would not mistake feelings of excitement and attraction for love. Yet he could not pub her completely from his mind.

The lights were dimming, and the orchestra began tuning their instruments. For Helga's sake, Elise's date had best arrive soon. As patrons milled around, trying to take their seats, Adolf scanned the room for Helga . . . and Elise. He did not want to see the other girl, but he did want to ascertain that Helga was in the theatre in time to see the beginning of the opera. He watched what entrances he could, hoping to catch sight of her and learn where she was seated. She knew where he was—would she look for him?

The theatre's broad double doors closed at last, the lights dimming so that searching for anyone, even Helga's bright-blond hair, was futile. The curtain rose as the sound from the orchestra swelled, skeins of colored cloth covered sections of the stage, depicting backgrounds of Paris. Bright lights lit the stage, flooding the dark stage floor with warm illumination for the day scene.

Adolf soon wished he had paid more attention to his French studies. The first act contained a scene in which the family condemns Julien, the artist, for proposing marriage to Louise, a well-born young woman. Although the libretto had not yet caught his attention, the scene almost angered Adolf. Even the family on stage did not approve of the artist's life.

The second act was much more to Adolf's liking. The artist

told his friends that if the girl's parents would not consent to their marriage, he would run away with her. He presented the plan to the girl, who at first balked at the idea, loving her parents too much to leave them. But by the end of the scene, the artist had convinced the girl to leave with him, and the act ended with the lovers running off together.

The music was not particularly suited to Adolf's tastes—it lacked the epic majesty of Wagner's work—but the setting pleased him greatly. Charpentier's depiction of the bohemian lifestyle matched that of his own daydreams. He decided that despite the fact that he did not entirely understand French, he was enjoying the opera very much.

With the second act over, the theatre lights came on again. Because the opera was not long, the intermission would be relatively short. Some productions did not include an intermission at all, but the Linz Opera House always did so. It boosted their concession sales, if nothing else.

As the people standing to either side of him filed out to the concourse and its concessions, Adolf remained where he leaned against the fluted column. He wondered what Helga would think of the play. Would she seek her freedom from her parents' tyranny as ardently as had Louise? Would her friends laugh and giggle at Adolf 's dashing looks and strong voice? Although he had not sung since Lambach, his voice could match the singer playing Julien—he was sure of it. Could Helga sing?

Stop! These were foolish thoughts. He refused to compare the opera to his own life. He was not an artist yet, but he would be. He was certain of it.

He nearly jumped out of skin when Helga's hand touched his shoulder. He had expected her to approach from the same direction as before. This time she had been sly and approached from another door.

Feeling his shoulder tense under her hand, she could not help but giggle at his reaction. "Did I scare you?"

Adolf twisted so that he could look behind him. "You surprised me."

She smiled. "I am sorry." She gestured down at the stage. "What do you think? Is it not a wonderfully romantic story?"

"It is," he said lamely. She waited, saying finally, "And that is all?"

Adolf was confused. "What do you mean?" His response had been brief, but accurate. Her question had been entirely vague, and he was becoming frustrated. He did not like to be touched, and she had laid a hand on his shoulder as if they were the best of friends. No, he would not make the same mistake as he had made with Elise. He would remain deliberately distant. He would be civil, but he refused to play the fool again.

Helga just shook her head. "Never mind." Why was Adolf being so curt with her? What had changed over the course of two acts? He was looking at her the same as he had before, albeit with less excitement. But he was not saying anything, just watching her.

She tried again. "What would you have done, Adolf? Would you have asked Louise to run away?"

He considered her question for a moment. "Well," he began, but paused. Was she doing exactly what he had done, picturing herself as Louise, with him as Julien? "Well, I do not think I would have asked," he said at last.

Helga's eyes dulled in disappointment. "You would not?" She spoke in a tentative, almost fearful tone.

Adolf shook his head. He was putting Johan's teachings to good use. They might not be kissing, but he could still leave her wanting more. So far, it was working. He could hear the worry in her question, the precipice on which her disappointment teetered.

"No, I would not ask," he said, lifting his chin. "I would demand."

Helga lifted her eyebrows in surprise. "'Demand'?"

Adolf nodded. "Yes. I would take her hand and say something like 'You must come away with me,' or perhaps, 'You are coming with me, and we are going to live happily ever after,' but either way, I would demand."

Helga decided his version was even more romantic than Julien's tactic of persuasion. She smiled, a smile so full of mischief that it might have been mistaken for Elise's. "And if she refused?"

Adolf shrugged. "I suppose I would have to live happily ever after on my own."

That was not the answer for which Helga had been hoping. "On your own? How terribly lonely! Truly, if you loved the girl with all your heart, you would not try to convince her to come away with you? You would only demand that she did, and if she said no, that would be that?"

Adolf sighed. He liked repeating himself even less than he liked being touched. "If she truly loved me, as you describe, and I loved her with all my heart, then I should not have to convince her of anything, should I? She should just come away with me of her own accord."

Helga realized that he was quite right. "I see." She smiled again, "You are a very interesting boy, Adolf. There is not much time before intermission ends, and I am not certain I will be able to find you after the opera concludes. Elise and I have our curfew, but I would very much like to see you again. May I have your address? I will write to you, and perhaps we can go to another opera some time."

Adolf was surprised, but pleased. He was experiencing the same fuzzy feeling he had when he had first met Elise, and so he knew he liked Helga, but seeing the smile that was so similar to her sister's reminded him that although the two girls were very different people, they also had their similarities. He was not sure he should risk his heart again, especially with Elise's sister.

However, all she had asked was for his address. Letters were harmless enough, and considering his handwriting, she probably would not understand whatever he penned in response anyway. That thought made him smile, and Helga, thinking he was smiling at her, smiled back expectantly.

"I am currently living in the town of Steyr," he said," at the Cichini residence. Have your letters sent there. I am afraid I do not visit Linz as often as I would like to any more. I have been focusing on my studies."

Helga nodded. "Of course, as you should. Still, as I said, you are a very interesting boy. I will enjoy exchanging letters with you, even if I cannot see you again soon. Who knows, maybe I will come to Steyr and visit you instead."

He chuckled. "I doubt there is anything in Steyr that Elise would want to do, unless she knows boys there, as well."

Helga laughed at that. "I would not be surprised if she did, but no, I would not bring her. Tonight has taught me two things. The first is that I am old enough to be without her company, despite what my parents might think."

That was a great relief to Adolf. "And the second?" "That you should not have to ask me to disobey my

parents and leave my sister behind. I should just do it." Helga understood better than Adolf had first given her credit for, it seemed. It was a revelation, and it was exciting to think that this boy had been the catalyst.

People had begun filling back into the theatre, most enjoying an alcoholic buzz that would sustain them until the opera's finale, which, if it was any kind of opera at all, would be rousing enough to hold the crowd's attention.

Adolf thought about what Helga had just said, and decided she was smarter than he had first credited her. He would look forward to her letters after all.

Helga smiled and reached out to take Adolf's hand. "I should get back to my seat, before Elise finds me here. She is still angry at you for leaving and will never understand why it would be her fault. I am very glad now that things worked out the way they did. If Johan truly had feelings for me, he would never have kissed my sister. I was as hurt that day as you were, I think. You are not like Johan, though. You are like Julien, an artist. A romantic. Like me."

Adolf did not say anything. He considered pulling his hand away, but her soft skin felt warm and comfortable.

"Enjoy the rest of the opera, Adolf. I will write soon." With that, she gave his hand a final pat and made her way through the crowd.

As Adolf watched her go, he decided that this time he would be the one in control. But even with that thought, he could feel his skin tingling in the absence of her touch.

It was a feeling that would linger throughout the night.

Chapter 7

FRAU CICHINI RAN her boarding house quite differently than Frau Sekira. Frau Sekira ran her house as a business, her interest in her tenants motivated by her desire to protect her assets. Petronella Cichini could not have provided a greater contrast, not only in her motive for lodging boys, but also in her attitude toward her residents.

Perhaps the only similarity between the two landladies was their austere manner. Both wore their hair in severe buns that stretched their brows impossibly tight. Frau Sekira likely did so in an effort to smooth her age-wrinkled brow, but Frau Cichini, was nearly thirty years younger. Her bun was still robustly brown, and her brow needed stretching no more than her figure needed a tight corset to keep her trim. A woman of middle years, she had married for money, a much older man who kept to the confines of his bed.

Her husband's infirmity had left his wife with no children of her own. Although she was well-provided-for, she offered lodging to young boys in Steyr, not as her occupation, but as more of a hobby, treating the boys as her pets. She was always very curious to know what Adolf had learned in school that day or what occupied his hours when he was in his room with the door latched.

Adolf was a private person. He had appreciated the fact that Frau Sekira had respected his independence. She had only interfered in his business that single night, after he struck Handel, and Adolf had **understood** that she had done such because she was protecting her business. Frau Cichini, however, constantly sought to meddle in his affairs.

"You received a few letters today, Adolf, one from your mother and one from a Ms. Faveshra? Well, I left them both on your desk." It was almost as if the woman had been waiting just around the corner from the front door all day for his return. He could hardly maneuver around her imposing presence to get to a bench where he could take his boots off. In fact, the thought had crossed his mind to simply track mud through the house to his room, but then he would truly never rid himself of this woman's attention.

Adolf had just returned from a particularly long day of school. He had no desire even to acknowledge Frau Cichini's question. He did not like Frau Cichini's use of his first name, and he certainly did not like her scrutiny of his mail. Ms. Faveshra was none of her business. The woman should have seen the letters were addressed to him and been content to leave them for him without comment. She was too curious by far.

"Thank you," he said, starting toward his room. "If you will excuse me, I have a great deal of schoolwork to do before dinner." Adolf hoped that his tone had not betrayed the shortness of his temper.

She followed him, chatting. "Is she pretty, Adolf? Does she smell like flowers? Her letters certainly do. How very urban of her. She is from a well-to do family, is she not? She must like a dapper man such as yourself very much indeed. She must think of herself as being very lucky." And while the woman did not exactly tease Adolf, he did not see how it was any business of hers to begin with. He wished she would at least step away from him. Instead, she kept inching closer.

Adolf paused in front of his door. Turning to face Frau Cinchini before she could advance any further, he said, "Hyacinths, she smells of hyacinths, and she is very, very pretty." Despite the blush rising in his cheeks, his eyes became hard and his voice formally stern. "She is also none of your business, madam. My correspondences are not your concern. I hope there is no cause to remind you of that fact again." As his words supplied greater confidence, his tone shifted toward arrogance. "I am your tenant, not your plaything. If I am to continue paying rent, I must do so under the condition that my privacy is honored. I hope I am clear."

Frau Cichini had never been spoken to in such a manner—not by a man of Adolf's youth, of her own husband's ripe age or any age in between. Accustomed to charming men and women alike, she derived a certain pleasure from living out the exploits of her youth through the tidbits she snatched from her young tenants' lives. More than once she had considered taking one of her young boarders to bed, but she feared that if she were ever caught, she would be forced to go back to the dregs of Austrian society. So although Adolf's demanding tone surprised her, she would appease him for now. He was not the most handsome boy to whom she provided lodging, but there was something in his speech and manner that was nonetheless attractive, albeit in a different way. She did not want to lose his presence in her home so soon.

She bowed her head slightly. "You are right, Herr Hitler. I apologize; I only thought to make pleasant conversation and perhaps fluff a young lad's ego. Clearly you have no need of such assistances."

Adolf nodded, missing her veiled insult. "Good. Thank you, Frau Cichini. Now, if you will excuse me, I have schoolwork to occupy me until the dinner bell." He could not be more satisfied by Frau Cichini's deference to his wishes, but he wished he could have been even more severe with the woman. She had no right to speak to him of Helga. She had no right to smell Helga's scent before him.

He was sure to latch his door shut once he was within his room. His space here was even larger than his room in Linz, although the bed was far less comfortable, and his windows looked out into an alley instead of Frau Sekira's small garden.

He set his schoolbooks on his desk, placing them next to the two letters Frau Cichini had indeed left there. He did not particularly like the fact that the woman came and went from his room as she pleased. It might be her house, but so long as he was paying rent, this was his room.

Most weekends he tried to absent himself altogether from the boarding house. He would return to Linz and either see an opera or visit his mother. Soon he would go to Linz to see Helga, which brought a smile to his face. This weekend he had stayed in; he had a history exam this coming Monday, a subject Adolf enjoyed. He had been looking forward to reading about the Franco-Prussian war...

An explosion of sound like chickens in a henhouse came from

downstairs: Frau Cichini and her Jewish friends gathered for their weekly cake and gossip. The Frau did not have many friends, her husband's age and physical condition precluding them from participating in society, but she had befriended a small group of Jewish women. They were friendly people and natural gossipers, so Frau Cichini got along with them quite well. Adolf hated the fact that every Friday afternoon, while most of the boarding house tenants were celebrating their freedom from the school week, his parlor was filled with Frau Cichini's Jews.

The women were flattered to be invited into Frau Cichini's home. They were a friendly sort of people to start with, but once they had befriended you, they insinuated themselves into your life. These gatherings had begun with monthly visits, and now Frau Cichini had these women over weekly. What gossip did they spread over their honey-cakes? What rumors did they foster and monger, those prattling kerchiefs with their upward inflections on almost every word? They were not to be trusted. So far as Adolf was concerned, "Jew" was just another word for "Judas."

It was a part of Austrian culture to regard the Jews as a bottom-class culture. His teachers in school practically had made that sentiment a part of their curriculum. It was no surprise that Adolf 's religion class would propagate such ill feelings toward the rival faith, but the history teacher echoed the same thoughts, as did the French teacher, the German teacher—even the gymnastics teacher, who complained about the physical inferiority of his Jewish pupils.

Yet many possessed wealth that at times admitted them into the upper spheres of Austrian society. At least, as upper as Frau Cichini's societal status managed to elevate them. The only thing these women shared beyond their status as social outcasts was that they enjoyed wealth. He did not understand why Frau Cichini associated with them.

Adolf hated all of it. He hated having to attend classes here in Steyr. He hated being away from Linz and Helga. He especially hated the cackles and squawking laughter from Frau Cichini's kitchen. Aggravation, frustration and hatred stirred rage he could neither vent nor resolve. He could do nothing but remember that moment and hope he would have the opportunity to avenge it.

Adolf took his blanket from his bed and stuffed its edge beneath his door. It was a surprisingly rational act, given his current level of irritability, the kind of cold, stoic act that gave the hard edge to his eyes. There was a reward in shutting out the world for right now. He could lose himself in the comforting words of his mother's letter, and Helga's letter would restore to him bliss worthy of enduring his present hell.

For a few moments, he simply sat with a letter in each hand. A letter from his mother was always a welcomed thing. He missed her and her letters made him homesick, but he was always happy to hear from her. The other letter, however, felt heavier in his hand. It had been nearly two weeks since he had seen Helga at the opera. Since that serendipitous meeting, Adolf had sacrificed more than one's nights rest or one day of classes wondering whether the girl would write to him after all. He was very careful not to let those thoughts consume him, as he had with Elise, but many times he caught himself wondering if Helga would write. Now there was nothing to wonder. Her letter was here. He set it aside for the moment and picked up the letter from his mother.

He opened his penknife with a snap. The blade slit open the envelope with a clean, effortless cut. Adolf was very careful closing the knife before extracting his mother's letter. There were nearly two pages of his mother's small but precise handwriting and a page of his sister Paula's larger and less refined script. Aunt Johanna had included no correspondence of her own, which was just as well. Adolf had never liked the disabled woman.

His mother's letter was very much like all the others she sent weekly. She was of course concerned first for his health, and then for his studies. She said she hoped he was putting his new opportunity in Steyr to good use. She appreciated his artistic ability and was proud of her son's talent for rendering landscapes and architecture, but she still championed his father's dream of Adolf becoming a civil servant. She wrote of Angela and how happy she was in her marriage. Her husband was a tax collector who provided well for her. Did Adolf not want a career that would also provide for a wife and family someday? Artists simply did not earn a stable living.

She made a point of mentioning how well his father's pension still provided for the family. If Alois had not been so dedicated to his career, the family would never have had the money to keep their house and board Adolf in Linz or Steyr. Adolf scanned such passages with impatience. He was not a dunce. He understood he would not have the opportunity to live in a boarding house without that civil servant's pension. He merely did not believe that he should dedicate his life to that career. No, he would use his opportunities to fulfill his own dreams. He would become

successful in his own right, on his own terms.

His mother's letter went on to assure Adolf that all was well at home. Paula was growing into a very polite and thoughtful child, who often mentioned how much she missed her big brother. Adolf smiled at that. He had treated her so poorly during his last days at home, and yet she still adored him. More than once after he had beaten her, he had regretted letting his temper get the better of him.

As Adolf came toward the end of the letter, he found that his mother was experiencing a strange soreness in her upper back, but she assured Adolf it was nothing to worry about. She had probably strained a muscle, but it was only a nuisance that she was sure would pass. She ended the letter as always, wishing Adolf well and hoping that he would write back if he were not too busy with his studies. He would write a response later that night.

He folded Paula's unread missive back into his mother's missive, deciding it could wait until later. His thoughts had already moved to Helga's letter. What had she written?

Adolf's palms began to sweat as the penknife blade passed into the corner of the letter's heavy envelope. With a surgeon's care, he ran the knife along the envelope's upper fold, a small smile playing at the corner of his mouth as he extracted the envelope's contents. In his haste to read the letter, he did not bother to close the knife again and instead set it on the bed beside him. Although the letter was heavier than his mother's, it consisted of only three pages in all. Helga had used an expensive correspondence paper that absorbed the rich black ink as if the paper had thirsted for her thoughts. Adolf 's dark eyes now drank in those words. Once again, he detected the faintest hint of perfume on the page.

Dear Mr. Hitler,

How rigidly formal that sounds! We must do something about that, I think. In fact, I insist you call me Helga, and I hope you will permit me to address you as Adolf from here on. There, that is much better already, do you not agree?

I hope this letter finds you well, Adolf. I must apologize for not writing to you sooner. I have not been terribly busy, but life has been very stressful just the same. I enjoyed the opera immensely, as I am sure you did as well. Louise displayed such courage when she ran off with Julien. I have tried to show such courage myself as of late. It has been difficult. Ever since Mama passed, Papa has been so very harsh in his words. If we have any sort of disagreement, he simply refuses to listen to my opinion. It is as if he fears losing control over us, although really that has been happening ever since Elise and I began socializing.

If Papa had his way, we both would be in a nunnery. Elise, of course, would never stand for that. I must admit that I have no desire to wear the habit, either. It took my sister and me almost a full year of arguing and being positively awful to the man before he at last relented and allowed Elise and I to go out, so long as we were in one another's company.

I am not sure I have the strength to endure another year of such arguments. However, Papa is very old, and I do not think he would notice if I slipped out after he goes to bed. I think Elise has been sneaking out herself, although she refuses to admit it.

Whether she has been or not, I intend to try myself soon. I will still have to be back by morning, so I do not think I will be able to visit you in Steyr just yet. Perhaps I am being too forward in thinking you would even want such a visit from a rebellious girl.

I hope your schoolwork is going well. I am sure it is, now that you do not have distractions such as my sister or me. Surely this letter cannot be too distracting, I will hope. I will also hope that I have occupied at least a sliver of your thoughts, as you have been occupying mine. You are a handsome boy, Adolf, so well-mannered and talented. I would like another opportunity to see your sketches.

Have you been working on anything new? Perhaps I will someday be lucky enough to pose for you. I am sure you could paint a much better portrait than that which Papa commissioned just before Mama died. That was nearly three years ago, and I would like to think I have done some growing up since then.

I would like to see you again. Perhaps you would accompany me to a late opera the next time you are in Linz?

Please, write back at your earliest convenience. Tell me of Steyr! And your studies and anything else you would care to share. I will wait for the post with great anticipation. I can only hope that wait will not be too long.

Sincerely,
(and expectantly)
Helga

As Adolf read the letter, a variety of thoughts and emotions filled him. His heart had quickened since he had first caught that faint trace of perfume on the heavy paper. He could scarcely believe she had written to him at all. As his eyes followed the delicate script of what Adolf knew must be a very light but precise hand, he again cautioned himself. He had mistaken interest for infatuation before, and should he allow himself to study Helga's words too thoroughly, he was bound to be hurt again.

Learning Helga's mother had passed away did not resonate with Adolf as it may have had with another boy whose father had died. Instead of thinking of his father, he found himself thinking of his own mother. How could he ever cope with her death? She had always protected him. She had shielded him from blows that had instead fallen upon her. She had spent long and cold nights by his bedside whenever he fell ill, which had been a frequent occurrence in his youth.

The more Adolf thought about his mother, the more he wondered if he would ever find a love like hers. Helga was a very nice girl, intelligent and eloquent in her thoughts, but would she rub his back until he at last found sleep? She was also very beautiful, a beauty different from what his mother possessed. Adolf was too young to understand that the differences between Helga and his mother would only increase his attraction to the blonde, cerulean-eyed girl whose perfume smelled of hyacinths. Yes, that is what that scent was.

He was glad she had enjoyed the opera. It was even more interesting to see that it truly had impacted her, that she had been serious when she had told him she wanted to be more like Louise. Well he would have no objections to being her Julien, so long as she came to him of her own will.

He was impressed that she had suggested visiting him in Steyr. Sneaking out was a large step in itself, and if she were willing to be so bold as to attempt such rebellious behavior, then he should certainly reward her efforts by acceding to her wishes and accompanying her to another opera. When, though? Not too soon. This situation was just as Johan had taught him, though he was still bitter and loathe to admit he had learned anything valuable from someone who had so readily betrayed him.

Betrayal. Even opening Helga's letter had been a step toward exposing himself to that circumstance all over again. True, he had no reason to distrust Helga. She had been just as hurt as he had been in those stands—perhaps even more so. Maybe their shared hurt was part of the reason she seemed so eager to trust him.

Should he mention Helga in the next letter to his mother? What would she think of his new friendship with the older girl? Not that Helga was older than him by much.

He was born in April of 1889. He was not sure in what month Helga had been born, but he knew it was 1887. They had discussed before how she was two years his senior, though the years meant nothing to either of them. It was said that girls matured earlier than boys, but Adolf was mature beyond his own years. In fact, he had just discovered the chore of shaving, although the hairs he removed were still very light and fine.

He was old enough to recognize Helga was herself in a time of very early blossom, and while she did not yet possess—or did not display—the same shapely curves that would set every young men's blood afire, she did have a distinct beauty of her own, decidedly more delicate than most girls'. The more Adolf thought about her, the quicker his pulse raced. Girls were troublesome, at times being outright difficult.

Angela had become an incredible enigma to him as she grew older. He remembered how his older half-sister used to bounce him in her lap or play soldiers with him so long as he later attended her tea party. As they grew, Angela had distanced herself from him. She would spend more time brushing her hair than she would doing things for him, like sewing small flags or uniforms for his toy soldiers.

Paula had been even more difficult than Angela. His younger sister had grown to become a pestering brat who ruined his games by intruding upon his battlefields with her dolly. He sometimes thought of the times he had struck her, but he did not quite regret his actions. Paula should have had the sense to listen to his commands. She should have taken dolly to Angela's room or her own. Maybe all three could have brushed their hair together.

He sighed and sat back on his bed, leaning against the yellow—plastered wall. Helga was very different from his sisters or his mother. He would be very cautious with her. He would be careful and deliberate, certain of his thoughts and feelings before he again acted upon them. He would never again be the fool Johan had labeled him.

He read Paula's letter. Her adolescent script was very different from his mother's or Helga's, and the letter was not nearly so long. It spoke of dolly's new haircut and the progress Mother was making on a new dress. It also expressed a sincere desire to see him, and Adolf wondered if perhaps he should plan a trip back to the Garden House in Leonding before he made his plans for a night in Linz.

Finding himself suddenly far more tired than he had realized, Adolf sat up and placed all three letters atop his desk. A stone he had carried with him since the family left their farm in Hafeld served as a paper weight. Tomorrow he would write his responses to his mother and sister. Then, perhaps, he would write to Helga. If his schoolwork was too much, Helga would simply have to wait. Yes, yes, that was the responsible decision to make. She simply was not his first priority. He would not be a fool again.

A week passed. Adolf wrote several letters in that time, but viewed each as a draft, ultimately depositing them into his trash basket instead of the post box. The letters all maintained an average length of nearly two pages. Having never considered himself a particularly adept writer, he was rather pleased with himself for managing even that volume. He meticulously employed his best handwriting, which, having always received poor marks in school, seemed quite legible now. What others might consider brevity, he decided was conciseness that kept him from saying too much, something he might later regret as being too personal.

His first draft had been largely concerned with his analysis of the opera. However, on his second read-through, he decided that since Helga had enjoyed the performance, any criticism of his might sound pretentious. In the end, he decided it best to simply agree with her and tell her how much he had enjoyed the evening as well.

His second draft was much more general in its contents. This time he remembered to express his regrets over her mother's passing. He even mentioned his own father's death, but neglected to present his feelings on the subject. He wrote vaguely of his studies and gave some depth and length to his description of his latest sketch effort, a large mill here in Steyr.

Ultimately that draft also found its way to the trash. By the time he was midway through the third draft, he discovered that his hand was not used to so much writing. His efforts of employing his finest handwriting were leading to hand-cramping. He wanted to finish this letter tonight; it was Sunday, and Monday was certain to bring a pile of schoolwork. If this letter to Helga were still weighing on his mind by then, there was no hope of focusing on his studies at all.

So he gave himself a break. The sun had set hours ago, and his oil lamp was running low on fuel. Its flame had begun to waver, no longer burning with bright vitality, long shadows flickering on the plastered walls. As he sat at his desk, his mind began to wander. How much longer could he remain here in Steyr? He wanted to be done with school. He wanted to move out of this boarding house and return to a city with culture. Linz, perhaps, although a grander dream had entered his mind that night at the opera: More than anything, he desired the bohemian lifestyle.

He had little interest in Julien's Paris, but there was an even better city for his dreams, and it was closer. He would finish school, or perhaps he would just quit. Either way, he would free himself and move to Vienna. What would Helga think of that? He would not try to convince her to accompany him, the way Julien coaxed Louise. He had explained to Helga already that if someone truly loved him, she would follow him of her own accord.

He extended his arms above his head in a hard stretch, twisting his neck to each side, waiting for audible pops before releasing his tension. He then cracked his knuckles and gave his hands a good shake. With luck, he had enough fuel to finish one last letter and his hand was rested enough to avoid cramping again.

His paper was not nearly so expensive as Helga's, and he owned no cologne to scent it with, but if she truly liked him, his words alone would satisfy her interests.

    Helga,
    I will thank you for the privilege of addressing you in such a familiar manner. I had always thought that girls of your beauty and station would prefer formality, but I am pleased to find otherwise.
    I am sorry you are having such difficulty with your father. I imagine losing your mother was rough on your entire family, but perhaps hardest for your father. When my father passed away, my mother certainly grieved longer than did I or my other siblings.
    You are not as old as Louise. Do not feel rushed in your efforts of obtaining freedom. Sneaking out in the night is a bold step. Let that satisfy your desire of freedom, for now at least. I would not endorse your nocturnal ventures if there were another way to attend an opera with you alone, without your sister. If you can find out what performances will suit your needs and then plan your escape, I will make arrangements to meet you at the opera house.
    My studies are going well enough. I will be very happy when I can burn pencils and books alike, but my grades have been adequate and, in some classes, exceptional. I do not like school, Helga. My teachers care nothing for original thoughts. They drill you with the same rote with which they were likely drilled themselves. They allow no space for creativity. If it were not for the subjects of history and art, I would think school was little more than a forewarning of hell.
    I should not be so negative, perhaps. You have not made any mention of your own schooling or your feelings toward

education. That you are educated is obvious. Your letter is evidence enough. Do you have a favorite subject?

I have had less time for sketching lately, but when I am not studying, I am drawing a mill not far from my residence. It is being renovated from water to steam-driven, and now that they have removed the waterwheel, the building looks monstrous compared to its surroundings. I will perhaps show you the drawing, if it is ready when next we meet.

Sincerely,
Adolf

There. He had managed to include everything that he should, without babbling or risking his ego in any particular manner. It was a perfect letter, and it was with great satisfaction that Adolf at last set his pen down. He folded the paper carefully, crisping each edge between forefinger and thumbnail, and inserted it into an envelope, itself a second draft of her name and address. The first had looked rushed and spindle-handed. He would mail the letter in the morning. For now, he placed it in the top drawer of the desk.

Adolf looked to his sketchbook and opened it to his rendering of the mill. His shading techniques were already vastly superior to those his classmates possessed. He had accurately captured the play of shadows and the building's proportions, noting the position of the river on which the mill had once worn a tremendous wheel. Now the river quietly lapped at the mill's foundation.

He had wanted to capture the mill's industrial decay, the manner in which the advent of engines had amputated the great waterwheel, no longer in balance with the mill's original design. He had decided to sketch the building because he wanted to redesign it himself one day.

Vienna. He wanted to run away. He wanted to leave school and leave Steyr. He wanted to depict the world's realities in paint and improve them in charcoal pencil. A sigh escaped his lips, and at last he stood, turned and went to bed.

Would Helga follow him?
What would Mother say?
Adolf sighed again, closed his eyes and dreamed of burning books—and pencils.

Chapter 8

TWO WEEKS PASSED before Adolf received Helga's reply. She had devoted nearly half a page of her expensive correspondence paper just to thank him for writing back to her. Again her letter was faintly perfumed, a lingering hint of hyacinths that made the young woman's words even sweeter. She agreed with his opinion of teachers, although felt that school itself was a necessary institution for any civilized society. She was also very interested in his depiction of the mill without its waterwheel and hoped she would have the opportunity to view that work soon.

According to the letter, "soon" meant either this coming Friday or Saturday night. Unfortunately, the latest performance at the Linz Opera House began just after 7:00 p.m., which was far too early for Helga to attempt her rebellious escape. If they were to meet at the opera, Elise would have to accompany them.

Adolf's eyes narrowed as he considered what effect that meeting would have on his emotions. It was no longer a matter of pain for his heart, but for his pride. Months had passed since he had left Helga in the soccer stands after Elise and Johan's betrayal, time that had put the entire incident into perspective. It now embarrassed Adolf to think of his behavior then. He had been betrayed, but the gravity of that betrayal had not been nearly so weighty as he had made it out to be.

After a moment of thought, he decided that seeing Elise again was perhaps the last step in actualizing the maturity he had gained since that cool spring day. Helga's letter promised that their seats would be far from Elise and her date, making it very possible they would not meet the other pair the entire night.

Adolf's response was brief, but genuine. He promised to meet the sisters at the Linz Opera House at 6:30 p.m. and said that he would be happy to view the performance together that Saturday, that there was no need for Elise and her date to sit elsewhere. He had run from Elise once. This time would be different. The only way to conquer his embarrassment would be to prove that he was no longer embarrassed.

The thought crossed his mind that Elise would see him with Helga and become jealous. She had been jealous of Helga when she was with Johan, had she not? Yes, he might enjoy some small amount of revenge. The thought excited him almost as much as did the idea of seeing Helga.

Adolf arranged for his transportation. Coaches were expensive, but trains often stopped in Steyr on their way to Linz, so he went by rail. He dressed in his Sunday finest and carried his rendering of the mill in a leather satchel, in which he also carried a change of clothing. There were no trains with passenger cars that ran to Steyr past ten o'clock, so Adolf would need to find lodging in Linz after the performance.

The train arrived in Linz just before six o'clock, giving Adolf plenty of time to walk to the opera house. The city was very different now that autumn was settling. The crowns of deciduous trees were fading from green to mottled yellow and brown; very few trees changed to the startling orange or red hues Adolf had read about in books about the savages. The weather was simply not extreme enough.

The days and nights were again cooling, but at a moderate pace, and rarely did the air fluctuate more than ten degrees from noon until night. Adolf hardly noticed the chill at all. His pace was casual, but his face flushed with expectation. He would not think of it as anticipation, for that implied a sort of hope for what would happen, a weakness of desire for what *should* happen, much the way he had anticipated Elise's reactions to his artwork. His expectations for tonight, by contrast, were more of a pragmatic appraisal of how he planned the evening, with little emotional involvement beyond what disappointment might result if those plans went awry.

He had just taken his place in the ticket line when he noticed Helga had already spotted him. The plan had been for Adolf to arrive early and purchase the tickets for all four of them. He had no idea who Elise's date was, but decided he must surely be good for the money. She was not with her sister now, and Adolf wondered if she might not be attending after all. He felt a small amount of disappointment that he would not be able to avenge himself on Elise, but he was glad that he would have Helga to himself.

Helga wore a welcoming smile that managed to draw Adolf's attention away from her dress of deep-green and white lace, which showed that she did indeed have a figure. She appeared pale in the deepening twilight, her golden curls piled atop her head decorated with a small white flower that matched the lace of her dress. Where she had found such a flower so late in the fall, Adolf could not guess.

"Surprise!" she said with unabashed enthusiasm.

Adolf's palms rarely moistened when he became nervous, but he could feel his underarms trickling small rivulets and his mouth was cotton-dry. Expectations of distance, indeed—his plans were already as substantial as the wind.

"Oh you *are* surprised," Helga said. "Happily, I hope. Have you grown since last I saw you? I think you have. Well, you look very handsome this evening. Come, you need not wait in this line. August Kubizek, my sister's date whom you will meet shortly, arrived early. Rather than subjecting him to small talk with Father, we decided to leave early as well. August purchased our tickets and is likely now endeavoring to intoxicate my sister, which he should accomplish all too easily if I know dear Elise."

Adolf swallowed and stepped out of the ticket line, smoothly offering his arm to Helga, which she took while she continued to talk. Adolf led them to a small bench facing the opera house.

As they sat, Helga kept her arm laced through Adolf's. Normally he would not enjoy being in such proximity with anyone besides his mother, but he found that he enjoyed Helga's presence immensely, and so he made no attempt to withdraw his arm, but rather leaned his head back and smiled at the night sky, just now beginning bloom with the evening's stars.

He at last answered her earlier question. "Yes, I am quite happily surprised to see you. You look beautiful, and I would say that you have grown also, if my mother and sisters had not taught me that a comment even remotely related to the topic of age is inappropriate for conversation with any lady."

Helga smiled at the compliment and the joke. "If you mean to say that I have matured in my beauty, I will accept that as a very gracious compliment. I am not so many years removed from being a girl that I do not still enjoy hearing comments complimenting that distinction."

Adolf smiled also, not only for her own compliments or smile, nor because she had enjoyed his compliment. No, Adolf smiled because she was very beautiful, and he was simply happy to be with her. Adolf's favorite composer was again being showcased at the Linz Opera House; Wagner's *Tristan und Isolde* was playing, one of the few works of the great Wagner that Adolf had neither seen nor read. He could hardly imagine a better evening.

Sitting near to him on the bench, Helga briefly wondered if her perfume was too strong. She had wanted him to notice the same flowered scent she had sent with each letter, but hyacinths had a soft fragrance, and fearing the air would diffuse the scent before they met, she had been perhaps too liberal with the product tonight."

Adolf recognized the scent and found it oddly comforting. "I am very glad you invited me here."

Helga gave his arm a gentle squeeze. She had been watching him in the manner of a young lady, from the corners of her eyes. He *had* grown—she could see it in the angles of his face. His brow seemed deeper, pitched on a straight incline that continued to the top of his nose, beneath which Adolf had recently begun sporting a light moustache. Adolf was not physically impressive, and his stature was slight, but his dark, intense eyes were alluring. All the strength Johan displayed in his body, Adolf showed in his eyes. He was not as handsome as some of the boys she had dated, but something about his countenance pleased her.

Without warning, she leaned over and kissed his cheek.

It was not the reaction he had expected, but he added the softness of her lips to the list of touches he did not mind. His surprise by her tender action was soon replaced by uncertainty of how he should respond. Just before his uncertainty could progress to embarrassment, Helga saved him from having to respond at all.

"We still have a few minutes, Adolf. Although the street lamps provide meager light, I think it is still enough to see your sketches. You did bring them, did you not? I have been very curious to see this mill of which you wrote."

Adolf wondered if the meager light was enough for her to see the color of the cheek she had kissed. "I did," he answered, extricating his arm from hers so he could open his leather satchel. Just as he reached inside, Elise's voice arrested his movements.

"Ah, there you are, Isolde." As she approached Helga and Adolf on their bench, Elise held her date's arm so tightly that the young man was actually being pulled off balance. "And have you brought Tristan or Marke with you tonight? Melot, perhaps, considering how effectively he killed your relationship with Johan. What do you think, Adolf? Which character would you enjoy Helga playing for us tonight?"

Helga's eyes narrowed at her sister's rude greeting. "And I suppose you fancy yourself as Brangäne, concocting love potions that result in tragedy."

Adolf understood that both sisters were referencing the opera they were about to see, but as he had no knowledge of the plot or characters yet, he could not begin to guess at the allusions they were making or how he should respond.

"I had not thought of that," replied Elise, "but the role of Brangäne does suit me, does it not?"

The sketchbook never left Adolf's satchel. He removed his hand and closed the buckles before standing and offering Elise and August a short bow of greeting. "Miss Elise, I am afraid you have the distinct advantage of having seen the performance we are about to attend, whereas I am still new to this particular opera. Please, do not spoil the experience for me." He smiled, quelling the emotions that had arisen when Elise had approached. "How fortunate for me to see you again, as I presented myself poorly the last time. I was hoping we could start afresh."

Surprised, Elise felt as though his words had been a reproach almost. If she responded less civilly than he, she would lose this verbal spar. Instead, she chose to graciously accept his offer of a truce. "Of course we should start fresh. We are both different from who we were before. I am with August now, and you are with my dear sister, after all.

"But I have not yet introduced you, have I?" Elise gave her date's arm another squeeze, which caused the young man to tighten his eyes in discomfort. "August, this is Mr. Adolf Hitler, currently of . . . Spetzburg? Steinhold?"

"Steyr," said Helga flatly.

"Ah, yes, that industrious little town outside our wonderful city here. Mr. Adolf Hitler of Steyr, this is Mr. August Kubizek of Linz, and soon Vienna, right Auggie?"

The young man, who had finally stopped wincing from Elise's grasp, smiled and offered his hand to Adolf, "Mr. Hitler and I had the pleasure of meeting once before, actually, in this very opera house."

Finally recognizing the man to whom he had spoken in the standing section, Adolf appreciated the humble tone the young man offered with his hand. He took August's palm firmly in his own and shook as he had often seen his father do, not with his friends, but with those with whom he worked. "Well met, again, Mr. Kubizek. I am briefly in your debt for purchasing our tickets. You have saved me from a good deal of standing, it seems." He nodded toward the ticket queue, which was longer now.

"Oh do not think to mention it again," August said. "It was merely a convenience of my early arrival. Once the ladies have excused themselves to powder their faces, we can discuss what debts resulted. I am sure it will not be long before that happens."

Helga smiled at the jest, while Elise again tightened her

possessive grip on August's arm. Adolf laughed and offered Helga his hand, "Well, I do not see much sense in continuing to wait out here—shall we find our seats?" Helga took Adolf's hand and rose from the bench, picking up Adolf's satchel and handing it to him

Elise said, "No, our early arrival is precisely why we do not need to wait here in the deepening night. We can instead go in and find our drinks before we find our seats."

August rolled his eyes. "We had to find drinks before we found the pair of you. It only stands to reason that the lady would require another libation to liberate her sense of direction. I suppose it is just as well—I would like to buy you all a drink now that we are all assembled."

Adolf decided that this August fellow's generosity and temperament were to his liking. The night was going better than planned. With his leather satchel again over one arm, his other arm occupied with the task of escorting Helga, Adolf was very happy.

He had no heavy overcoat to check, but he did leave his satchel in the care of an elderly man whose responsibility was to guard the coats, frocks and other accessories that were too obtrusive to be kept at one's seat.

"Are you thirsty, Adolf?" Helga asked. "It is no surprise that Elsie already has August in line to buy her a drink. I do not want anything for myself, but I would not blame you if you wanted something to relax you, although you seem much calmer than when last we met."

Adolf shook his head. "No, perhaps at intermission, but for now I am content to enjoy your company. The last time we met was so unexpected that I was indeed nervous, but I do not feel there is anything to be nervous about now."

Helga smiled and slipped her arm through his. "Good. I think Elsie enjoyed the thought of making you uncomfortable tonight. She will be so very disappointed when she realizes her efforts are futile."

"I only hope she does not take her disappointment out on August. He seems a good sort."

"Yes, he was very polite with Father, and while he has been very kind to Elise and me, he is also smart enough to tell my sister when she is wrong, which is something most boys do not do."

"I am sure you have the same problem, Helga. Pretty girls are very hard to say no to."

Helga blushed at the compliment. She knew she was a very attractive young girl, even if her figure was not yet as enthralling as her sister's. They maintained that they were twins, but everyone always guessed Elise to be the older girl. "Well," said Adolf, "should we wait for your sister and

her escort to acquire their drinks, or should we find our seats?"

"August has our tickets, although I doubt the ushers will ask us to present them. Our seats are at the rear of the upper balcony, but at least they are not standing room." She winked.

Adolf smirked at that. If he had not been in the standing section, Helga might never have caught sight of him at *Louise*, and this night would never have happened.

"We will wait for them," he decided. "There is plenty of time to find our seats."

Helga smiled and drew Adolf out of the growing crowd of people moving to their seats. "I am sorry I have not had the opportunity to see your drawings yet. I do not mean to sound presumptuous, but I believe tonight will go well; however, Elise and I do still have our curfew, and we will not have much time to return home after the opera, so I do not think I can see your drawings then. What are your plans for tomorrow? The weather is supposed to be warm again, and if you are not busy, perhaps we could take a walk through the park together?"

Adolf had planned to spend the night in Linz, and then travel to his family's house the next day. However, the letter he had sent his mother only stated that he would visit sometime that weekend. He had never specified a day or time. "Yes, if we went in the morning. I must leave sometime in the early afternoon if I am going to make it back home to see my mother, and then back to Steyr before dark."

Helga squeezed his hand. "Wonderful!"

Her hand was softer than his and cooler. Not that Adolf's was particularly rough—he had not done any form of physical labor since the family sold their farm in Hafeld. He enjoyed gently pressing his fingers on her smooth skin. She squeezed back, just as gently, and he wondered if his warm hand excited as much as hers had him.

He smiled broadly at her. Conversation was becoming increasingly difficult as B flats and G sharps attempted to find their tune in the orchestra pit. The sound drew the attention of patrons who had been socializing and swelled the crowd's own sound as people began flowing up broad staircases and down carpeted corridors. Beyond the heavy double-doors, standing open to show a view of the voluminous stage curtain, red-vested ushers directed people to their seats.

August and Elise almost missed Adolf and Helga standing against the wall, nearly behind a broadly fanned fern, in their effort to remain clear of the inflow of traffic. "There you are!" called August as he stopped and aggravated older patrons behind him. "We did not think to find you in this mad rush."

Adolf should have seen August and Elise coming, but he had been so immersed in his thoughts of Helga's hand that he had missed the pair. Helga had caught sight of August, but his smile had told her that she had seen him as well, and so was content to wait for them to draw closer.

"Yes, I think I was daydreaming." Adolf was surprised to feel Helga squeeze his hand. He must surely be blushing and thought twice about his decision not to imbibe any fortified port until intermission. If he had gotten himself a drink as August and Elise had, he might at least blame the blush on the libation. "Good of you to spot us."

August smiled. "My dear Adolf, you I might have missed, but Helga certainly caught my eye. I do not think either Faveshra sister is easily lost in a crowd."

Elise and Helga laughed goodheartedly at the joke and stepped back into the traffic flow. Soon it would bottleneck—the ushers were checking stubs after all.

Adolf followed the girls and August, but he did not laugh or even smile. He was not sure what had insulted him more, the fact that August all but admitted he was attracted to Helga, or that Adolf himself could ever be just part of the crowd.

August had no idea his jest had insulted Adolf so deeply. His hand on each girl's shoulder, he directed them to turn up a grand stairwell. Their seats were far from the stage, but still better than the vantage from which Adolf and August had last seen an opera.

All the time they were walking to their seats, Adolf's dark eyes grew harder, his fists clenching beneath his shirtsleeve cuffs. As he followed his party up the stairs, he thought about striking August, perhaps in the back of his knee or the small of his back. He might have liked to punch August square in the back of his wavy-brown head, if he were not a stair too tall for Adolf's reach. Yes, the small of his back would be just right, a staggering blow straight to bastard's kidney.

But the punch would surely topple him forward, and he might then injure the girls. Perhaps it should be the back of the knee, after all. It would cripple the leg and topple August backward down the stairs—unless the people behind him caught August before he knocked them down the stairs as well. If August twisted in his fall, he might take Adolf with him. That would not do.

As Adolf considered the repercussions of his intended violence, August stopped on the stairs, turning and offering his hand as if beckoning for Adolf to hurry and take a space beside him. He saw the intense look on Adolf's face.

Adolf was taken completely by surprise, and saw that August had been also. Adolf suddenly understood that he had become far too jealous of August far too quickly.

August understood what had happened also, but only laughed quickly and again waved Adolf forward. "Come along and catch up before we are separated. I still have all our tickets."

As they were intent on reaching the top of the staircase in their heels, the girls did not notice August's words. Adolf shook his head, but relaxed his features into a smile. August still did not know how much he had insulted Adolf, but at least the fellow was not so offensive that he should be sucker-punched. Adolf was glad he had only thought of punishing the other boy and not acted.

In a voice low enough that only Adolf heard him, August said, "I am sorry if I offended you, Adolf. You actually stand out almost as starkly as Helga and Elise, although it is more a function of your demeanor than your beauty." August winked, smiling.

August's words surprised Adolf greatly. "You did offend me, but I believe you did not mean to. Thank you." He should have then apologized to August for presuming the comment was truly meant to be belittling, but Adolf never apologized so readily to anyone.

August, not expecting any sort of apology, was glad to have that miniature rift closed before it could begin to widen, which would be disastrous for their evening. No, now he could focus his attentions on other things, like the attractive outline of Elise's backside as she ascended the stairs in front of him. Pity, they were almost to the top.

As the usher directed them to their seats, Elise made a scoffing sound. "This row? These are our seats here?"

August blinked, looking a bit put out. "Yes, well, they were the best I could do for the four of us, paying for us all up front as I did."

Helga smiled. "I feel like a bird looking down from a tall tree. These seats are just fine, August."

Adolf only shrugged. For August and he, these seats were a thousand times better than trying to jostle for space in the standing room section. "Do remind me later of what sum I owe you, August. The seats are good."

Elise did not say anything, but sat with a dramatic whoosh of her light-blue skirts. Helga narrowed her eyes and shook her head at her petulant sister, and then took Adolf's hand as she sat between him and her sister. August filled the last seat next to Elise, but his date ignored him entirely, choosing instead to open a small mirror from a powder case she carried in her purse. As she worked to reapply the makeup she had already spent hours preparing at her house, Adolf happened to notice that she occasionally tilted her small mirror to look surreptitiously at August.

The air was becoming increasingly charged with anticipation and the orchestra began to ready for the overture. The heavy double doors finally were shut, and the lights dimmed. The first note rose from the orchestra pit and silenced what dwindling conversations had lasted into the darkness.

What followed was an almost visible difference of the music's effect on those who had seen this opera and those who were experiencing it for the first time. Adolf was in that latter category, and although he was a true fan of Wagner, he was entirely unprepared for the first chord, which ended in dissonance and left the audience with a sense of tense foreboding.

In the relative darkness, Adolf felt a light trace of almost imperceptible pressure on the back of his hand. It was not the feeling of some insect crawling on his flesh, and it was not the tickle of some angel's feather either. Rather it was a methodical touch: Helga's index finger was barely circling over the bones and tendons and veins of his hand, occasionally disturbing the fine hairs that grew from his fair skin. Her eyes were still watching the opera, but her finger's single point of contact was rapidly becoming the center of Adolf's world. It provoked him to turn and look into her brilliant, cerulean eyes.

She smiled and dropped her middle finger down, continuing to trace with those two digits spaced perhaps another finger's width apart, although they remained just as gentle in their contact. Adolf continued to smile, and Helga continued tracing and smiling back, until at last she lifted his hand and kissed the one space at the center of the back of his hand where her fingers had neglected to touch. If Helga's fingers had been soft, her lips were ethereal. He felt only the faintest moistness in her soft exhale of breath.

Adolf did not know what he should do. His own breath had caught when he felt that whisper of connection, the excitement it stirred within him amplified by the low light and harmonic innovations of Wagner's work. When she had kissed the back of his hand, she smiled so ... so sweetly, seductively, perhaps, except for the innocence in Helga's features. It was a look Elise could never replicate.

For her part, Helga was pleased with Adolf's reaction. He had obviously enjoyed the tenderness, and yet he did not take it as an invitation to kiss her or do anything else besides enjoy her attention, which had been her intention from the start.

So the two sat and enjoyed the opera while also enjoying the tantric explorations of their fingers on the exposed skin of their hands or arms. When they tired of tracing and touching one another's appendages, they resolved to a compromise of holding hands. Adolf was quite sure he had missed some key moment in the opera, but he did not mind the cause for his distractions, and decided that he should enjoy all opera in Helga's hand.

"You know, sister, this music was outlawed by the church." Elise, having spurned August for purchasing such horrible seats, had been quiet for too long, and seeing the intimate flirting between Helga and Adolf, she felt the necessity to interrupt.

Helga knew her sister enjoyed pointing out instances of even the most minor rebellion, as it was Helga who always insisted they follow their father's rules to the letter. Lately,

Helga had begun to understand Elise's perspective. So far as this performance was concerned ... "Elise, it was not the music itself, but the combination of the chords Wagner employed. They were banned by monks singing Gregorian Chants. Really though, I do not think there is anything devilish about the sound, though it is powerful in the measures Wagner used."

Adolf had been lost in a naïve fantasy of mounting ecstasy, allowing the music and his proximity to Helga to swell his emotions. Since Helga had turned to address Elise, Adolf used the opportunity to move Helga's hand from his lap to instead rest in hers. Not only did it allow Helga to turn easier to her left so that she could talk to Elise, but it saved Adolf from any possible embarrassment that might have resulted had their hands remained in his lap much longer.

August leaned across Elise to say, "Very powerful. The meter of the chants lends greater weight to the harmonic suspensions. You feel the tension in this opera, like—"

"Would you be so kind as to save your conversation until the intermission?" A hoarse voice whispered from just behind Elise's chair, abruptly silencing August. The girls attempted to contain their onset of giggles.

Adolf then surprised himself, leaning close to Helga so that his breath was in her hair as he whispered, "The man is lucky to hear anything at all. I believe August was making a cogent point."

Helga whispered back, "I think you are right on both accounts. This is more fun, anyway."

August had been embarrassed by the elderly gentleman's reproach, but seeing Helga lean in to either whisper to Adolf or perhaps kiss his ear, he decided that a similar tactic might help thaw Elise's chill toward him.

"You are absolutely stunning in this light, Elise," he said, leaning toward her.

Elise reached out and patted August's thigh, and though she turned her head, she did not lean closer for her whisper, making it much less of a whisper. "I could easily take that comment the wrong way, if I did not already know I am stunning in any light, August."

Her whisper was so loud that Helga, Adolf and half-dozen other patrons heard it. The elderly gentleman sitting behind Elise went so far as to admonish the pair with an equally loud "shhhhh."

Watching August's situation, Adolf smiled; Helga's squeeze told him that she must be similarly amused. Elise whispered again, although this time Elise leaned close and spoke softly enough that no one heard what she said.

The opera was incredible, but not as much for the story as its music. Oh, the plot was moving along nicely, and it was certainly a twist when, instead of choking on poison, Tristan and Isolde declared their love for one another. The composition itself, however, held this opera's true majesty and spectacle. The crescendos hastened the beating of his heart until emotions of exhilaration and suspense coursed through him and, given the rapturous looks of others in the audience, everyone else present as well. This was only the end of the first act!

Soon the orchestra was again silencing the audience as the curtain rose on the second act. It seemed that this production had elected to save intermission until after the act. Adolf was aware that he was still holding Helga's hand, but her touch seemed far more natural now. Helga seemed similarly accustomed to the contact, and she no longer traced her fingers on the back of his hand. She did nothing at all to cause distraction, simply held his hand. Even Elise seemed content to merely sit and enjoy the performance without talking.

It was easy for Adolf to imagine himself as Tristan, with Helga playing Isolde, of course; Elise could play the role of Brangane.

As the captivating measures of the second act's love duet swelled with emotion, Adolf found that he had never felt more alive. His pulse quickened, and his eyes widened as his mouth fell slightly agape in rapturous awe of the music; in a moment of quick-silvered clarity, he noticed the same expression on Helga's face.

Her eyes found his, as shining and wide as her own. Without another thought, she leaned in and kissed him squarely on his surprised lips and did not stop kissing him until she felt him soften from surprise to sensuality. Then she sat back again, a small smile upon her lips.

It had been a moment of temporal hiatus for Adolf. Already firmly in the throes of Wagner's genius, all the emotion the opera had built was now passing through the conduit of his lips against hers, and in that virginal connection, Adolf knew he had at last achieved bliss. He had never imagined that kissing a girl would make him feel so entirely . . . supreme. He had found the center of his young universe, and it was Helga's lips.

Hyacinths. She still smelled of hyacinths, but she tasted so much sweeter. He wanted to kiss her now. He was elated that she had kissed him, but should he not have been the one to do the kissing? She had taken the initiative, and he wanted it back. But just as he caught her eye, the audience erupted into another round of thunderous applause. So fixated on his desire to kiss Helga again, Adolf had missed the climatic wounding of Tristan. The curtain fell on the second act, and patrons were already standing, continuing to applaud, but also anxious for the intermission.

Adolf again thought his opportunity to kiss her had come, but Helga's attention was stolen by her sister, who was prodding Helga to stand so they could leave their seats sooner.

Having realizing Adolf's intention before Elise had distracted her, Helga smiled as she stood, drawing Adolf up with her.

She was again taking the initiative, and although Adolf stood with her, he felt a moment of irritation. He was the man. She should be following his lead.

The crowd's migration from their seats to the concourse seemed to take nearly as long as had the entire second act. Adolf did not mind crowds, but it was difficult to hold any sort of conversation that could be heard above the clamor of voices and feet. He kept Helga close at his side, even being so bold as to put his hand on the small of her back as he guided her through the masses.

When they reached the concessions stand, Adolf ordered a glass of water. The others would all be drinking, but Adolf felt drunk with life. After looking to Helga, who smiled at him, he said, "Make that two."

Looking over at the other couple, Adolf asked, "Elise? August? What are you drinking?" Both would likely assume Adolf had ordered some kind of Russian Vodka that was becoming so popular, or some other clear spirit.

The pair was in line behind Adolf and Helga. Looking pleasantly surprised at Adolf's courtesy and generosity, he said, "I was thinking of cognac, an x.o. if they keep a decent one behind there." They did, although it was more expensive than Adolf's generosity had realized. Still, he nodded, and then looked to Elise. "And you, miss? What will you have?"

Elise was even more surprised than August. "I enjoyed their

Riesling earlier. I will try the Spatlese this time. Thank you, Adolf—you seem to understand what expenses dating a Faveshra sister entails." She smirked at August.

August's face darkened as Elise continued to embarrass him. "Well, no offense to Adolf, but perhaps next time he should buy the seats, and I will buy . . ." It began as a joke, but August knew even before he finished that his frustration had affected his judgment, and his words trailed off awkwardly.

Adolf was not sure if the unfinished comment was meant to offend him or not, but he decided that it did. "August, I have already told you to remind me just what I owe you for the seats."

"Of course—I did not mean to imply otherwise. I meant to say that I simply cannot seem to please Elise tonight."

Adolf nodded, but Elise narrowed her eyes.

Helga accepted the drinks Adolf had ordered for the four of them, and Adolf paid a sum that might have indeed purchased all their tickets if they had been in the standing room section.

Elise took her glass of white wine ignoring August entirely when he asked if she liked it.

The four of them moved away from the concessions stand and found an open area in which to stand while they enjoyed their drinks. Helga stayed very near to Adolf, although she no longer held his hand; neither was his hand on the small of her back, not now that they were standing in public.

Elise, still intent on torturing August, gave her attention instead to Adolf. "What do you think of the opera so far, Adolf? Is not it genius? Much better than his *Rings* cycle, do you not think?"

Adolf, who favored Wagner's version of the Nibelung saga over all other opera, began his reply with a simple shake of his head. "No, I do not. The music is certainly compelling, but the plot leaves something to be desired, in my opinion." Which was not truly a fair statement, since Adolf had missed much of the plot in thanks to Helga's frequent but most welcomed distractions.

August nodded as he swallowed the last of his cognac. That

drink had been nearly as expensive as the other three combined. "I believe Adolf has a point. Really, the plot is very similar to *Romeo and Juliet*. Tristan dies, and then Isolde dies of her grief. It may not have been directly from poison, but poison began all the trouble. Love is the poison in this instance, but it still results from a potion that they drink. It is almost cliché, really."

Looking irritated, Elise swatted his arm. "August, you imbecile! Adolf has not yet seen the opera, and now you have spoiled its ending for him! Honestly, is there anything you cannot ruin tonight?"

August understood his error, but the severity of Elise's reproach was perhaps too much for the young man. He looked at the empty glass in his hand, and then shrugged. "Apparently, no."

Elise smirked in satisfaction, but Helga reached out and put a pitying hand on August's arm. "There now, that is hardly true. Elise is only teasing you, August."

Adolf said, "If that is truly the opera's plot, you may have saved me from undue attention, which I can now instead apply to the lovely Miss Helga's company."

Helga blushed at the compliment and withdrew her hand from August's to instead put her arm around Adolf's waist.

August shook his head. "Still, I apologize, Adolf." He then looked to Elise, saying. "And I am sorry for spoiling the opera for you, if that is what I have done, Elise. I know the seats are not as good as you would like, but I hope you will let the matter rest, before I begin to think that you agreed to accompany me tonight for reasons other than the simple enjoyment of my company."

It was as close to insulting Elise as August dared, but it still struck too close to truth's mark, and so Elise's response was perhaps too extreme. She was only halfway through her drink, but she had already imbibed at least two glasses before the opera began, and alcohol could be a powerful agent in blood so young as theirs.

"I beg your pardon," Elise began, "but do you mean to imply that I am some prostitute who accompanies young men for their money?"

Adolf, thinking that statement was also near to the truth, could not help but laugh abruptly, which arrested everyone's attention. Trying to decide how best to explain the outburst, Adolf said, "Sorry, I was just thinking that August would have expensive tastes, if that were the case." It was not exactly an insult, but it was hardly a compliment.

Helga's mouth fell open in astonishment, but then she too was laughing.

Elise's eyes narrowed further, while August, still insulted by the very suggestion that he would ever accompany a girl under such circumstances, shook his head, turned and began to walk away.

Elise actually had taken Adolf's words as a compliment, although she would never admit such. No, instead she was left in relative disbelief that any man could simply turn and walk away from her company. She had, after all, only wanted to tease August. Obviously she had gone too far.

"Oh, this will not do," Helga said. "The intermission is nearly over, and if we return home with you, and not August,

Papa will think we traded one boy for another, and we will not be able to see either of you again. Do something Adolf! Go talk to him!"

"Me?" asked Adolf. "What should I say to him? Elise was the one to start this. She should go and talk to him. It is her attention he craves."

"Not now..." Elise said, a surprising note of disappointment in her voice.

Helga shook her head. "No, Adolf, he will be embarrassed if I speak to him, and I do not think he will even look at Elise right now. It must be you! Hurry! This drama needs to be resolved before Act III begins. Just tell him that Elise is drunk. If she is not yet, she is close enough to at least claim such."

Adolf knew the general direction in which August had headed, but already he had lost sight of the fellow amidst the crowds.

"Hurry!" Helga repeated, sounding somewhat urgent.

With that last prodding from Helga, Adolf sighed and set off after August. It was no easy task catching up to the taller boy's stride while dodging between patrons of varying states of age and intoxication. At last he was even with him, just as August was about to pass beyond the realm of re-admittance. Adolf reached forth and was able to forestall August with a firm grip on the older boy's shoulder.

"Wait, August." Adolf said. "Just a moment, please." August felt Adolf's grip and stopped. "Wait for what?

That girl is impossible tonight. I have taken her out before, and she has never complained so much."

"Well, I still owe you money, for one thing," said Adolf, thinking pragmatically.

Money was the last topic August wanted to discuss at that moment. He could care less if he saw a penny from Adolf. He simply wanted to be as far from the opera house as his two legs could carry him. Without bothering to answer Adolf, he began to turn again toward the exit.

Adolf followed him. He resented having to debase himself thus, but Helga had asked him to speak with August, so speak to him he would."All right, August, just wait another moment. No one thinks you are cheap. Elise has only been teasing you. She likes to make men uncomfortable. If she cannot do it with her beauty, then she finds another way. Believe me, I know better than most people, I think."

August narrowed his eyes at what Adolf's words implied.

Realizing the misunderstanding, Adolf shook his head and rubbed a hand over his eyes. "No, August, I did not mean it like that. Oh I will admit, I fancied her myself, once. I even went so far as to think she was my first love, but then I saw her kissing a man who was my closest friend at the time. I was young, and foolish."

August could not know that Adolf's infatuation had been only a few short months ago and not the years Adolf made it sound. Still, it was comforting to know that Elise did not actually think he was cheap. He knew well enough that she enjoyed teasing as much as she enjoyed flirting. They were often the same thing for her. Perhaps the fact that tonight it had been mostly teasing, and not nearly enough flirting, was what truly had him bothered.

"Forget what you owe me, Adolf. Stopping me from walking out on Elise is worth far more than the cost of those seats. You are right. Besides, I have already spoiled this opera's ending for you, for which I am truly sorry. I was not thinking." He shrugged, and then left that topic for the more immediate concern. "Now I need to decide how to return with any dignity. I will not go back with my tail betwixt my legs, Adolf. My ego has suffered enough slights tonight."

Adolf, thinking it was more than generous of August to forget his debt, turned his mind to the other man's predicament. "We all know the circumstances; there is no shame in simply returning. You do not need to apologize. If anything, it is Elise who should apologize. Come, there is not much time for us to return to our seats."

While Adolf counseled August, Helga was left with Elise. "Honestly, there are times I think you are the living incarnation of that Greek demigoddess, Discord."

Elise only shrugged. "We deserve only the best. Father would never purchase seats in the balcony level. If the man I date cannot provide at the very least what Father could, what is the point of dating him?"

Helga felt like slapping her sister. "The point? Honestly, Elise, you are impossible. August is only seventeen. Papa has had years to amass his wealth—of course he can afford better seats for us than August and Adolf. You had better apologize to August when he returns. Do not let him apologize to you, for he has done nothing wrong."

"So you say," replied Elise. "I am only thinking of my future, Helga. Oh, August is handsome enough, but if he cannot provide for me in the manner I deserve, then he hardly deserves my company, does he?"

Although Helga understood her sister's argument, she could not begin to agree with it. Love was always more important than wealth. If Elise was not attracted to August, and found nothing admirable in the man's personality, she would understand. Scorning him for purchasing seats in the upper mezzanine, though? Elise's behavior was unconscionable.

"Look, here they come," Helga said. "Please, apologize to August, and tell him you were only teasing him. The night has gone so very well, otherwise. Please do not ruin it for us all."

Elise smirked, "Perhaps for Adolf and you. I have seen you looking at him with those saucer eyes of yours."

Helga blushed and smiled at that.

Elise sighed. "Oh, all right. I shall make an effort at being civil for the rest of the night. Do not expect me to date him again, though. He actually walked away! Can you believe that?"

Helga, thinking it was likely in August's best interest that he never saw Elise again, nodded.

"Well it will not be much of an apology, that is certain."

Then Adolf and August were too close for further conversation between the sisters.

"Just in time," said Adolf as they reached the girls.

August said nothing.

"My apologies, August." She did not sound very apologetic, but managed to soften her tone somewhat as she continued. "I did not think you would take my taunts so seriously." And then she was very firm and not apologetic at all "However, so we are clear, I am no man's whore, nor will I stand to be likened to such again."

August grit his teeth. Elise's apology was not precisely that for which he had hoped. But he kept his word to Adolf and offered his own flag of truce. "I am also sorry, Elise. Your taunts may not have been meant as barbs, but they wounded my pride just as readily."

Helga patted August's arm, and then said in a light tone, "Well, now that all that is settled, let us return to our seats before we miss the curtain." Helga was anxious to return not only to their seats, but also to the relative darkness of the theater, to her private world with Adolf.

Elise would surely marry for money and status, but Helga was far too romantic for such aspirations. That was not to say that she was in love with Adolf, or that she planned to marry him, but after that kiss, she certainly had much stronger feelings for him than she had known.

Adolf's thoughts were occupied with the prospect of finding another opportunity to kiss Helga. He had enjoyed that kiss very much, but it still bothered him that she had taken the initiative of kissing him before he had kissed her. The man should always take the lead.

Soon the couples were back in their seats, and the opera began its final act. Helga reached over to find Adolf's hand, but before she could do so, he settled his arm across the back of her chair. Before he was entirely aware of what he had done, his hand was on her far shoulder, pulling her to lean into his chest, where she eventually laid her head against the crux of his chest and shoulder.

Holding her was even better than touching her hand. Although her perfume was hyacinths, her golden tresses smelled of rose petals. The more he thought about her scent, the less attention he paid to the performance.

That was just as well. He had missed Melot mortally wounding Tristan at the end of the second act, and so he found it difficult to understand why the music had turned so dramatically sorrowful. He wanted nothing to do with Tristan mourning over his fate. He could care less about the shepherd's piping and whether or not Isolde would arrive in time to save Tristan. Adolf had his girl under his arm, and that was far more exciting than any opera could ever be.

He noticed that August and Elise were as close together as he and Helga, and they did not seem to be watching the opera either. Well, so much for Elise's taunts and insults. Indeed, so much for August's indignations, also. If a couple that had been fighting all night could spend the final act kissing one another, then nothing was preventing him from doing the same. But how could he capture Helga's attention?

Resting comfortably against him, Helga's eyes were intent on the opera. Unlike Adolf, she had no difficulty imagining herself as Isolde, with him as Tristan. Knowing how the opera ended might have dissuaded some girls from such comparisons, but because Helga was well educated and had studied the libretto, she understood that Tristan and Isolde's love had always belonged to the night, and that death was simply a metaphor for an eternal night. In death, the pair would be together forever. What could be more romantic than that?

Adolf had no such thoughts. His had long since stopped paying attention to the plot. His thoughts were fixated on how he might catch Helga's eye so that he might then kiss her.

At last as the shepherd finally changed his tune from the mournful dirge to the tune that announces Isolde's impending arrival, Adolf made his move. His lips kissed the very top of her golden head, lingering a moment as the scent of rose petals again suffused him. As he drew back, Helga lifted her head from his chest and looked up at him with a shy smile.

Her soft, plush lips eagerly met his, falling slightly open as his tongue instinctively flickered to meet hers. Adolf had never before experienced such passion. He pulled her tighter against him, and she responded with a supple fervor that bordered on indecency for so public a place. True, the theatre was very dark, and other couples were similarly engaged . . . Adolf soon found that kissing Helga was only the beginning of his desires.

The opera continued, and soon the final aria resounded throughout the opera house. At last he realized he could not just kiss her forever, and remembering what Johan had told him, he pulled away first.

His discipline was rewarded with the sight of the blissful expression on Helga's face. "That was amazing," she whispered. The look in her eyes told Adolf that she had not been referring to the opera.

He kissed her again, although much softer this time. The rest of the audience was applauding the opera's conclusion, but it felt as though they might have been cheering for Helga and him. As the performers took their final bows, Adolf sat with Helga, quite content.

Chapter 9

OH HE HAD spent the night with August, but not in the boy's parent's apartment. He and August had snuck into the Faveshra household once the sisters' elderly father had gone to bed. It had not been proper behavior for the young men, and it was even less proper for the young ladies to have invited them.

After the opera, August had offered to walk Elise home, which had of course prompted Adolf to extend the same courtesy to Helga. The four walked the few blocks to the Faveshra household in relative silence. By then the night had lost much of its warmth. The veiling clouds that had blocked the heat earlier had now pushed westward, revealing a dazzling array of stars in the heavens, but also bringing the reminder that autumn was moving closer to winter with its biting wind.

Helga had remained very close to Adolf throughout the walk. They walked with their arms around each other, in an almost cadenced step. Invigorated by the cold, but kept comfortable by Helga's warming presence, Adolf had never felt better, his chest broad and powerful and his eyes sharper. With Helga under his arm, all felt right in the world. He was happy to keep her slower pace; he wanted to continue walking with the girl as long as possible. It was a shame the sisters did not live further from the opera house. Was Helga beginning to lag in her steps, as well?

The two couples eventually reached the Faveshra household, which was nothing like Adolf's home in Leonding. The Garden House was a large Cape-styled structure that stood alone on a plot of land, surrounded by gardens. The Faveshra household, conjoined to its neighbors had a narrow frontage and a small communal yard. The marble front steps boasted a certain opulence of the neighborhood. The street was lined with homes of similar shape, with steps of similar material, although some varied in the color and quality of the marble.

The couples paused at the base of those front stairs and, standing a few feet apart, seemed ready to make their farewells.

Adolf was smiling as he looked down at Helga, who was looking up at him with either the street lamp or the star's light in her eyes.

"Thank you for such a wonderful evening, Adolf," she said softly and sweetly.

Before Adolf could respond, Elise giggled loud enough to draw their attention. "August, you . . . you rogue!"

Helga held a quieting forefinger to her lips and glared at her sister.

"Oh, Father cannot hear us," said Elise, although with significantly less volume. "He could not even if he were awake,"

"No, but our neighbors might. Sometimes I think you purposely invite scandal," answered Helga, in an even quieter tone. "What if you woke poor Josef? You know how difficult it is for him to fall asleep."

"You worry too much." Elise shot back. "Besides, you have only August to blame. Can you believe he asked to come inside?" She winked at her sister in a most mischievous way.

August, thankful for the darkness that hid the embarrassment on his cheeks, shrugged. "If your dear sister had not all but suggested such herself throughout our entire walk home, I never would have presumed to—"

"Oh honestly, August. If you are going to betray me to my sister instead of acting like a man and taking responsibility for your own words, I shall greatly regret having made any such suggestions."

Helga shook her head at her sister. "You do enjoy pushing any boundary you can find, do you not, Elise?"

Adolf, emboldened by the excitement of the evening, gave Helga a gentle squeeze and said, "You had said you wanted to sneak out to meet me—perhaps instead August and I should sneak in?"

"Sneak out?" began Elise, looking incredulously at her sister.

"Adolf!" interrupted Helga, but a small smile was already playing at the corners of lips still full from the night's kissing. "Well . . ."

Now it was Elise's turn to interrupt. "Well then, it is settled. We cannot risk you being seen entering with us now. Father and Josef may be asleep, but I am sure more than one set of eyes are watching us now." She gestured at the lamp-lit street around them, "Even at this hour. No, Helga and I will enter first. Follow that alley there and see if you can climb the gate to our yard in the rear. Wait until I set a candle in one of our windows, and then enter through the back door. Take your shoes off. Our tiled floor will echo your steps throughout the house if you do not."

Helga seemed ready to protest again, but before she could begin to voice her objections, Adolf leaned down and kissed her lightly. It was enough to silence the girl and draw a smile from her.

"Right then, off we go," August said a few moments later, sounding a tad breathless.

Adolf lingered a moment longer, gazing into Helga's eyes, but at last he released her hand. "See you soon."

Helga was incredibly nervous about the whole affair, but it was all rather romantic, certainly exciting. She followed Elise up the steps, all the while watching as Adolf and August disappeared down the dark alleyway. "Father will send us to the nunnery if he ever learns of this."

Elise smiled mischievously in the shadows of their stoop. "Then he had best not learn of it. Come, they'll be waiting." With that, her key clicked the lock open. The house was dark, lit only by the dying embers of the evening fire in the sitting room.

"I hope no one mistakes us for burglars," said Adolf in a strained whisper as they felt blindly down the alleyway, using their hands to guide them along the brick walls. Doing such kept them out of the center of the alley, in which pooled trash, sullied water and piles of animal excrement. Linz was considered to be a clean city, especially compared to places such as London or Berlin. But an alley was an alley.

"My dear Mr. Hitler, burglarizing is precisely what I had in mind for the evening."

Adolf raised an eyebrow in the gloom. "Burglarizing?" August laughed as quietly as he could. "Well, I suppose I cannot steal what is likely to be more than freely given. Regardless, sneaking about in the night like this, I cannot help but feel as though I am some romantic thief, come to take Elise's honor in the deep night. Think of the opera. Tristan and Isolde both reserved their passions for the evening's darkness."

Adolf was not sure he would have viewed their actions in quite that manner. "I will just be happy to be out of this cold and back in Helga's warm embrace."

At last they reached the end of the alley. It did not connect to another street, but provided access to the communal yard this block of houses shared. August had no trouble vaulting the locked gate, but Adolf, a few inches shorter, found the task to be more difficult. He made far more noise as his shoes scrambled to find purchase on the wrought-iron bars, balancing precariously above the iron spikes that topped the gate. Adolf was not as strong in his upper body as August; when his footing slipped halfway over the gate, he very nearly impaled himself. He threw his weight forward, tumbling headfirst onto the lush grass on the far side of the gate with a resounding thump.

Adolf and August flinched at the sound, loud in the darkness. A few houses down, a dog began barking. Soon three or four more were baying into the night. Never fond of dogs, Adolf hoped that the mutts were on chains and their barking would end as suddenly as it had begun. After a moment, they quieted.

The boys crouched in the shadows, waiting for the candle to appear,

August whispered, "It seems the night will turn out even better than I hoped. Thank you again, Adolf."

Adolf could barely make out August's features; nor could he understand the hushed whispers. "Thank me? For what?" he asked, just as quietly.

"For stopping me when I was going to leave Elise there at the opera."

Adolf could only smile at the irony. "Yes, well, having already made that mistake once myself, I am happy to have spared you from that embarrassment."

"Oh?" asked August, unaware of what had transpired. "Let us just say that Elise has a knack for causing men to abandon her company."

August's eyes widened in the darkness, "Adolf, you sound as though you speak from intimate history."

Adolf snorted softly. "Not nearly so intimate as you are about to be, I am sure. I had thought I loved Elise once, but it was an entirely foolish notion. I am happy things worked out as they did."

"Indeed," answered August. He was not precisely decided on how he should react to such information. "What are you doing?"

Adolf was pulling off his shoe. "Getting ready."

"A premature action, do you not think? What if the candle never shows? Or if we should suddenly need to flee?"

"Of course the candle will show. As for needing to flee, how quickly do you think I could pass that gate? If we should be discovered, I do not think fleeing will be of much use. Besides, we have not done anything wrong, precisely."

August just shook his head. "We are prowling and, at the very least, trespassing. I will keep my shoes on for now—I suggest you do the same."

Adolf shrugged, and as he was about to put his shoe back on, a single candle illuminated a window in the house diagonal from where the boys waited. They looked at each other for a moment, excitement clear on both their faces.

"Well, August, I believe that is our official invitation." Adolf pulled off his other shoe and began walking toward the lighted window. August, shaking his head, followed.

The thrill of sneaking about in the darkness coupled with Adolf's excitement to see Helga again to create a feeling of near invincibility. They had only been apart for a few minutes, but the time felt like ages to Adolf. As he mounted the steps, he thought about August's talk of burglary. He meant to have sex with Elise, which really should not have been any sort of surprise. Was Helga expecting the same? Intercourse had never crossed his mind. He was aware of the fundamentals, but the specifics of such an act were fairly foreign to him, except for what he had experienced with Friar Roald.

The door opened before he reached the top step. Seeing that he carried his shoes in hand, Elise permitted him to enter. Helga was waiting a few steps from the door, wearing a decidedly nervous smile, which he returned with no trouble.

August was forced to halt and remove his own boots before he too slipped through the dark house. The sisters did not dare turn on any of the lights. Instead, each carried an old shuttered lantern that cast a mere sliver of light.

Elise took August's hand, and then spoke very softly to Helga and August. "We should meet back here before the sunrise. It would not do to have the boys trapped here all day."

Helga nodded in agreement, moving tentatively closer to Adolf. "Well before sunrise, sister." She was relieved when Adolf shifted closer to her.

Elise rolled her eyes. "Well then, I bid you both a good night."

August only shrugged at Adolf, offered a slight bow of his head to Helga, and then followed after Elise.

"You are shivering," said Helga in a very quiet whisper. And before Adolf could respond, Helga had put her arms around him.

He was indeed shivering, but her arms warmed him from the inside. He placed his arms around her almost reluctantly, but in truth he was only nervous. He had never known such intimate contact beyond his family's hugs, and this was a much different embrace. Soon nervousness was replaced with surprise as his hands felt the smooth cotton fabric of her nightgown. In the darkness, Adolf had not seen that she had changed from her dress.

She stepped away from him. "Come, I have a blanket in my room that will warm you better than I can."

Before Adolf could protest and explain that he much preferred her to a blanket, Helga was leading him through the kitchen and up a flight of stairs. He ascended behind her as quietly as he could, unabashedly staring at her well-rounded posterior as she climbed the steps ahead of him in the dark. Her nightgown displayed her curves superbly.

Soon, they were tiptoeing down a long carpeted hallway, trying to avoid the occasional creaks and groans of the floorboards. While the house was narrow, it was also deep. The light spilling from under a doorway on the left suggested August and Elise's destination. Helga stopped at the opposite door and opened it as quietly as its brass hinges would allow.

Once inside, the door closed quietly behind them, Helga at last opened the lantern shutter, bathing the room in warm yellow light that caused both of them to blink as they waited for their eyes to adjust.

"Well, what do you think?" asked Helga, still quietly, but no longer in an almost inaudible whisper.

Adolf took a moment to look about him. The walls were papered with intricate floral designs that matched well the bedroom set, a large, handsome mirror adorning the wall furthest from him. Helga's bed was larger than Adolf's own, both at home in Leonding and at Frau Cichini's residence. Her dresser was similarly oversized, nearly twice as big as his. How could she possibly fill so many drawers?

"It is well furnished, and that mirror is magnificent. I do not think even my mother has one so large." He moved toward it, Helga following him.

As they stood near one another before the mirror, Helga looked at their reflection. She smiled with mild pride, and then looked at Adolf directly. "It was a gift for my sixteenth birthday last year. Elise was incredibly jealous."

Adolf's smile was far shyer, and it only added to his nervous tone, "I am sure she was."

Helga ignored his manner, and thought to make him more comfortable by carrying on. "She should not have been. Her mirror belonged to our mother. If Elise did not resemble her so much, Father would not have given it to her when she passed."

Adolf only nodded, unsure whether or not the statement merited an offer of sympathy.

"Elise is never happy with what she has," said Helga. But then she was moving, crossing the length of her room to open a closet. Inside hung dresses of varying cuts and colors, as well as coats, frocks, shoes and even a stack of boxed hats.

"Here," said Helga as she pulled down a folded blanket. "Wrap this about you and come sit with me. It seems we will have ample time for me to see your drawings after all." Adolf slung his satchel off his shoulder so that it landed with a soft bounce on Helga's bed. He then allowed her to drape the wooly green blanket about him, protesting as she did. "This is not necessary. I was chilled outside while we waited, but now that I am inside, I will warm up quickly enough."

Helga agreed, "No doubt, but are blankets not that much cozier? Come, sit and show me your work."

She was right about the blanket. Despite being wool, it was finely spun and not so course or itchy as were most wool products. He sat next to Helga, on her right, close enough that their thighs pressed together, and reached around her shoulders, so that the blanket covered her as well. It was indeed much cozier.

She was looking at him with her cerulean eyes, and, in the flickering light of her lantern, he admired her fair, unblemished skin. She wanted him to kiss her. He knew it by the look in her eyes. So he did, lightly, using the blanketed arm about her shoulders to draw her even closer.

She returned his affection by lifting her small hand to gently cup his cheek as she kissed him back. It was not so passionate a kiss as they had exchanged in the darkness of the opera, with the fervor of the music and atmosphere to embolden the both of them. This kiss was tender, lingering in the silence of Helga's room. It might have lasted forever, if Helga's hand had not fallen away as she withdrew with a smile.

"Adolf, you can be so wonderfully gentle. No boy has ever kissed me the way you do."

"No girl has ever made me want to kiss her in such a manner," said Adolf through a smile that was as much from his enjoyment of the kiss as it was from the pride her comment gave him.

"Show me your drawings, Adolf? I would very much like to see them."

The abrupt change in subject surprised Adolf. For a moment, he felt a flash of disappointment, but he turned away and extracted his sketchbook from his satchel.

Helga caught his expression as he turned, and when he opened his sketchbook across both their laps, she laid her hand on his arm. "I am not like Elise, Adolf. I would never have been so bold as to invite you in here."

Disappointment was shifting to a look of confusion, but Helga quickly continued. "That is not to say I am not very glad to have you here. I truly enjoy your company, immensely. I just do not want to give you the wrong idea."

"Wrong idea?" asked Adolf.

"Well," Helga began to blush, "Most young men who find themselves in a young lady's bedroom in the middle of the night also find themselves expecting certain events to transpire."

Now Adolf understood quite clearly what Helga was too much a lady to say. "I would never—"

She cut him off with a finger on his lips. "Yes, you would. It is perfectly natural. I like you very much, Adolf. I just do not want to proceed too quickly in that direction. I want to know you better, and for you to know me. Please, show me your drawings?"

He felt conflicted. "Of course." he said at last. The first page held his sketch of the Abbey Lambach, with its Byzantine frescoes and strange swastikas adorning it. His eye for detail was as evident in the sketch as his talent for portraying proportion.

Helga smiled in awed appreciation of the piece. "It is magnificent. Where did you see this? I have never seen anything like it here in Linz."

Adolf had mixed emotions about the piece. It was one of his better efforts, and so he was proud of the work. It was the memory of the place that disturbed him still. He tried to keep that discomfort from his voice as he answered, "It is the Abbey found in the town of Lambach. I lived there for a short time before my family moved to Leonding."

Helga sensed there was something Adolf was not telling her, but instead of pressing him on the subject, she turned the page. "Have you moved a lot?" She gazed at a rural setting with tall mountains that rose from the rolling hills of the sketch's foreground.

Adolf nodded. "Since I was a baby, I am told."

"That must have been difficult. You must miss the friends you have had to leave."

"Sometimes—" began Adolf, but then he shrugged, upsetting the blanket across their shoulders so that it fell from Helga. He again put his arm around her to draw the blanket back into place. "I lived in Passau, Germany for a time. I was young, but I had made good friends there. I was only six when we moved to Hafeld, Austria. Near the Salzkammergut Mountains, which is where I drew this sketch."

Helga's eyes lit with recognition, "I know of Hafeld. It is not far from Linz, and my father often enjoyed apple brandies from its orchards. I would not be surprised if there was a bottle to be found in this house now."

Adolf smiled, "My father had always wanted to live on a farm, so we did. The ground was bad, though, and instead of producing crops, it produced rocks. So we sold that land and moved instead to Lambach."

Helga noticed again the change in Adolf's tone as he mentioned that town. He became quieter, and his eyes tightened at their corners. "You did not like it there," she offered in the wake of his silence.

His dark eyes hardened into two smoldering specks of coal. "No, I was . . . mistreated there."

Helga frowned, not understanding what he meant; but it was obvious that the topic bothered him, so she moved on to another question. "So where did you live after that?"

"Leonding. My mother, aunt and younger sister still live in our house there. I moved to Linz on my own to be closer to school. My mother thought that would improve my grades, which it did—I was simply happy that I did not have to walk nearly four miles to and from school any longer."

"Four miles, no wonder you are so trim." Her eyes were complimenting him even more than her words.

Adolf regained a hint of his former smile at that. "Well, that was quite some time ago. After my father passed away, I was allowed to move to Linz proper. That was how I came to know Johan. We stayed at the same boarding house."

"Ah." Helga turned another page. "I met Johan at a spring festival. He seemed like a nice-enough boy, and he was certainly handsome. At the time, I liked that he was older."

Adolf frowned at that admission.

Helga lightly kissed a corner of his frown. "That is not to say I do not like younger boys, also. In fact, at the moment I would say that I like them a great deal more."

"Kind of you to say so," replied Adolf, though without much conviction.

She kissed him again, "Well, I like *you* a great deal more, at least." That brought his smile back.

She turned the page to Adolf's sketch of the factory in Steyr. "Oh my . . ." she began. "Your shading is incredible. You have made it look as though the waterwheel is still attached to the building by how you faded the brick around the outline is in comparison to the brick to which the wheel was attached."

Adolf was pleased with Helga's keen eye. She understood the nuances of his drawings in a way most people might overlook. "Can you see what I was trying to explain in my letter? The factory looks unbalanced without its wheel. It is as noticeable as a man with only one arm. The original architect had planned for the wheel's presence when he designed the oversized factory windows. Now, with the wheel gone, the face of the building is monstrously out of proportion to its exterior elements."

Helga nodded thoughtfully. The windows did seem ridiculously large without the wheel to balance them. "I would like to see the real factory," she said at last. "Would you mind if I came to visit some day?"

Adolf shook his head. "Of course I would not mind, but there would be little to occupy us in Steyr besides seeing an old factory. I very much doubt there is anything that would convince Elise to accompany you on such a trip."

"No, I do not suppose there is," answered Helga. "But," she continued, as she looked up from the sketch to instead gaze into his lantern-lit eyes, "I think it is time I began traveling on my own. I am nearly old enough to marry. If I do not find my independence now, I may never have any at all."

Adolf nodded and did his best to stifle a yawn. "Excuse me," he began, but was interrupted by a yawn that might have been an echo, if it were not actually louder than Adolf's own. The two laughed quietly at one another.

"It must be very late by now," she whispered.

Adolf nodded again, and then failed to suppress another yawn. "Mmm, well past midnight, I would wager."

Helga gently closed the sketchbook and set it off to the side before she rose and walked to her desk. From it, she took a small alarm clock. "I do not expect to keep you up all night, especially if you plan to visit your family tomorrow."

"Today, you mean," said Adolf with a grin.

Helga walked back to sit beside Adolf on the bed. "Father is generally up just after the sunrise. If I set my alarm for just after four, we can have you and August safely gone before anyone knows you were here."

"Yes, I think that will be ample time to make our escape."

"Adolf, you make it sound as though I have you as my prisoner here."

Adolf grinned, "If this were a prison, I think there would be a lot more criminals in the world."

Helga rolled her eyes and finished winding the alarm. She then closed the shutter on her lantern, content to let what oil remained to burn itself out. Her house had electricity, but she still preferred the lantern's softer light. She then crawled beneath her covers and nestled herself between the still-cold sheets, looking back at him. "Well, will you not join me? Or do you intend to sleep upright there on the edge all night?"

"I…" he began, but then paused as he felt nervousness threatening to crack his voice.

"Oh, Adolf, you are sweet. Come lay with me. I will not bite. Besides, you still have all your clothes on. You can lie atop the covers if you would like."

Holding Helga's hand was one thing. Kissing her was another thing, but sharing her bed with her? But then, what else had he expected when he snuck into her home? He removed his shirt and trousers, exposing his small clothes in the meager starlight filtering into the room. He then veritably jumped under the covers to avoid exposure to the room's chill.

"There now, is that not better?"

It was Adolf's turn to roll his eyes at Helga's almost motherly tone. He settled himself between the cotton sheets that were much softer than any to which he was accustomed. Helga's bed was larger than his, and there was plenty of room for him to lie comfortably without crowding her too closely. For a moment, he thought of what his mother would say about this situation.

The feel of Helga's nightgown against his bare skin halted such thoughts, and he was very surprised to find Helga's head nestling into the crook of his arm and chest as she lay against him. "Adolf, you are the most wonderful boy I have ever known. Thank you for everything tonight."

She kissed him then, perhaps lighter than any of their kisses that night had been. And as she settled back onto his chest, Adolf sighed, a very happy and contented sound. That kiss would linger on his lips and mind until they both drifted to sleep.

"Goodnight, Adolf." "Goodnight, Helga."

The alarm bell startled Helga and Adolf awake in almost the same instant, perhaps because both of their internal clocks had been waiting for the sound. It was still mostly dark outside of Helga's bedroom window, but the predawn light was just enough to see Helga's face and notice the line in her cheek where she must have slept on a wrinkle of his undershirt. She was beautiful.

"Good morning" were the first words from her raspy morning voice, and he could not help the instinctive kiss he gave her.

"A very good morning," he answered quietly.

She smiled and pushed herself up. "I wonder if Elise was smart enough to set an alarm. I will go and check on her while you dress."

Adolf suddenly realized he was in a fairly indecent state of morning rigidity. He turned on his side and nodded. "Yes, that is a good idea."

She did not notice his embarrassment, although she was aware of its source, having woken at least once earlier in the night from an accidental prodding.

"I will not be long. We do not have long, remember." And with that, she left the comfort of their covers to venture forth to Elise's room.

Adolf was left where he was, lying in sheets that still smelled of her. How had he come to this? Last night he had been firmly set on not falling in love, and yet now he was lying in Helga's bed. He was not sure if what he felt for Helga was love, but the evidence was certainly mounting toward that conclusion.

At last he cast aside the covers, feeling his skin prickle upon contact with the cool air. He dressed quickly, changing from the small clothes he wore to those he had brought in his travel satchel, and then donning the same fine clothes he had worn to the opera. He was lucky not to have torn that clothing in his effort to climb over the gate—which reminded him that the way into the house was likely also the way out. Well, he would cross that gate when he got to it.

Helga returned just as Adolf had finished buttoning his overcoat. "They said they would meet us in twenty minutes."

"Twenty minutes? What sort of clothes does August have to put on?"

Helga's blush battled with the smile on her face. "Dressing has very little to do with their delay," was all she offered.

Adolf's mouth dropped, and a short laugh escaped him. Then, as he was gathering his sketchbook back into his satchel, a thought crossed his mind. "Helga, I have not disappointed you, have I?"

This time it was her turn to laugh. "My dear Adolf, had you tried to initiate that in which Elise and August are presently engaged, I would have been disappointed. No, you are as wonderful as ever. I have told you, I am not like Elise. In time, I will desire deeper expressions of our affections for one another, but I have little interest in participating in carnal acts that are not firmly rooted in love. Do you understand?"

Adolf, feeling foolish for having posed the question, just nodded.

Helga crossed the room and kissed his cheek. "You are sweet and honorable." She stepped back and looked out the window. Already the east was passing from indigo to an orange pastel. "Unlike my sister, I have been saving myself. The more I know you, the happier I am that I have done so."

Adolf was not entirely sure what that meant, but she had said it with a smile, so he was content to assume it was a good thing. "Did you still want to take that walk in the park later this morning?"

"Yes, I would like that very much. What will you do until then?"

Adolf shrugged. "Wander, I suppose. It will be good to stretch my legs about the city. I do not do nearly as much walking in Steyr. There simply is not enough worth seeing."

"Wander? Adolf, it is hardly past four in the morning. I cannot even offer you breakfast. Are you sure you want to wander aimlessly until I can again escape this house? You may have hours to pass before I can meet you. Would you not rather get an early start on your travel home?"

"I would much rather enjoy your company again before I head homeward."

Helga smiled. "Good. I did not really want to convince you otherwise. Come, I can at least offer you a fruit from the kitchen while we wait for Elise and August. Remember, we must be very, very quiet."

Adolf nodded and followed Helga. They reached the kitchen without detection, and Helga offered him an apple and a peach. The peach he began eating; the apple he dropped into his coat-pocket for later.

"So where should we meet?"

"Shhhh—" Helga held up her finger, listening intently. "I thought I heard . . ."

Now Adolf heard it as well, heavier footsteps on the floor above.

"You must go!" Helga's eyes had gone whitely wide. "But—." Adolf began. He did not even have his shoes on. "I will meet you near the stands where we first met as

soon as I am able. If I am not there by nine, assume that I am not coming. Now go!"

"Who the hell . . ." came a loud and gravelly voice from upstairs.

"Go!" said Helga in a desperate whisper. She opened the kitchen door and all but shoved Adolf through it. He still did not have his shoes, but Helga was smart enough to toss them out after him. The door then closed, but Adolf could hear more yelling from the second floor. It was obvious that Mr. Faveshra had woken and likely discovered poor August and Elise.

Having no desire to be caught himself, Adolf made for the deeper shade of the tree under which he and August had first waited just a few short hours before. He had just finished tying his shoelaces when the backdoor was flung widely open again. With his shirt and coat clutched in one hand and his trousers held up by his other, August came running from the house.

Adolf shifted around the side of the tree trunk so that it would be impossible to see him from the house. "Over here!" he cried out as the boy raced by.

Hearing the familiar voice, August veered and dove into the shadows beneath the old oak tree. He nearly tackled Adolf in his effort to escape the sight of the enraged elderly man.

Adolf recovered, steadying August to a sitting position. "Finish dressing!" he said in a fierce whisper. He then poked his head around the tree trunk and saw Mr. Faveshra standing on his back steps, a fireplace poker in one hand and his nightcap in the other. The man was large and looked powerful, despite his age. He was searching the communal yard to see in which direction August had fled.

"Is he still there?" asked August, panting as he tried to regain his breath while still dressing with the utmost alacrity.

"Yes, you fool! Why were you still there?"

August finished buttoning his shirt and peeked around the trunk. "Elise had promised he would not wake for at least another hour! At least!"

"Well he is certainly awake now," said Adolf.

"Awake? He is insane! He nearly took my head off with his first swing of that iron."

Mr. Faveshra remained on his back steps for another minute, and then, after slapping his hand with the long poker, he returned to the kitchen, closing the door behind him. Just as Adolf thought all was clear, the back door opened again, and August's boots were each thrown savagely into the yard.

"Well, that was rather decent of him," said Adolf. "Decent?" said August incredulously.

"At least you will not be out a pair of boots."

"You think I am going to go and get those? He is probably watching them like a farmer who stakes out a sheep for the wolves. It is a trap!"

Adolf had not thought of that, but it made cogent sense. "Well we cannot stay here. Once the sun rises, this tree will not give us enough shadow to hide in."

August looked around, considering their options. Behind them, the fence was too tall to scale, and there was only another yard on the opposite side for the houses on the other side of the block. The only exit seemed to be the two gates at either end of the yard.

"We will have to split up. That way, if he does see one of us, there is at least a chance he will not see the other. Knowing one boy spent the night in his house will be bad enough. If he learns that there were two, I doubt there will be much chance of us seeing either sister again. Not that there is much chance I will be invited back to see Elise as it is. I am certain he recognized me from when I picked the girls up last night. Last night!" cried August in despair.

"You run that way," he pointed to the west gate. "It might give you the chance to snatch up your boots as you go. I will head out the way we came in, and with any luck, he will not catch site of either of us. Why did you have to linger so long?"

"It was worth it," said August with a roguish grin. "Tell that to Elise, now that she has to face her father's

wrath," answered Adolf, even as he was hoping that Helga would not also be punished. Of course, that could only happen if he were seen. The longer he waited, the more likely that scenario would be come.

"On the count of three, we run. If you can, meet up with me around the other side of the block behind us. All right?"

August nodded and readied himself.

"Three!" said Adolf, and without pausing to look whether or not Mr. Faveshra was watching from his window, he bolted straight for the gate over which he had climbed to enter the yard.

August, surprised by Adolf's failure to say the preparatory numbers "one" and "two," put his head down and ran as swiftly as his bootless feet would carry him. He snatched up those items as he passed in front of the Faveshra's back door and did not stop to see if he or Adolf had been spotted.

Adolf did not bother looking back to check August's progress, either. He ran at a full sprint and tried to time his jump so that momentum might compensate for what his height and strength lacked. It was just enough to plant his hands between the long spikes that topped the gate, but as he tried to swing his legs over, his pant cuff caught on one of the spikes. The sudden pull stopped his momentum and destroyed what balance his arms were trying to keep. He ended up falling head-first over the gate, much in the manner he had upon entering, except this time he heard his trousers tear where they had snagged on the spike.

He landed in the alley with a jarring thud, but after a brief inspection he found nothing broken or particularly bruised, so he continued his escape into the early-morning light. Once he was clear of the alley, he paused to inspect the damage to his trousers. It had torn a good five or six inches up his inseam, and his leg stung where the spike had grazed his skin. "Wonderful," was all he could say. Then Adolf walked to where he hoped August would be meeting him.

It was only another minute before August came around the street corner, now properly attired in coat, shirt and boots. He was walking briskly, not bothering to hide the furtive glances he cast back over his shoulder.

"Come," said Adolf as he met August. "We cannot stay here. What if he calls the authorities?" Their jokes earlier that evening about August's intent to steal something from the Faveshra household no longer seemed so funny.

"No, we cannot," August agreed. Noticing the tear in Adolf's trousers, he said, "Are you all right?"

"I will be fine, although I do not know how I will explain this tear to my mother when I visit later today."

"Do not worry about that," said August. "My home is not far. We can go there and get cleaned up and fed, and I will see if I have a pair of trousers you can borrow. You are not that much shorter than me, I suppose."

"Thanks," said Adolf, although without much enthusiasm. This was all August's fault, after all. "Lead the way."

They made it back to August's apartment just as the sun cleared the horizon.

"My parents are likely to be just waking up," August said. "With any luck, we can sneak in and make it appear as though we both spent the night here after the opera."

"We probably should have," said Adolf.

"But Adolf, just think of all the . . . excitement you would have missed!"

"Are you not at all concerned about the trouble Elise is going to be in? Helga too, maybe." Adolf betrayed his true worries with that last bit.

August only shrugged. "I told you, it was Elise's idea for us to stay the night there, and it was she who convinced me not to leave when Helga woke us. Whatever trouble she is in, she has earned."

"And Helga?" pressed Adolf.

"And Helga what? You did not force your way into her bedroom. If her father discovers you were there, then she has as much right to punishment as Elise. I doubt that will happen. Either way, there is no good in worrying about it now."

That hardly satisfied Adolf, but it did not make the statement any less true. He would find out soon enough whether Helga had been punished for Elise's indiscretion.

Until then, his only concern was finding another pair of trousers.

Chapter 10

"A BIT BAGGY, BUT they'll have to do. Thank you, August." Adolf pulled at the excess material that made his already lank frame seem almost morbidly gaunt. His own trousers were already folded neatly and in his leather satchel. Luckily the trousers he borrowed from August matched the color of his coat.

August suppressed a smile at the almost comic sight of Adolf. The younger boy was always so meticulously dressed that seeing him in such ill-fitting garments was amusing. But August knew better than to make any joke regarding Adolf's appearance, which he had learned the hard way at the opera last night, when he made the off-handed jest about Adolf being unremarkable in a crowd.

"Would you care for anything to eat? I am not sure what I have to offer, but there are usually some sweet-cakes or muffins for breakfast."
"Either would be fine," answered Adolf. He had not eaten since he had left Steyr yesterday, and after being up half the night, along with the excitement that had followed, his stomach was empty, even if his worries about Helga had suppressed his appetite somewhat.
"Come, let us see about those cakes and muffins," said August, leading Adolf from his small bedroom.
The Kubizek household was modest, and while Mrs. Kubizek kept an orderly home, it was clear that they were not a wealthy family. Downstairs from their three-room apartment, Mr. Kubizek ran his upholstering business, to which August was an apprentice, although he dreamed as often of being a musician as Adolf dreamed of being a painter.

More so, perhaps, as recently Adolf's thoughts had shifted. Ever since he had sketched the old mill-factory without its waterwheel, he no longer drew for the capturing of the scene, but rather sketched so as to improve the structure. He would look at a building and redesign it, or demolish it entirely and start from scratch. He would tell August of those plans—and Helga, of course, if he was able to see her again after last night.

His mood darkened again at that thought, but August did not notice. He had just led Adolf into the kitchen, where Frau Kubizek was already cooking a few links of sausage on the stove. "I thought I heard another voice in that room. What have I told you about having friends over without telling me?" The woman's voice was scolding in an endearing way. She was not exactly upset, but taking the opportunity to gently embarrass August in front of his friend.

"Mama, this is Adolf Hitler. He came with us to the opera last night. He lives in Steyr, you see, so instead of having him rent a room in Linz for the night, I invited him back here. I am sorry that I could not tell you, first."

Frau Kubizek narrowed an eye at her son. "And have I not told you that girls only lead to mischief? Well I hope you were not up too late. Your father will be expecting you downstairs with him shortly." She wiped the sausage grease from her hands onto her broad apron and looked over her son's newest friend. "Well, Herr Hitler, welcome to the Kubizek home. Would you care for a breakfast sausage?"

Adolf was startled from his pensive mood as Frau Kubizek addressed him so formally. "Yes, Frau Kubizek, thank you for offering." These were good people to receive him and offer such hospitality!

The Frau was similarly pleased by the formality of the young boy. His trousers were a bit oversized, which was odd considering that his coat, shirt and tie were so meticulously tailored.

But it was his crystal-blue eyes that arrested her attention. She could not help being startled by their intensity and the dominance they held over his other features. What sort of boy had August brought home? But he was very polite, and his voice was confident. What sort of family did he come from?

"Would you also like some bread, Adolf?" August asked as he pulled a chair for Adolf. "And will you have milk or water to drink?"

"Water, please," answered Adolf, not wanting to impose on the Kubizek household's hospitality any more than necessary. He sat in the offered chair and pulled himself up to the table.

"Sit, August, I will get it for the both of you. Here, the sausages are done." Frau Kubizek pulled the links straight from the frying pan with calloused fingers that had long since become impervious to heat.

The sausages were still sizzling in their own grease when Adolf used his penknife to cleanly slice precise portions of his link. August used the crude edge of his fork to crush his link into similarly sized bites. Adolf lightly blew on his food, taking his time and being careful not to burn his mouth. August, accustomed to rushing through his breakfast so he could work with his father in the workshop downstairs before school, ate his links without hesitation and appeared no worse for doing so.

Adolf wondered what time it was. He could not stay here with August much longer. He needed to meet Helga soon so that he had time to walk to his mother's house. What if Helga came early to the park, and he missed her? What if she were waiting there for him already?

"When do you think you will be in town again?" August returned to sit with his friend until Adolf finished his meal.

At first August was not sure if Adolf had heard the question. He was just about to repeat himself when Adolf turned and shrugged. "Next weekend, perhaps." Adolf furrowed his brow, and then shrugged again, "I am supposed to put my studies first, but they are so dull. I would like to come home and see my . . . mother each weekend. Perhaps we could resume our posts at the theatre on the evening before I trek home?"

"Yes, that would be good," agreed August.

"Are you going to change your clothing, August?" Frau Kubizek interrupted. "Your father will be waiting."

Adolf understood that he was keeping August from work, and now that the sausages had cooled, he made quick work of what remained. "Thank you, Frau Kubizek. That was excellent."

"You are welcome. A polite boy like you? You are welcome any time."

Adolf could not help but to blush faintly at the praise. Being polite, it seemed, was all any woman wanted from him—Helga, Frau Kubizek, even his own mother. Despite his disgust for civil servants and all their soulless protocol, he believed strongly in observing formality and acting with proper protocol. He had abandoned that propriety last night, and look where it had led!

"Thank you, Frau Kubizek. If you will excuse me, I should be heading on my way. My mother may be disappointed when she learns I have already had one home-cooked meal today, but I will doubtless be hungry again by the time I reach her, so all will be well. Thank you again!"

Frau Kubizek smiled at the young boy's gratitude. August led Adolf back into his room so that Adolf could recover his travel satchel before departing. With that slung over Adolf's shoulder, August then led him down through the family's upholstery shop in a hope that he might introduce Adolf to his father also, but the old man was in the back room. Clouds of horsehair dust billowed out of the open door. August reconsidered his plan. He could introduce Adolf to his father another time. His own clothes were soon to be covered in that dust, but it would not do for Adolf to be subjected to those particles.

Instead, August led Adolf past the various couches and chairs displayed for customers and let him out the front door. "Good luck, Adolf," August said, "I am sure everything will turn out well enough. You will be in touch?"

"Yes, we will plan something for next Saturday evening, if I have no plans then with Helga."

August was satisfied by the answer. He would not expect to be in Helga and Adolf's company again anytime soon. He wondered briefly if he should ask Adolf to obtain news about Elise, but ultimately decided against doing so. He would send Elise a letter. Whether she received it or not would be up to the discretion of her father, meaning she would not receive it at all. He could then at least claim he had tried to contact her. It was not as though he was particularly in love with the girl.

Adolf soon found himself feeling quite ridiculous in his oversized trousers. What a foolish, foolish mess he had let them get into. That would be the last time he allowed himself to be persuaded toward an idea he inherently knew to be a bad one.

It was now well after seven, and the sun was climbing to warm the city streets. Autumn was upon them, but chilly mornings still turned into sunny afternoons. The heat of his steps also helped to keep him warm enough.

Before he realized it, he was at the park. Already he could see the tall soccer stands between the beech trees that marked the park's perimeter. A group of boys similar in age to Adolf were already gathering on the field. They wore no uniforms, so Adolf doubted that there was an impending match. A few months ago, he might have enjoyed the game, but since then his views had changed. It was nothing to do with his physical ability. Despite his fits with infirmity in his youth, Adolf had grown into a young man of passing athletic ability. No, his interest in politics and art had simply diverted his attentions to other aspects of society. Sports were played by brutish men who did not have the intelligence to think on loftier subjects, such as art or politics.

Politics he did not know very much of, aside from what his teachers had taught him, but so far the subject interested him greatly He had learned that it was a more complex and interesting subject to pursue than he had first guessed. As a civil servant, his father had always been a staunch supporter of the monarchy, but Adolf 's exploration of the subject had developed in him a contradicting sense of nationalistic pride and a dislike for the Hapsburg crown.

His new political stirrings jockeyed with his devotion to art; he had just begun to reveal his drawings and sketches to others, but he was still far from sharing his political views. Helga and August would make for an excellent audience, but he was not ready to present the subject to either. As he walked through the park and looked for any sign of Helga's golden hair, he wondered if he would have the chance to share those thoughts with Helga.

His thoughts were so preoccupied by Helga that he did not even notice Johan and Samuel were also in the park. Samuel noticed Adolf, and after pointing him out to Johan, the other boy burst into a raucous fit of laughter so loud that other folk stopped to see the cause. Before Adolf knew it, Johan was still laughing and pointing. People turned to look at Adolf.

Adolf knew full well that the oversized trousers he still wore from August's were the source for not only Johan's laughter, but the continued scrutiny of the surrounding public. Adolf found himself ashamed and incensed by his embarrassment.

Samuel stood beside Johan and grinned with satisfaction. After all Adolf's bold words at the dinner table so many months ago, Samuel at last had the last laugh—well Johan was having it for him, actually, but that was fine enough.

Johan had ignored Adolf entirely since their last heated exchange over Elise—or had it been Helga? Johan could not remember which sister was which any more. Either way, what fortune had brought Adolf to the park in such ridiculous trousers? They were bunched at the cuff and cinched at the waist. Johan knew how meticulously Adolf normally attired himself. Seeing him in his ill-tailored trousers was sheer comedy.

Ignoring his humiliation was Adolf's only option in this social circumstance. Despite the fire in his cheeks and the anger in his clenched fists, Adolf crossed the park to where Johan and Samuel stood. "Laugh all you want, Johan. If you knew the reason I am dressed this way, your amusement would sharply turn to jealousy."

Johan raised an eyebrow at that statement. "Truly? Well, now I wonder what experience you could possibly have had that should make me jealous!" He turned to Samuel. "I do believe Herr Hitler is referring to whichever of the Faveshra sisters to whom I happened to acquaint him. I very much doubt it was any lass he found on his own."

Adolf did not like what Johan was implying. What did it matter if Johan introduced him to the Faveshras? He looked at Johan and realized the boy had been jealous of him. Johan had lost Helga, and now she was his. But how had Johan learned of his relationship with Helga? He must have been guessing—a mere leap of logic. Such jumps often landed on dangerous grounds.

Adolf drew himself taller, saying, "The last I saw of the Faveshra sisters in the context of your 'introductions,' *your* date was in shock, and mine was too loose for my tastes. I do not think you know half as much about girls as you think you do, Johan. If you did, you would know that a girl of Helga's quality was never meant for a boar like you. You will end up with the Elises of the world."

Johan blinked. He could hardly believe Adolf had the gall to say such things. "'The Elises of the world'?" Johan thought for a moment, and then began to laugh. "If that is my lot, then I have no complaints!"

Adolf glared at him. "No, you would not. You are ignorant of love and romance. A boar, Johan. Your interest is in rutting. Tell me, what girls are you meeting today? Another set of sisters? Cousins, perhaps? With whom will you set up this cur?" Adolf looked to Samuel. "He will only try to steal the girl away, although your sort deserves such." Johan was in disbelief at Adolf's audacity; and the first time in years, his own temper was tested. "To hell with you, Hitler. I never lost Helga to you. I lost interest in Helga after my fun with Elise. Both sisters were rare specimens, but in the end I was happy with my choice. You speak of love and romance as if you are a knight in some opera. You are a fifteen-year-old boy, and you think you can lecture me on love? Really Adolf, which of us is the ignorant one here? No, I never lost Helga to you. The last I saw of her, she was crying alone in the stands, probably because you were not man enough to stay with her. Were you crying, too, on your lonely walk back to Frau Sekira's?"

Adolf exploded with the intensity of his response. "I left because I had no further business there! The girl I believed to have been my date was kissing you. The friend I thought had brought me to better acquaint myself with that girl instead stabbed me in the back.

I trusted you, Johan. You betrayed that trust. You have no thought for anyone but yourself. You used me. You will regret it."

The threat should have been entirely hollow—Johan was nearly twice Adolf's size—and yet in the manner Adolf spoke, and with that intense glare to his eyes, it was obvious that there was nothing hollow about the statement.

Samuel smirked. From where he stood, Adolf was in the weakest position of the three of them. No matter how his brave words, he still looked ridiculous in his trousers. It was time to remind the arrogant fool of that fact. "So, this Helga you go on and on about, is she a witch? Or a terrible cook? She is either starving you or shrinking you from the waist down, it seems."

"Funny, the Faveshra sisters had quite the opposite effect on me," said Johan with a grin. If his womanizing ways truly bothered Adolf that much, Johan might as well continue to get under the other boy's skin.

Adolf constrained his anger and the desire to physically strike the larger Johan, countering again with words. "I simply suffered a minor accident early this morning, and my trousers were an unfortunate casualty. These are the only pair I could borrow, and they still look better than those threadbare tweeds you have worn since your first day at Frau Sekira's, Samuel, so you can wipe that insolent grin from your face. I could be dressed in rags, and I would still stand above you."

Samuel laughed. "Perhaps, Adolf. Or perhaps the trousers belong to another man. Tell me, Adolf, are you one of those chaps more interested in fellows than ladies? How else could you come to wear another man's trousers so early in the morning? I doubt your acquaintance with the Faveshras had anything to do with your garb."

Samuel's insinuation was a powerful insult, and Adolf's patience had endured enough. What if Helga arrived just then? If she did, then she would dispel Samuel's theory, but at the cost of her own reputation.

"Only a Jew would make such an accusation," Adolf spat. "You, swine, know nothing about a real man's relationships. You know more about plodding about in your own filth with cloven hooves while flies bite your hairy backside. You are below even the goats, who can at least swat flies from their own arse. No, you could only speak such perverseness because the good Christian God did not endow you with any true proof of manhood of your own."

Delighted, Samuel could hardly believe Adolf's vehemence. This was becoming even more fun by the minute. "I hit too close to the mark, did I? Your best defense is to insult my religion? Come now, Hitler. You can do better, I am sure." Samuel knew this Hitler boy's type, and the racial slander no longer had the same effect on him, simply because Adolf had used it too many times before.

Adolf was surprised when his insults provoked no response. There was then only one way to deal with the ignorant swine: Slaughter it. Boar was too wild and tough for Adolf to take down on his own, but Samuel was no boar. He was a swine. Adolf might not slaughter Samuel now, but he would make sure that if his insults did not hurt, his punches would.

The strike was decisive in its speed and brutality. Adolf's balled fist caught Samuel on his jaw with a crack of flesh against flesh. The blow sent the Jewish boy reeling backward a step, but after the initial shock wore off, anger came to Samuel's own eyes. Adolf did not squander the advantage his first strike had offered him: He followed his punch by spitting at Samuel, a distraction that gave Adolf time to throw another punch, this time in Samuel's belly. The boy staggered to the ground.

"Nothing to smile about now, is there?" Adolf fell atop him, pinning the boy's arms by the weight of his knees while he sat back on Samuel's chest. "I should beat the Jew right out of you and punish you properly for your insolence. I warned you fairly at Frau Sekira's. You are below me, Samuel. Always!"

Johan could not believe Adolf's sudden ferocity. His natural instinct had been to back away from the surprising violence, but once Adolf spat at Samuel, and it became obvious that Adolf intended to fight dirty, Johan interceded on Samuel's behalf. He grabbed Adolf's collar and threw him backward onto his backside, while Samuel tried to straighten himself and recover from the pain Adolf's blows had caused.

Adolf had no patience left. He could have beaten Samuel as his father used to strike Alois or his mother, even himself. He could have beaten Samuel until his tears were washing the blood off Adolf's scraped knuckles, but with Johan present, Adolf could never fight both boys. He had already regained some of his pride. That was enough. He picked himself off the ground, dusted off the loaned trousers and looked hard at Johan and Samuel.

"I have no more time for this," he said with harsh intensity. "You have both had your laugh—and seen the consequences. Have it louder and longer if it pleases you, although I doubt Samuel will find anything funny for quite some time now. Either way, neither of your opinions is worth another minute of my time." With that arrogant pronouncement, Adolf turned and walked away from the soccer stands.

Johan recovered from the shock of Adolf's violence and began laughing again as Adolf walked away. Samuel just stared through angry, teary eyes. Neither could believe Adolf's foolish air of superiority. He was dressed as a clown, but acting like a king. How did you take seriously such a person?

But Adolf existed in his own world, and in it he was, indeed, a king. He was certainly a class above Johan, and he was practically a species above Samuel. The Jews were hardly a people at all. They were gypsies and worse. The more Adolf encountered people such as Samuel, the more he believed his teachers had been right.

He continued on to the end of the park from which Helga was most likely to arrive.

He was almost happy for the encounter; if nothing else, it had provided Adolf with the opportunity to fulfill his threat to Samuel. He may not have whipped the boy, but he had certainly given him a good beating. What stories would circulate Frau Sekira's dinner table that night! Adolf's anger faded as he imagined Samuel's bruised chin over the next few weeks.

He could hardly believe the Jewish boy would have the bravado to insult him in such a manner. Did the boy really think Adolf would let such a comment pass? If Johan had not been present, Adolf would still be beating the Jew, and the beating could have been even more brutal. But then he might miss Helga's arrival, or Helga might find him engaged in such violence. That thought gave Adolf a moment of pause to reflect on his actions. She would not have approved. She believed he was kind, and gentle, and more concerned with beauty than with violence. She would think him a completely different person. Perhaps he was, and how long would it be before she came to know that side of him as well?

The park continued to fill with pedestrians of varying age and class, and Adolf at last decided that he should conserve his energy for the long walk to his mother's house. He found a park bench from which he could see both entrances at either end of the park. As he waited, he saw many mothers escorting their young—and likely eligible—daughters through the park that morning. Some were also accompanied by young gentleman, and some wore officer's uniforms, which reminded Adolf of his father's own civil service uniform.

What a useless display of uniforms! Did the military have nothing better to do than allow its officers to parade about with young women? The inefficiency of the military was upsetting. What idle government allowed these peacocks to strut with their swords at their hips, rather than training to use them in their hands? The soldiers of course were trained, and trained well. Adolf however gave no credit to that training in his own ignorant criticism. He only knew that any man who joined the military was a pawn. They were a step above the civil servants of the world, perhaps, but they served just the same. He then decided that not only would he refuse to ever become a civil servant. He would never serve in the Hapsburg Empire's military. He would rather be jailed.

Time passed quickly amidst such serious thoughts. Church bells had begun to toll, and Adolf's thoughts were interrupted as he felt compelled to count the number. Had he missed the first bell, or even a second? He did not think so, but neither could he be sure. No, it must be nine o'clock and still no sign of Helga.

He was just tensing himself to stand and search for her, when he caught a glimpse of her golden hair bobbing toward him—was that a basket she was carrying? He stood and made his way across the pathway toward her. His relief was great, but mitigated by his staunch faith that she would join him here. Like every opera he had ever seen, he and Helga needed only to believe in one another, and all obstacles might be overcome.

"Are you all right?" was his first question as he reached her.

She smiled and nodded. "Oh yes, I am just glad I made it here. When I heard the bell, I was afraid you might leave immediately, thinking the situation hopeless."

He offered his arm and began leading her deeper into the park. "Hopeless? Hardly. I had the very firmest belief that you would find your way here."

"Are you not the confident optimist! I nearly disappointed you. Father was incensed when he discovered August in the house. Had he found you, I would be packing my things, as Elise is now."

"The nunnery?" asked Adolf, assuming the worst.

"No, Elise made a deal with me while Father was debating what he should do. She would not tell Father about your presence if I helped to convince him to send her to live with my two aunts, who are currently traveling in Italy. I think Father half expects her to put her talents to better use and find herself a decent man abroad. He nearly suffered an apoplectic stroke when he learned that August is just an upholsterer's apprentice."

"Quite the bargain," reasoned Adolf as he led Helga to another vacant bench.

"Indeed," replied Helga as she sat. "So we are safe, for now. With Elise gone, you will have to meet Father yourself before I am allowed to go out for a date again. I doubt even he would go so far as to send Josef as my chaperone."

"That would be cruel, I suppose." Adolf's answer sincerely pitied the cripple. It was bad enough that the boy's illness made him little more than a parasite, unable to benefit society because of his disability, but to force him out into the public was just poor taste. Better he live a sheltered life at home, Adolf thought. Perhaps he should introduce the young man to Aunt Jo. Then he would have an Aunt Jo and an Uncle Jo—a crippled couple. The very idea made Adolf laugh.

Helga frowned. "There is nothing funny about my stepbrother, Adolf."

Adolf blinked in immediate embarrassment. "No, it is not that." He paused, considering, "Well, I mean . . . never mind. It was a tangential thought. I apologize. Now answer me this. How did you manage to come here if you are not supposed to be out without escort? Are you attempting an impersonation of Louise so soon?"

Helga smiled and set the basket she had been carrying on the bench between them. "No, nothing so dramatic, though I suppose I was at least clever. While Elise and Father were arguing, I disposed of what eggs we had left in the kitchen. I am supposed to be out buying more."

"Then you cannot be gone long, or he will be suspicious, no?" Adolf took a moment to look over his shoulder.

Helga thought he was searching for signs of her father. She had no idea he was actually looking to see if Johan and Samuel were still in the park. He caught sight of neither boy, but that did nothing to assuage his anxiety.

"You are right. I am sorry, but I really only came to tell you not to worry."

Adolf was disappointed and relieved at the same time. Helga took his expression to be one of confusion, as if he had expected to hear one thing, and she had said another. Then it dawned on her what might be missing.

"And to tell you," she went on, looking straight into his disappointed eyes, "that I am very grateful to you for everything. I had a wonderful, magical time at the opera, and though we did not sleep very long last night, I do not think I have ever rested better. Thank you, Adolf."

"You are welcome," he offered somewhat lamely, although the praise pleased him.

To his disappointment, she kissed only his cheek. They were in public, in broad daylight, after all. He could not expect the sort of kiss they had shared in the seclusion of the opera's relative darkness, especially not with Adolf wearing his ridiculous trousers. Helga could care less about Adolf's appearance, but Adolf cared enough for them both.

Helga stood at last, lifting her basket. "I should go now. Father will already scold me for dallying. If I wait any longer, his desire to scold will progress instead to suspicion."

Adolf nodded and rose with her. "Can I at least walk you back home?"

Helga shook her head. "No, I do not think that would be wise. I very much doubt that father caught sight of you, or else his questions to me this morning would have been very different. I do not think he would recognize you, but still, it is not smart to take the unnecessary chance." Seeing the disappointment on his stark features, she linked her arm through his. "You can, however, walk me to the park's limit. I will be happy for each step I can take with you—even if you look as though your trousers are going to fall at any moment. Where did you get those?"

The joke was not taken as lightly as it was given. Adolf's tone darkened to the point that Helga was nearly frightened. "I tore my trousers in my effort to climb over the gate to your yard." He felt foolish explaining the state of his appearance, something in which he normally took so much pride. "It was the only way in."

Concerned, Helga cried," You were not hurt, were you? The spikes atop those gates are very sharp!" How suddenly reserved and shameful he had become!

"Only my pride." His admission was in those same dark tones.

"Well that should be healed easily enough." She countered his dark demeanor with light, a broad, bright smile that conducted a current of comfort to the furthest reach of Adolf's self. She stood on tiptoe and kissed his cheek again.

The contact returned a smile to his face, and although the park gate was not far, Adolf again felt as though everything was well and right after all. He only wished he did not have to leave her company again so soon. "So, when may I call on you?"

Helga considered the question. "Well, we may write to one another as much as we'd like. I think that for now we should wait at least two week. Elise will be gone by then, and hopefully I will be able to soften father's view toward young men. Then I can introduce you properly."

That sounded reasonable to Adolf, even if he were already longing to kiss her again. "Very well."

They were rapidly approaching the park exit; a few more steps, and they would make their grand farewell—except that it was not grand at all.

Helga let go of Adolf's arm, but looked into his eyes. "I will write—and I will miss you."

Adolf nodded. Their farewell had been cut short in Helga's kitchen. Now it felt constricted by their presence in public. "I will miss you, too," he said in earnest, but he kept his distance. Instead of kissing her as he so greatly wanted, he took her hand and it that to his lips.

Helga, unsure of whether she should feel embarrassed by this display of affection or whether she would do something incredibly un-ladylike and kiss him properly, decided on giggling affectionately.

"Until next time," said Adolf, trying his best to avoid feeling foolish for using so gallant a farewell while looking so comic in August's trousers. His satchel slung over his right shoulder, Adolf shoved his hands into his pockets, trying to add bulk to his frame as he began the long walk to his mother's home.

It was still rather early in the morning. Helga could not have spent more than fifteen minutes with him from the time she entered his sight until the time she left it. He would be at his home in just over an hour, and what would he tell his mother? He would tell her he caught it on the sharp edge of a fence, which was close enough to the truth.

He never liked lying to his mother, but he could hardly tell her that he ripped his trousers while vaulting a young lady's fence. In fact, he was still debating whether he should tell his mother of the young lady at all. What would she think of her son dating at his young age?

Angela had been married not even a year ago, and her husband was by all accounts a gambler and a drunkard. But dear Roald was a civil servant, just as Adolf's father had been. His mother knew that the man's career could provide for her stepdaughter even if he gambled and drank much of their money away. Adolf possessed a distinct distaste for both of those habits, and simply did not like his stepsister's husband at all. The fact that he encouraged the belief that Adolf should become a civil servant did not help.

What a waste of existence! Adolf would never serve a society as fundamentally corrupted as the Hapsburg Empire. It was the sentiment of many youths his age at that time, but it had taken a firmer hold in Adolf, perhaps because of his personal experiences. Half his childhood had been spent getting used to new towns and new schools. And for what?

As he walked the streets of Linz, he noted structures mentally redesigned. That house there should be remodeled to resemble the newer, modern structures at the far end of the street. What new building was being put up next to the city hall? Would it have the same columns and broad stairs? Before he knew it, Linz's streets were behind him, and he walked through the more subdued atmosphere of the surrounding countryside. His family's home at the Garden House was already in sight, and from the smell that wafted from the house's chimney, his mother was already cooking. After spending the past few weeks adjusting to life in Steyr, and the excitement of last night's exploits, he found himself very happy to at last be home.

"Adi! I missed you!"

Adolf smiled and knelt so that his little sister could hug him, dropping his satchel on the floor and opening his arms to the pigtailed girl running toward him. "I missed you too, Paula."

She hugged him as tight as an eight-year-old girl could. She had forgotten or forgiven her brother's beatings. Like most children, she was simply excited to see her big brother. Behind the girl, Klara watched her children and smiled a motherly smile. "You look well, Adolf. You have grown at least another two inches, I think."

Adolf, once released from his little sister's embrace, stood and walked to his mother. She kissed his cheeks and forehead, before smothering him in a hug of her own. "Ma . . ." managed Adolf.

Klara at last released her boy and pushed him out to arm's length, her hands on his shoulders, as if fearing to release him before she could make a more detailed inspection of his state. She nodded. "At least two inches. Maybe three. What are these bags under your eyes? Are you sleeping? Have you been eating well? Those trousers look two sizes too big on you. You are still so very thin . . ."

Adolf, embarrassed by the attention even if he enjoyed the affection, laughed. "Yes, Mama, Frau Cinchini cooks almost as well as Frau Sekira." As for the bags under his eyes, he had only a few hours of sleep last night, but he could hardly explain that to his mother. The evening had not ended at the opera, and he certainly could not tell his mother of the adventure that had followed.

Klara just nodded at her son's answer, and then brushed her index finger over the light growth above his lip. "And what is this you have here?" she teased.

"Mama . . ." began Adolf in the tone of a child who knew he was being teased.

Klara smiled wider, and then pinched his cheek. "I think it is very handsome. Are you hungry? Would you like something to drink? You must be tired from all your traveling. Sit, I will bring you a snack. Dinner will not be ready for another hour-and-a-half or so."

Adolf shook his head. "No, Mama, I am fine, really.

How are you? You look well."

Klara all but pushed her son into Alois's old chair. "Sit." She looked to Paula. "Go tell your Aunt that Adolf is home."

Paula nodded and set off for the second floor.

"How is Aunt Johanna?" asked Adolf, not particularly concerned.

"We are all doing well, Adolf. But what about you? Do you like it in Steyr? How are your studies? Of course I read your letters, but I want to hear the details from you now that you are here. You truly look well. You have such color in your cheeks!"

Adolf smiled. Despite his lack of sleep, he thought that if he looked as well as he felt, then he must appear very well indeed. He had spent the morning with Helga, and although he had been reluctant to part from her, he was happy to be at home with his family. "Thank you, Mama. School is still difficult. My teachers insist on stuffing my head with the most trivial details. They do not approve of creativity or independent thought. Indeed, I often feel as though they are trying to smother what intelligence I possess with the sheer volume of the facts and figures they expect me to remember."

Klara nodded as she rocked in the chair beside the fire. "Most students feel that way, Adolf. Just be thankful you are able to attend school at all. Neither I nor your father had that privilege."

"I know, Mama. I am trying my best."

Klara smiled. "I know you are, and I am very proud of you for it. Now tell me, what else is new? You seem . . . happier, than usual."

Adolf could not help the blush that rose in his cheeks. He was not good at keeping secrets, and although he was embarrassed by the topic, there was no reason he should not tell his mother about Helga. "I am . . ." he began, but just then his aunt made her way into the room.

"Hello Adolf." Johanna leaned heavily on her cane.

Adolf did not stand to greet his aunt, nor to hug or kiss her. He remained in his father's chair and simply inclined his head to the disfigured woman. "Hello, Auntie, you look well." It was a hollow compliment, the sort Johanna was accustomed to receiving. She was not surprised that Adolf did not rise to greet her. Just the same, it did hurt her feelings.

She tried to manage a smile, but gave up that pretense when a jolt of pain lanced up her hunched back.

"Sit with us, Jo. Adolf was about to tell me why he is so happy." Klara had long since learned not to offer aid to her sister, who did not like being the center of attention.

Adolf did not wait for his aunt to settle. He did not even look at her as she crossed the room with unbalanced steps and contortions of effort on her aging features. He had no sympathy, no interest in acknowledging her struggles. He simply continued where he had left off. "I am indeed happy, Mama. I have met a most wonderful girl. We went to the opera last night, and today we had a very lovely walk in the park." What would his mother say if she knew he had also spent the night with her?

What a lovely, if brief, walk it had been. He had been so relieved that she had met him in the park after what had happened in the predawn light at the Faveshra household.

A genuine smile pulled at the corner of Adolf's mouth as he thought how joyous their meeting at the park had been.

"A girl? Adolf, you are much too young to be seeing a girl. You are not even out of school!" The words were chiding, but said in a kind enthusiasm.

His mother's reaction was no less than what he had expected. "Do not worry, Mama, she understands very well that my studies are my first priority. She gives school as much importance as you."

Klara was glad for that. At least the girl sounded intelligent. "Then she is a smart girl, at least. How did you meet her? What is her name? What opera did you see?"

Adolf laughed. His mother was very good at stacking questions one atop another so that it became difficult to answer any of them in their proper order. "Her name is Ms. Helga Faveshra. She lives in Linz with her father and sister. I met her through . . ." Adolf paused, not willing to call Johan a friend. "Through a past acquaintance."

"Helga Faveshra," repeated his mother. "The name is not familiar. Perhaps your father would have recognized the name. Did she recognize yours?"

Adolf shook his head. "No, I do not think so."

Klara smiled. "Well go on, what does she look like? What opera did you see?"

Adolf began to blush again as he considered Helga's beauty. "She has long, curly blond hair and bluish-green eyes, depending on the light. She is perhaps a few inches shorter than me, and many consider her to be very, very pretty."

"I am sure she is positively angelic," said his mother with a happy smile of encouragement.

"And what was the opera?" asked Johanna, at last settled as comfortably as she could in a deep-cushioned, crushed-velvet chair.

"We saw *Tristan und Isolde* along with her sister, Elise, and Elise's date, who I think is going to be good friend of mine."

"Oh?" inquired Johanna.

"Yes, a Mr. August Kubizek. We had met once before, at another opera, actually. It was mere coincidence that he was Elise's date last evening, but he seems to be a good man from all I know of him."

"Another opera? Adolf, how do you find the time to study? And is not the opera expensive?"

Adolf's expression darkened as he turned to look directly at his aunt. "Attending an opera once every few weeks hardly affects my daily studies. Living alone in Steyr, I have ample time for my schoolwork. As for the expense, well, I see most opera from the standing-room section. That is where I first met August."

Johanna nodded.

Klara, sensing the tension her sister's questions had built, rose from her seat. "Well, I think it is all wonderful news. I am glad things are going well for you, Adolf. Just remember the promise you made me before moving to Steyr."

"Yes, Mama. My studies come first."

Klara smiled at her boy. "Good. I need to check the roast. Please take your things and wash up before dinner. You look as though you could do with a quick scrub."

Johanna nodded in agreement. "Yes, your mother is right."

Adolf's eyes narrowed at his aunt's agreement.

"Adolf, if you attended the opera last night, where did you stay after? Surely you did not return to Steyr, just to travel back here to Leonding today?"

It was easy to sense the trap his aunt's question had laid. He deftly avoided it with a half-truth, which, in his aging adolescence, he was discovering were his favorite kind. "August was kind enough to offer lodging. As I said, he seems a good man. Not only did he pay for my seat last night, but he refused to allow me to spend the night in a costly room when he had his parents' large apartment to offer."

"A generous fellow, indeed." answered Johanna, coldly and somehow suspiciously.

Adolf did not respond, merely rose from his father's old chair and retrieved his travel satchel. Without bothering to excuse himself, he made his way to his old bedroom.

It had been less than a year since his father had died. And yet so much had happened in that time. Angela had married. He had moved first to Frau Sekira's in Linz, and then to Frau Cichini's in Steyr. He had believed he had fallen in love once, but he now knew those paltry feelings had been a pale fantasy compared to the emotions he was now experiencing. As he lay on the bed and kicked off his boots, he could not help but wonder if all fifteen-year-old boys' lives were as exciting as his.

Adolf could not bring himself to fold his friend's trousers. He simply rolled them into a ball, and flung them into the far corner of his room. No amount of washing would remove the horsehair entirely. Perhaps he would do August a favor and gift him a new pair of trousers. Where he would get the money, he did not know. He had no desire to find employment. He was a student, and so he studied. One day he would be an artist. He would continue painting and sketching, his father's civil service pension would provide his means.

He finished undressing, and then gave himself a quick sponge bath with cold water. He dressed in casual clothes once he finished washing, and remained in his room. He had no desire to return to visiting with his aunt or Paula.

His baby sister had grown so much in his absence! She did not seem nearly as bratty as she had just a few short months ago. She had been excited to see him when he entered, but she was mostly shy and reserved after that. The old Paula would have been incessantly pestering him to play with Dolly and her. Now she was not even knocking at his door. What had changed in the child?

Like his father before him, Adolf had little comprehension of the lasting effects of corporal punishment. He had gone to live in Linz because it was that much closer to school. At least, that was the primary reason in his memory. He had largely forgotten the grief in his mother's eyes when she learned he had beaten his little sister.

"Adi, dinner is on the table!" his mother's voice sounded through his closed door. He then heard something unusual, the clear sound of his mother coughing violently.

Rushing from his room, he found his mother in the kitchen, leaning over the back of her chair as she tried to catch her breath. Her face was almost as red as the bright apron she wore.

"Are you all right, Mama?" asked Adolf, his hand reaching to rub her back gently in an effort to soothe her.

Klara straightened herself and took a last deep breath before turning her grimace into a smile. She waved her son to come and sit. "I am fine. Just a cold I picked up a few days ago at the market, I think. It has not gotten much worse. I just get a pain in my back sometimes, and then I cough for a bit. I am sure it will pass in another day or two."

"You have been saying that for a week now." Johanna slowly hobbled from the living room into the kitchen.

"Mama," chastised Adolf. "You should see the doctor if this has lasted so long."

Klara busied herself pulling the cover off the roast and setting it on the counter. She had already cut the meat, a job Adolf would have expected to be saved for him now that he was the man of the house. "I am sure I am getting better, Adolf, and I do not feel otherwise ill. I will be just fine. Now sit, and help your sister cut her beef."

Although Adolf was no longer accustomed to being told what to do, he did not object in the face of his sudden concern for his mother's health. He forked a pair of thin slices onto Paula's plate. She really was very cute with her hair tied back in two pretty blue ribbons. It was the same plain brown hair as his mother, not as dark as his own hair. He wondered if Paula would ever match Elise's beauty. She certainly would never compare to Helga!

"So what have you been studying, Adolf?" Aunt Johanna asked as Adolf carefully cut his sister's portions for her. "What's something new you might teach me?"

Adolf hated vague questions, but his aunt seemed to excel in them. Something new he might teach her? The woman had never gone to school. How could he teach someone who had never been a student?

"Well, we have been studying the work of a Frenchman, Descartes. If two functions are charted over the course of their projected calculations, their figures can be displayed on a quadrant consisting of an x and a y axis. You see, each axis has both positive and negative sectors, allowing for the calculations of hypothetical mathematic expressions. By following the apparent trends of these 'graphs,' we can estimate what the next number in a sequence might be or project the sales profits for the local customs house, if you prefer a more tangible example."

As Adolf spoke, he fixed his Aunt with his piercing gaze, relaying the various terms with precise enunciation and a confidence that belied his poor understanding of his own words.

Johanna listened attentively. She was an intelligent woman, even though she was self-taught. Forced to remain in her room for the majority of her life, she had taught herself to read and lived vicariously through the works of various novelists. Jules Verne was her favorite author, although she read a variety of genres ranging from philosophy to the Romantics. It was from philosophy that she recognized Descartes' name, but what did he have to do with math? Quite a lot, from what young Adolf was explaining.

"That is very interesting," she offered at last, sounding genuine. It was always a contention of wills with her nephew. She had offered him a challenge, and he had met it. Now she felt like an ignorant fool.

His mother was even more impressed by the brief lecture than Johanna had been. "See what studying brings you, Adolf? What a mind you have!" She had no idea what his words had meant, of course. She listened only to the sound of them coming so intelligently from her son.

Adolf smiled at his mother, pleased by both her praise. "I told you I would try hard. I still want to be an artist, and I will be," he said with cold conviction, "but that does not mean I cannot first make you proud of my schoolwork."

He savored the pink slice of salted beef seasoned with rosemary, parsley and basil, which he loved. The potatoes and carrots, boiled in the roast's juices, were excellent. He ate well in his boarding house, but never as good as when he visited home.

For a moment, he was very homesick. He did not like Steyr, and it was even further from Helga than his home here in Leonding was. If only it were not for school, he could move back home and enjoy the three things he loved most in this world—his mother, his art and his Helga, although he was not certain that was the order in which he would rank the items on his list. Steyr held none of those things, except maybe the freedom to see Helga when he wanted—when he could manage, at least. If he had been living at home, could he ever have gotten away with staying at Helga's last night? No, was the answer. Plain and simple.

So he would remain in Steyr a while longer. He would continue to attend classes, and learn frivolous theories about coordinates and y-theories. Soon, though, he would execute his plan to revolt and leave the technical school that was so intent on making him into a civil servant. Oh he would leave school, but not before he was certain he would not break his mother's heart.

His mother, Helga and his art...

Chapter 11

"IF YOU ONLY knew the plans they had for us..."

Walking beside Adolf, August was surprised by the other boy's sudden attempt at conversation. They had been making their way down the Klammstrasse Promenade, with no particular destination in mind. They just enjoyed roaming through the city. Adolf had been unusually quiet so far, and his tone now suggested that it had been because he was brooding as they walked. August had been quiet, but that was more his nature than it was his mood.

Since the incident at the Faveshra household nearly two weeks ago, Adolf had visited August twice. Both times they had gone for rambling walks, during which their path meandered as much as their conversations. Adolf always led, and August was content to listen to his new friend vent thoughts that ranged from art to architecture, to the Hapsburgs to German nationalism. Today, however, Adolf had only directed their footsteps and hardly said a word.

"Plans, Adolf? What plans? And who is planning them?"

Adolf's eyes seemed to focus, looking as intense as they always did when he was preparing to voice his thoughts. "Society, August. Teachers, priests ... The Hapsburgs ... everyone. They have built ant hills to draw attention from their cavernous burrows below, interconnecting, intersecting, forming a society in which we are all just drones."

August, sensing his friend was far from finished, knew to supply the single word Adolf required before he went on to make his next point. It was a pattern he had begun to notice with his new friend. Adolf would relate an idea by providing a metaphoric example, and then he would supply a general term at the end of his metaphor that required explanation, allowing for further analysis of the main topic itself.

"Drones?" August said.

"Yes, drones. Drones, August! Look around you!" Adolf's dark eyes flitted from building to building while his hands gestured with broad sweeps in an effort to encompass the city. "This is all ridiculous. There is no care given for aesthetics. No consideration for artistic creation. That building there has columns, while the one next to it is being built only with arches. If they arched those columns, they could carry the theme of the building beside it. It would be a more natural transition for the eye, but they did not care to think of that."

He slowed his steps and peeled his eyes off of the surrounding buildings to again look August in his eyes. "Schools are the same. They care only that when finished, we will provide a certain function. They do not care for our mental aesthetics. They drill us with information they deem necessary, and if we do not remember that information in the manner in which they expect us to remember, then they fail us. They condemn us! They tear us down, just as that building there is being demolished because housing has gone up all around it, and now its plot should also   be used for housing. Because I attend a technical school, and all the students around me are training for civil service positions, I am expected to learn by rote everything a civil servant is to know in precisely the manner they expect me to know it."

August only nodded, knowing Adolf was far from finished. His new friend always articulated his arguments in so compelling a fashion that August often found himself agreeing with points he would normally have dismissed out of hand.

Adolf had learned to sense when he had someone's full attention, and saw August was as enthralled by his lectures as had been a few of the boys in his classes. More so, since his travels with August had given him ample time to explain his thoughts in detail.

"They care nothing for creative intelligence," he continued. They do not respect an artist's mind. Where they see protocol, I see enslavement. Where they see regulation, I feel strangulation. Where they see history, I see only their version of it. Mine would be very different."

"Different? How?" Adolf had not said anything particularly

profound just yet; August had heard this argument before, although in a different context. He agreed with everything Adolf said, but it was just as interesting to let him say it all again as it would be to change to another topic—not that August ever had much luck in changing topics.

"There would be no Hapsburg Empire, for one thing. There would be Austria or Germany; people would cheer for their nationality, not the Hapsburg name.

"Look, August," Adolf said, gesturing around them. "I would construct these building with as much thought to their appearance as to their functionality. People would walk the streets and see art.

"The teachers blame the Jews for our societal problems, but I blame the institutions themselves. Teachers give no credit to originality. They cannot stand a stray thought. And yet, how else are opera composed? How are books written or portraits painted if a person can not sit and think, and then find a medium to express those thoughts, whether through music, writing or art?"

August's own enjoyment of music, and his dream of one day being a great composer, had him smiling wide and nodding in response to Adolf's every word. His friend's tone was gaining momentum, a cumulative ascension of tones and volumes that began to sound as rigid and militaristic as he often claimed his teacher's approaches were. The difference, August supposed, was that Adolf could not agree with what the teachers believed was pedagogical necessity; his beliefs were formed by an artist's mind and so existed on a higher plane of consciousness—a purer plane, perhaps. August wondered if he should point out the irony.

Adolf continued speaking. "I will have no part of it, August. No part of it at all. A few months longer, and I will leave school. I will go to Vienna and study art as I should have been doing all along." He stopped walking altogether and looking up at August, spoke as if he were twice August's size. "And you are coming with me."

The last part surprised August, both in its seriousness and the force of delivery. "Father would never allow me to study in Vienna.

He would certainly never allow me to go to school and study music. I was grateful when he took me out of secondary school to begin my upholstering apprenticeship. I would rather choke on dust all day than sit through another lecture class. No, an upholsterer is all I will ever be. Father would never permit me to do otherwise."

Adolf had no patience for August's doubts. "Then I will convince your father that you must attend music school."

August had never been able to convince his father of anything. The chance that he would allow his son's younger friend to sway his opinion was almost comical. "I hope you can," said August lamely, not sounding nearly as enthusiastic as Adolf had expected.

"You doubt me? My dear August, I am hurt. Well I am certain enough for the both of us, and that is all that will matter. Come, we should start to head back. I have a date with Helga tonight."

It was amazing how quickly Adolf had shifted from a tone of fullest confidence, to a manner that suggested utter nervousness. August always found himself surprised by the suddenness of the change, but he had also come to understand that this was where he best contributed to their friendship, when Adolf showed his weakness and August was there to offer support.

"It has been two weeks already?" August said, surprised. "Well I am sure it felt like an eternity for you, but really, I can hardly believe it has been so long. Well never mind. You are a lucky man, Adolf. Where do you plan to take her, the opera again?"

He began to wonder what their date that evening would be like. He was supposed to meet Helga's father. What if he had caught a glimpse of Adolf vaulting the fence in the predawn light? What if the sight of Adolf was enough to jog the old man's memory?

"We are going to a concert in the park," he said to August. "A small band is giving a free performance."

They began walking again, making all left turns so that soon they were facing the direction from which they had come, albeit on a parallel street. "That sounds excellent," August replied. "Especially the price. It is going to be cool tonight, but you are certainly dressed for the occasion. I had wondered why you were so smartly suited today. I should have guessed you had a date." walked astride one another down a long and quiet street, it was August's turn to give an opinion for a change.

August thought for a moment before answering. The last time he had met Elise and Helga's father, he had been fleeing down a flight of stairs, retreating in such haste that he had not even been able to pull on his boots. That memory had been so vibrantly ingrained in his mind that he had almost forgotten his first meeting with the old man.

He had arrived early at the Faveshra home, having walked brusquely in his nervousness about the impending double-date. The girls' father had answered August's tentative knock. A tall man, possessing the grizzled strength that came with working his trade, Mr. Faveshra's height added a certain severity to his eyes, which looked down on an angular face that was dominated chiefly by its broad, square jaw. The man had been utterly intimidating, but none of that was particularly useful to Adolf.

"To start with, do not mention my name." August chuckled. "I suppose you will do much better than I did. You speak better than I, and you certainly dress better. I am sure you will make a good impression."

Adolf rolled his eyes at August's first comment, but he nodded at the compliments his friend gave him. But August had yet to tell him anything worthwhile. "Yes, yes Gustl, very kind of you to say so." Adolf had taken to calling August by this nickname just last week, but it sounded as natural now as if he had been using it for years. "But what about the man himself? Is he stern? Intelligent? He must be intelligent to have daughters such as his. I cannot imagine a coarse thing about him. Is he cultured, Gustl? Does he enjoy music? Or art? You must have seen their sitting room, or maybe the den? I have only seen the kitchen and Helga's room . . ."

"Well," August began, unsure of exactly how to answer Adolf's avalanche of questions—if he could answer them at all. The truth was that he was not particularly observant, certainly not in the same way as Adolf. His friend's eyes seemed to capture, consider and critique everything upon which they gazed. August's attention was rarely so focused. August did not remember seeing many paintings in the house; nor did he remember the presence of any musical instruments, not even a piano. There were books on shelves, but he could not remember any of the titles. A shrug was the best answer he could give his friend.

That did not satisfy Adolf. "Well, did he say anything to you? Did he ask you any questions? What did you talk about?"

"We did not talk long . . ." August shrugged again, "I suppose we talked about plans for the evening. He never asked about my profession. He commented on the weather, and . . ." August laughed as he remembered. "And the Summer Olympics in some American city. St. Louis? He wanted to know if I enjoyed swimming. I thought it was an odd question to ask in autumn, but when I told him I did not know how to swim, he changed the topic to the girls. Elise and Helga came down shortly after that."

Adolf thought about what August had said, wondering if his friend had inadvertently given him the information he needed: Having read about North America in the Karl Marx novels he had enjoyed, he felt he could carry on a conversation on the subject. The Americas were young nations, still searching for their own national identity. They were rising against an empire, too. Adolf imagined America as a wilderness, a land of savages and little civility, of cowboys and Indians and immigrants. He could never understand people of so many nationalities living together in a new nation, but he did understand the desire for that definitive nationality.

Helga's father also seemed a fan—or at least a follower—of sports. That knowledge did not particularly encourage Adolf, but at least he could be ready for a question on the subject. He wanted badly to impress the man.

"I see," Adolf said. "Is there anything else you can think of, Gustl? Anything you said that you wish you had not? Anything to which he reacted unexpectedly?"

August considered only for a moment before shaking his head. "No, not that I can think of. He was fairly quiet. The Olympics was the only topic in which he seemed interested. Perhaps you should find an old newspaper from this past summer and read up on the games."

"That is ridiculous. I have neither the time nor the interest. The games are good for nationalism, but sports are greatly overrated. Do you not think?"

"Well . . ." August began, but stopped when Adolf's dark eyes flashed with such intensity that August knew it would be best to simply agree. "Of course. What good is running fast or jumping far?" He knew Adolf would answer the rhetorical question.

"Exactly. Sport produces nothing—it is fleeting and meaningless. What is better, to be the world's greatest artist or the world's fastest man? The artist creates works that endure long after he is dead. The man who runs fast may be the fastest now, but what will he be in ten years? Twenty? An old man who used to be fast, but can no longer keep up with the younger men. He may set a record, but records are always broken. Art endures."

August nodded his agreement.

They were just about back to August's home. Relax," said August at last. "As long as you are not caught with your trousers halfway down your knees, he should like you just fine. My parents like you, and they do not ever like anyone."

Adolf managed to grin. "All right." They stopped in front of the upholstery shop. "Well, it was good to stretch the legs and get my blood flowing before I go there. I suppose I will be back again next weekend. Will you be free?"

"You know you are welcomed to visit any time. Good luck Adolf. Give Helga my regards. If things should go poorly with her father, give him my regards as well."

Adolf laughed and said that he would. He left August, happy he had taken the time to visit his friend first. Talking with August had helped settle his anxieties. It would be the first time he called on a girl at her house and the first time he took Helga on a date alone.

When he arrived at the Faveshra home, he took a deep breath, wiped his palms on his trouser legs, and then strode up the broad granite stairs that led to the Faveshra household's front door. Adolf lifted the brass knocker and let it fall twice on its striking plate. Then he waited.

To his relief, it was Helga who answered the door.

"Do you not look handsome!" were her first words. "It is very good to see you. Come in, Father is waiting in the den. I must warn you, he is not in the best of moods. My aunts sent a letter yesterday that informed him that while Elise had reached them safely, she had already begun to form relations with some of the Italian boys. I cannot imagine why he would expect less of her, but it has soured his view of young men."

Adolf should have been discouraged by Helga's words, but he was too enthralled by her appearance to worry about her father's temperament. She was dressed in crushed velvet of deep green that clung to her, cinching tightly above her waist and flaring at her hips to flow down to her trim ankles. Her golden hair was piled in curls atop her head, revealing the nape of her graceful neck, and was offset by a simple silver necklace she wore as a queen would wear diamonds. She was beautiful.

"Well do not just stand there, come in!" she said with a laugh and a lovely smile. Adolf obliged her and entered a home of modest wealth and sensible taste. The floors were clean hardwood that glowed from a recent oiling, as did the doors, chests, cabinets and other wooden furniture in the house. A painting hung over a vase of flowers sitting on a table in the front hall, although it was by no artist Adolf could recognize—which was not surprising. For all of Adolf's desire to be an artist, he had not yet studied much art.

He followed Helga down a hallway, turning at last into a room that opened from a pair of glass-paned doors. The strong smell of tobacco wafted from the room, its pungently sweet scent only adding to Adolf's nervousness: It reminded him of the cigars his father had enjoyed so much. The room was warmly lit by a small fire. A short couch ran the length of one wall, and the fireplace dominated another. The third wall was covered with bookshelves, each row seeming to hold even more books than the next. The man certainly enjoyed reading.

"Papa, this is the boy I have told you about. Adolf, Adolf Hitler."

Mr. Faveshra, who had been facing the fire, seemingly ignorant of Adolf's presence until his daughter offered the introduction, now stood, rising to a height that was well above six feet. Adolf could not remember ever feeling so small or uncertain.

"A pleasure to meet you . . ." Adolf managed to say without his voice cracking, offering his hand as he spoke.

The older man firmly grasped Adolf's hand. "Otto, you may call me Otto." It was meant to be a friendly gesture, but the severity of the man's ice-blue eyes and broad jaw still managed to intimidate Adolf. "Helga tells me you are going to school in Steyr?"

Adolf nodded. "Yes, sir. For the moment, at least.'" "Sit with me for a few minutes. Helga can bring us a

brandy." Otto Faveshra motioned Adolf to take a seat on the small couch and turned his chair away from the fire so that he could face his daughter's date. "'For the moment,' you say? What about after that?"

Adolf sat on the comfortable couch, finding its cushions to be firm but not stiff. He wondered what Helga had told her father about him already, and decided he might as well explain his plans to be an artist. He hoped Helga would return with the drink soon. His nervousness only increased without her reassuring presence.

"My father was a custom's officer," Adolf began. "His intention was for me to follow in his footsteps, and so I have been attending a technical school." Adolf paused then, feeling as though he should try to be straightforward and honest with this man. There was no reason he should not be proud of his own dreams, so he continued. "However, I am not my father. I have no desire to be a civil servant. My interests lie elsewhere. I plan to study art and architecture and to become an artist."

Otto listened as Adolf's nervous voice erratically rose and fell as he spoke, but he also noticed the intensity of the young lad's eyes as he spoke. Whatever nervousness he might feel at meeting his young lady's father for the first time, he more than made up for with his conviction in his goals.

"You have too much spirit to be wasted as a civil servant. Still, artists do not always earn a good living for themselves, much less a family. You dress well, so I assume your family has money, but what will you do ensure your future financial stability?"

Just then, Helga returned with a tray bearing two crystal snifters and a matching decanter. She set the items on a low coffee table in front of the couch and poured equal measures for her father and Adolf.

Meanwhile, Adolf was considering just how to answer the older man's question. At last the answer dawned on him. "I will start in art, but I will make architecture my career."

Otto nodded his approval as he accepted the libation his daughter handed him. He waited for Adolf to take his own glass, and then toasted him. "Those are fine aspirations for a lad such as you. Aside from art, what other interests do you have? Politics? Sports? Did you read about the Olympics this past summer?"

At last the question of which August had warned Adolf—Not that the warning had helped. Adolf had very little good to say about sports in general, and he knew nothing of what had occurred at the Olympics that year. "Politics are interesting. I only know enough to know I that do not know much at all. I enjoy the opera, and reading; between those interests and my art, I find it difficult to make time for sports."

Otto sipped his brandy. "Understandable. One can keep only so many interests, after all. I myself found the Olympics fascinating. It is beginning to feel as if the countries are competing as much as the athletes are. It is bad enough that Austria loses almost every event, but to make matters worse, they lump Hungary in with us. We did win a bronze medal, at least. In swimming!"

That last statement struck a nerve in Adolf. It had nothing to do with only winning the bronze medal in swimming. He could care less about the achievement. It was what Otto had said about Austria being lumped together with Hungary. It was because of the Hapsburgs that such a conjunction of nations existed. Adolf was not Hungarian. He shared almost no cultural similarities with that nation.

"I can believe it." Adolf eventually answered. "Many of my friends swim well. It is not surprising that an Austrian won the bronze—he was Austrian, yes?"

"The fellow's name was Wahle, Otto Wahle, which, I am not too proud to say, is probably the only reason I remember him. In any event, his is certainly an Austrian name. We only had two athletes competing in the games, and the other was a Hungarian fellow . . . Zoltan something. He won gold in two different swimming events, but—"

Adolf cut Helga's father short with an upraised hand. It was a gesture of authority, despite the age difference between the two men.

Surprised, Otto paused so that Adolf could tell him, "The Hungarian won two gold, and the Austrian only won bronze?" His short bark of laughter was a mixture of disappointment and disgust. "Perhaps it is the Hungarians who should be upset that they are so tightly joined to us."

Helga could hardly believe what Adolf said. She looked from him to her father, who sat with his mouth slightly agape, mouthing the word "Hungarian." "Adolf, how can you say that?" Her tone was chastising, but she said it with levity.

"How indeed," began her father. His eyes had gone wide, and it was clear that Adolf had insulted the man's pride in his country and his countrymen.

Adolf pulled on his brandy slowly and deliberately, savoring the spirit. By the time he set down the glass, he had drained more than half its contents, and a hue of color began to brighten his pale complexion. "Honestly and simply?" He looked first at Helga, and then at her father. "How many medals did the Germans win? The British?"

Still taken aback, Otto answered, "A German fellow was the top foreign athlete. He won gold in three swimming events. That is hardly better than that Zoltan fellow though, and Otto Wahle was not far behind him!"

Adolf chuckled at the older man's enthusiasm. "No, but he *was* behind. I do not know much about the Olympics. I did not follow them so closely as you have, but I would be willing to bet that three medals in swimming is not remotely close to how many medals the American athletes claimed. The United States hosted these games, and they supplied the most athletes for the games." He took another sip of his brandy. "And here we sit, discussing a bronze medal as if it is some wonderful achievement. It does not surprise me that a German led the foreign athletes; my friends in Passau all swam like fish. Austria is not known for its sports. We are a cultured people who enjoy music, whether it is a symphony or an opera. We enjoy art and commerce. If we are going to compete in these . . . games, we should at least send more than one athlete, and we should win gold, not silver—and certainly not bronze. But I still believe sports are largely just a waste of time."

Helga was afraid to say anything by this point. The look in her father's eyes was nearing a homicidal rage, but Adolf possessed his usual confidence that was always on the verge of arrogance. She could see her father's blood pressure steadily rising in the color of his cheeks and decided it was time to change the topic.

"Some say that sports are an art themselves. Have you considered that, Adolf? The spirit of an athlete is not so very different from that of an artist. Both seek audiences and enjoy performing so much as they enjoy the performance itself. Oh, you painters may not consider yourself performers, but if one looks closely at a painting, the brush strokes are as important as the picture itself. The picture may be your performance, but the strokes show what you were performing."

Adolf finished the contents of his glass, and then rubbed a finger over his light mustache. "I had never thought of that." he admitted finally.

"And why should you? Sports are a competition. Art is ..." Otto Faveshra shrugged, and then finished his brandy.

"A competition with oneself." finished Helga, thinking quickly. "You compete with your idea and with your critic, and perhaps most of all with your peers. Art may not be measured in time, distance, weight or scientific calculations, but it is measured by the heart and the mind. It is not a sport, but it is a form of competition all the same."

Adolf appreciated Helga's support. She was right in most respects, although seeing art as a competition was another matter entirely, one that bore considering. Adolf competed with himself, he supposed. He always wanted to improve his work. In truth, he always wanted to improve the work of others, too, although that desire manifested itself more in his architectural aspirations than in his paintings or sketches.

"I suppose so," admitted Otto at last. The tense look in his eyes had subsided, due either to the brandy or his daughter's well-spoken argument.

A strange sound then caught Adolf's attention, a slow, squeaking sound that seemed to be progressing from one end of the hallway to the other. The noise was so foreign to Adolf that he could not hide his puzzlement. He looked first at Otto, and then to his daughter.

Helga frowned. "I am sorry Adolf. There is still one member of my family I have not introduced you. My younger stepbrother, Josef, usually does not like meeting new people, and he rarely leaves his room." She looked to her father, "You should grease that wheel for him."

Otto would do no such thing. "He is old enough to grease it himself. So he cannot walk. His hands and arms work well enough."

Helga could only shake her head at her father's response. "He can, but it is difficult for him. Besides, it means a lot to him whenever you give him your attention."

"Hard for him—" Otto began, but then let his words trail off in silent fury. The boy did not need to know any more about the Faveshra family's private issues.

Adolf caught a glimpse of the wheelchair-bound boy through the open doorway. His squeaking left front wheel whined over the home's hardwood floors. Each time his frail arms pushed the tremendous wheels of his chair, the effort made the boy's face tighten. He did not look into the sitting room as he pushed himself, head down, toward the kitchen.

Helga shook her head and looked at Adolf with shame, not for her brother, but for her father's behavior. "You will meet him some other time, I am sure," she offered lamely.

Adolf only nodded. Living with the disabled could be such a burden. Aunt Johanna always required special considerations and care. It was ridiculous. The woman simply was not fit for survival. She could not contribute to the greater society, nor could she support herself or make a suitable wife so that a man could support her.

In a sense, Adolf found himself siding with Otto. Perhaps the boy's struggles would strengthen his muscles and his mind. It was probably the only hope Otto had for his son. How else could the boy overcome his infirmity? What use would society have for a wheelchair-bound boy who was taxed just by the effort of moving from one end of the house to the other? The boy looked to be nearly Adolf's age, fifteen. Soon he would be a man but, like Adolf's Aunt, Josef would remain a burden.

Even now, this crippled boy was robbing him of Helga's attention. It was not exactly jealousy that spawned such intolerant feelings for this sickly boy. How could Adolf ever envy this boy? No, no, Adolf's sentiments were a cause of his overall belief in the new paradigm that Darwin fellow created. Not the evolution part ... that was madness. Perhaps the Jews arose from apes, but the blessed Christian folks were most definitely made in God's image. No, Adolf believed in survival of the fittest, and this Josef fellow simply was not fit. He did not envy Josef; he believed Helga's concern was a waste of time.

Adolf was his own best example. His past may have been vexed with a number of childhood maladies; he had been weak, but that he had survived and even flourished proved his conviction that only the fit survive, and he was surely one of the fittest.

"We should be going if we are going to make the concert, Papa." Helga did not know how else to break the awkward silence punctuated only by the distant squeak of Josef's chair.

Otto looked from Helga to Adolf, and then back to Helga. "Very well." He was still gruff, but happy to be changing the topic. "I would hate for you to be late, dressed as pretty as you are." He managed a smile. Elise had already shamed him more times than he could stand. Josef was not only a cripple, but also a constant reminder of his mother, rest her soul. Helga was his princess.

Otto decided he liked this young Hitler fellow. He seemed sharp enough. He was dressed well and spoke with an assurance beyond most his age. Otto turned his attention back to Adolf, "And as for you, young sir, I am glad we had the chance to talk. While we may not agree on things such as the value of Austria's Olympic accomplishments, you have at least proven yourself to be an intelligent and well-spoken *boy*." Otto put no small amount of emphasis on the last word, winking as he did so. He continued quite seriously, "I trust you will take great care of my daughter."

Adolf no longer felt nervous or intimidated. He smiled and nodded, "The greatest care, I assure you."

"Just so," said Otto. To Helga, "Is that coat heavy enough? Why not pack a light blanket and some fruit to take along in a basket? I would like a word alone with Herr Hitler before the two of you leave."

Helga glanced nervously at Adolf, who offered the slightest tweak of a smile before shifting his attention back to her father. Helga continued, "Very well, Papa. Please be kind to him. He is always so very kind to me." She began to blush at that and she walked from the sitting room.

Otto Faveshra rose from his chair and set his empty brandy glass on the fireplace mantel. After deciding Helga was out of earshot, he beckoned Adolf closer.

In a softer tone than Adolf thought the man capable of, Otto said, "You were the lad who was Helga's date the last time I let her go out, correct?"

Adolf suddenly feared that his deepest concerns were being realized. Otto had seen him in the early predawn light. His mouth felt dry, and he licked his lips as he nodded.

"Then you know Helga's sister, Elise? Well," Otto paused for a moment, as if unsure if he should continue. It was never easy to admit that your daughter was engaged in . . . that your daughter was not behaving as a proper Christian girl should. Still, he went on, "Well, she decided that the night should continue after the opera. Whether her date coaxed her into making such a ridiculous decision, or whether . . . well that does not matter. My point is that on the night of that date, I discovered her young gentleman friend in this house long after it was appropriate. Now, I am not saying this to give you any ideas. Helga is very different from Elise, and I know that. I want *you* to know that if I should discover that another such scandalous incident has taken place, my punishment will be even harder on Helga than it was on Elise. Helga at least knows better. Elise takes too much after her mother, God rest her soul."

Otto had managed to grab Adolf's attentive fear after all. "No sir, I would never endanger Helga's reputation that way. Nor would I care to invite your wrath, sir." He spoke truthfully on both accounts.

Otto looked into Adolf's hard eyes and nodded. "Good. Because if I discovered you here the way I came upon that other fellow, I promise you would not leave this house alive. Am I perfectly clear, Herr Hitler?"

Adolf swallowed, having no doubt of the potency of that promise. "You are, Herr Faveshra. Again, I assure you, you have nothing to fear. My intentions are honorable, and I refuse to compromise my own honor any more than I would compromise Helga's."

Otto put his hand on Adolf's shoulder. "Well spoken. Let your actions prove to be as intelligent as your answers, and you will be welcomed in this household. Now go, and show my daughter a wonderful evening. She is probably waiting at the front door."

Adolf could not help but flinch at Otto's hand on his shoulder, but the man did not seem to notice. Adolf still did not like being touched—unless it was Helga touching him. Or his mother, of course. "Thank you, sir. I will surely try. Enjoy your evening."

Outside the Faveshra household, almost directly after Helga pulled the front door closed behind them, she leaned and kissed him quickly on his lips. "I missed you," she said, with brightness in her eyes that the stars might envy.

Adolf, surprised by her sudden affection, especially after his conversation with Helga's father, smiled lamely. "I missed you, too." Taking the basket from her, he said, "I will carry that." He took her hand with his free hand.

Helga smiled at him appreciatively, and they began to walk toward the park to watch the concert—the same park in which they had spent Saturday morning two weeks ago.

Helga squeezed his hand. "I hope my father did not threaten you. He can be intimidating at times."

Enjoying her gentle grip on his hand, he said, "He loves you and wants to protect you. I do not blame him for that. He was kinder than I would have been in his position."

"Because you love me more?" she asked with a coy smile and another squeeze of his hand.

The question took Adolf by surprise. He had thought he loved Elise when he first met her. He would not have hesitated even a moment to profess that love. Now, despite the fact that he cared twice as much for Helga, he could not readily admit those feelings.

"Because you are worthy of such concern, yes." Even as he spoke, he knew it was not at all what Helga had wanted to hear.

The air was crisp, quickly bringing color to their cheeks and nose. Adolf wondered how his palm could still manage to sweat in the cool temperature of the night, but it did. "Your father is a reasonable man," said Adolf once they had passed the first block. "He is concerned for your safety and wellbeing. I can appreciate how he feels."

"Well, it is good of you to say so. He must have liked you. Most of my dates leave his room trembling." She laughed lightly. "Not that I have had so very many dates—not half as many as Elise—but you understand what I mean."

Adolf nodded. "And you are sure the dates were not simply nervous about taking out a girl as wonderful as you?" As they neared the park, they began to see other people making their way through the park's arched gates. Regretful that he would soon lose his privacy with Helga, Adolf was not particularly anxious to join the swelling congregation of blankets and baskets on the lawn. This was the last of a series of very popular concerts in this park—the fact that the series was free had no doubt added to its success—and it seemed that every person who had attended every show

was there to watch the season's finale.

"Ahh, I suppose that is possible. It is certainly sweet of you to say so." Helga gave his hand another gentle squeeze. "So how have you been? Is your mother well?"

Enjoying her squeezes, Adolf kept a casual pace, in no rush to see their end.

Her question pleased him. Could she be so perfect as to care genuinely for his mother's wellbeing? "She is doing better. There was a pain in her back, but it passed as suddenly as it came. My sisters are well, too." It had been years since he had told anyone he had an older stepbrother. Alois Jr. had stayed away from home, even in the years after his father's death.

Helga was glad to hear Frau Hitler was doing better. She did care about the woman, even though she was yet to meet her. The fact that Adolf cared so much for his mother was an attractive quality. Despite his austere mannerisms in public, it proved that Adolf had a very sensitive and caring facet to his personality, a quality Helga had rarely seen in a young man. "And what about you, Adolf? How are *you*?"

Adolf considered her question. His studies had grown difficult again, and he was not spending half as much time reading books as he was wandering around Linz with August. Added to that had been his anxiety over Helga's welfare and, of course, their upcoming date. But right now, with Helga in his hand and the night before them, he felt buoyant. His steps were light, and the crispness in the air heightened his sense of clarity. The moment was sublime.

He spoke carefully, slowing their steps as he did. "I am happy, Helga. I am very happy." He was smiling so broadly that he felt foolish, but for once, he reveled in the feeling. It helped that Helga joined him.

"Well I am glad to hear that. I am happy too, Adolf." She could not help but think his smile was as cute as his enthusiasm.

They fell into the line of people slowly entering the park. Twilight was becoming true darkness. Already Adolf could hear the band warming up their instruments on the small stage erected for the performance. If August had been present, his keen ear might have commented on the sharpness of the brass and woodwind sections.

The pair found a vacant patch of lawn and spread out the blanket. As other couples and families settled onto their own swathes of grass, Helga drew another blanket, thinner and lighter, from the large basket she had packed. She soon had it draped around Adolf and her shoulders. She was not particularly cold—and doubted that Adolf was either—but the privacy and closeness the blanket offered merits Helga nonetheless appreciated.

"You smell good," said Adolf after a few moments of silence. The comment surprised even him. He was generally far more eloquent in his compliments.

Helga was just as surprised. The simple declaration seemed truer than flowery flattery. She did not care to paint her features as Elise often did, but she did at times indulge in a single squirt of the perfume her father had given her for Christmas last year. It was the same scent she had worn to the opera and had lightly misted onto each of her letters. Hyacinths, her favorite flower. Instead of thanking him for the compliment, she kissed his smooth cheek, letting the warmth of her lips linger on the coolness of his pale skin. As she drew back, he looked down at her with eyes that set her heart fluttering within her breast. His eyes were so clear, so intensely deliberate in their gaze, that she could almost see the intelligence within him. Even in the relative darkness, his eyes glinted as they spoke words neither would hear if their eyes had not also been listening.

The concert band was a small ensemble of flutes and clarinets, violins and violas, trumpets and even a pair of tubas. A percussion section stood behind the brass, great bass drums and snares, symbols and chimes. The music was a medley of military waltzes interspersed with Austrian folk songs that soon brought blood to the crowd's veins, and many people stood to dance on the field. Adolf watched couples rise around him, but instead of asking Helga to dance, he only hugged her closer.

He thought that he could escape the fate of those fellows whose dates coaxed them into trying to perform a skill they did not possess. Then Helga suddenly kicked her polished shoes beneath the blanket in excitement. "Strauss's 'Wine Woman'!"

Guessing what might happen next, Adolf was filled with apprehension. He was not a particularly good dancer. In fact, he felt dancing was a highly indecent activity, especially the waltz style. Strauss's waltzes, of which he heartily disapproved, were often militaristic, keeping to a regimented three-quarter time signature that allowed for little deviation or improvisation. Adolf disliked those waltzes because they seemed tailored to the empire's military officers. This waltz, on the other hand, was intended more for villagers dancing around the town well. It was for bumpkins and peasants more than it was suitable for bohemians.

"Dance with me?" came Helga's excited request.

"But . . ." Adolf began, and then saw the sudden twinge of disappointment around Helga's cerulean eyes as she guessed he was about to decline. It was too much for him to continue his words. She was not desperate to dance, but he could see that it would make her happy. It was reason enough to at least try.

He rose, unfolding his legs and bracing himself for the moment of cold air that would replace the blanket—and Helga's warmth. He then offered his hand, which she accepted. After quickly folding the blanket, she kicked off her shoes.

Adolf removed his own boots as well, using the heavy leather to anchor the opposite corner of their blanket. He wished the waltz had not been one of Strauss's. He preferred the lighter music of Joseph Franz Karl Lanner, who employed as many folk aspects to his music as he did courtly formality. His style was varied greatly from Johan Strauss, whose waltzes tended to be more of a militaristic march. Luckily for Adolf, who hated anything that related the military to nobility, such as a marching waltz, this particular song had folk roots of its own, and so the beat was kept lively and gay.

Adolf's mother had once tried to teach him the steps of square advancement, moving on each beat in the foot pattern of step-step-stop. It was a simple dance, owing a large part of its history to Austrian villages who found the lively steps and whirling movements to be easier and far more fun to master then were traditional dances. Many countries had deemed the waltz improper, saying the close proximity threatened people's morals. Churches had banned the dance, but its simplicity gave it a strong foundation that ranged from common peasants to the nobility. By the early 1900s, the waltz was easily the most popular form of dance in Western civilization.

Adolf was engrossed in keeping an ear to the strongly accented first downbeat of each stanza, making his best effort at keeping in time, and so avoiding stepping upon Helga's small feet.

She smiled at the expression of terrible concentration on his face. Even through the thick padding of his coat, she could feel his muscles were tense. Her hope was that if she kept smiling, he would eventually relax and enjoy himself.

Adolf wanted to be sure that Helga was enjoying herself, but she moved like water, whereas his movements were poorly coordinated and lacking confidence. But she continued smiling at him, so he continued moving, oftentimes following her lead—which only added to his embarrassment and discomfort—but trying to establish something she could follow, instead. As Helga continued smiling, Adolf's embarrassment slowly faded. By the end of the "Wine Woman's Song," Adolf had given up on moving his feet in time, and instead simply stood, holding Helga so close in his arms that her hair, piled in golden curls, tickled the tip of his nose.

This is wonderful, he thought he heard her whisper into his coat. It was. They remained as they were while the band prepared for the next song. Around them, couples were beginning to settle back onto blankets. Helga and he stood in the meager light of the yellow gas lamps and imagined his body was shielding Helga not only from the cold breeze that had begun to rustle the leaves, but also from the curious stares of people watching them stand so scandalously close in public.

"Let us cover up again," said Helga after a time, although she kissed him sweetly before making the suggestion. She apparently had no more concern for their audience than Adolf. Still, the kiss surprised him. They were, after all, one of the few couples still standing and therefore exposed to a multitude of eyes.

They sat, and then Helga lay back on the blanket. Drawing Adolf next to her, she covered them with the smaller blanket under which they had sat earlier. Her head was soon resting on his chest, much as it had that night in her bed. He wanted to envelope her entirely. She was so close to him, but after two weeks of separation, she still was not close enough.

She felt the same way. Covered as they were by the top blanket, no one could see Helga's hand slip past the buttons of his coat, soon passing his shirt buttons as well. When at last she came to his undershirt, her hand drifted anxiously close to his belt line, but as soon as she lifted the bottom of his under-shirt, her hand again began questing northward, at last resting on the flat of his stomach. Her hand was cold, which was to be expected, but after the initial tickle, it soon warmed and felt . . . right. Adolf wished he wore no clothes at all.

Should he reciprocate such intimacy? Her dress had buttons up its back, and the bottom of her skirt reached well to her trim ankles. Her creamy flesh was constrained in velveteen fabric, so he was denied such ready access as she had managed. He would have to be content to make contact with what skin was exposed, and so he kissed her cheek. Then, instead of moving to her lips, as he normally would, his kisses trailed her jaw line, until at last they landed on her neck, where her skin was usually hidden by her hair. However, with her tresses piled in curls atop her head, her graceful neck was exposed and inviting.

Her gentle whimper encouraged him to move his kisses up behind her ear, and her fingers suddenly dug into the flesh of his stomach. Not in pain, but arousal. His own response was a familiar throbbing. Adolf had never been so intimate with a girl. Not even sleeping next to Helga in her own bed—that night had been downright platonic compared to this.

The band was now playing a march, so few in the audience were dancing any longer. Those closest to Helga and Adolf's blanket were making their best effort to keep their attention on the band and not on Adolf and Helga beneath their blanket.

Helga could hardly believe the sensations of pleasure that sparked from his contact. Scintillating shivers coursed from her neck to her toes. Her hand beneath his shirt was now gently rubbing above Adolf's naval. It was not until she tried to move her hand lower that Adolf stopped his own efforts, recoiling from her. Although Adolf had only moved beyond her hand's reach, his sudden reaction put a distance between them as wide as a great chasm.

"Adolf?" She was surprised and somewhat frightened. His eyes were wide, his breaths deep and ragged. Had she inadvertently hurt him somehow?

Her hand, so close to passing beneath his belt, had reminded him of another time a hand had pressed so closely against his abdomen. It had been years since the incident with Friar Roald, a time he rarely remembered. His memory, and the ensuing reaction, had surprised himself as much as anyone would.

"I..." he began, his voice hoarse and strained with embarrassment. "I am sorry," he managed. He wanted to explain his sudden reaction, but he could not find the words.

Helga watched him closely, still afraid that this was somehow her fault. "It is all right," she said slowly, without confidence. "I should not have..."

"No, no, it is not your fault." His tone was almost pleading. "I do not know what came over me, I—"

She had never heard him speak in such a manner, and it only added to her confusion. She reached out, tentatively, and rested her hand on his. "It is all right. You were making me feel so good that I only wanted to..." Now it was her turn to blush furiously. "I wanted you to feel it, too."

He nodded and took hold of himself. He ruthlessly forced from his mind those hazy memories of Friar Roald's private study.

Adolf tucked his shirt back into his trousers and fixed his buttons. It was lucky that the blanket still covered them, as more than one neighbor had cast a nervous glance toward the couple after Adolf's sudden commotion. After a moment, he inched back to Helga. He did not offer any further explanation of what had driven him away so suddenly, and she did not have the courage to ask questions. She simply rolled against him so that her head again rested on his chest, and now, instead of resting her hand on the flat flesh of his stomach, she gently rubbed his arm.

Many of the previous concerts in this park had gone late into the night, but the cold was driving people back to their homes sooner. Adolf did not say another word or attempt to touch Helga with even a hint of affection. He simply lay there, staring up at the stars above, while he tried to synchronize the rhythm of his own breathing with Helga's. He did not want his breathing to upset her comfort.

And Helga continued to lay there with her head on that narrow chest, wondering what exactly she had done wrong to startle the boy that made her feel so very ... good. She wondered if she had overstepped a boundary, and if Adolf hated her for it. Elise had always been the one to tell stories of her intimacies with men. None had ever included a reaction such as Adolf's. But he seemed relaxed now, and she enjoyed simply being near him. He did not wear perfume as she did, but he smelled good, too. Or maybe he just smelled *right*.

So the two of them lay there together, kept warm by a wool blanket below, a down blanket above and of course, the warmth of one another. The band packed away their instruments, and still they remained. Neither of them spoke another word, until they finally stood up of one accord and walked home.

They shared an awkward goodbye on the stone steps, although Helga was smiling again, and Adolf was able to kiss her goodnight. He promised that he would write soon At last he began the long trek back to his mother's house. She and the rest of his family would long be asleep by the time he reached home, but that was just as well. He was not in a mood for talking, and his mother would want to know all about his date. She would be very proud to learn he had danced with Helga.

Perhaps in time he would understand what had happened. For now, he had a long walk ahead of him in what was going to be a cold night. He would be even colder in his loneliness, for though he had spent another magical evening with Helga, Adolf left the Faveshra residence feeling utterly and entirely alone.

Chapter 12

HER HAND HAD felt so pleasingly cool. Small fingers splayed on his stomach, a touch that infused excitement into his flesh, and not only where her hand rested. Hyacinths, and something else... her. It had to be her scent beneath the perfume and powder. Her head was pressed to his chest, her golden hair tickling his chin, but he only smiled and smoothed the wind-strayed strands with kisses.

She was on her side, one arm snaked beneath the undone buttons of his shirt, her hand resting just below his chest. She had drawn one of her legs over his, and though she was constrained by her long velveteen dress, it was enough for Adolf to feel the weight of her thigh. More than enough. She was everything.

The band still played, but Adolf had long since stopped listening. He was trying to measure his breaths so that he kept an even rhythm to the rise and fall of his chest, but it sounded too loud in his ears. He strove to keep his composure, dismissing the nervous anxiety that was vying with the intensifying sensation of excitement—young lust, awkward for its innocence, inasmuch as its intensity.

Johan's advice had never covered moments of such intimacy. Helga had been Johan's, first, but had Johan ever been this close to her? Had he tasted the space just behind her ear with just the lightest brush of his lips? Had he heard her soft whisper into his chest?

No, for all his talk of advice and instruction, Johan had never known Helga as Adolf now did. Yet his lips had only touched the surface of her soul. In the privacy of their blankets, amidst the public gathering in the park, Adolf had never felt so close to Helga. Not even the night he spent in her bed compared to what he was feeling now.

Her hand moved, her fingertips trailing south from where they had rested so comfortably. They were seeking, moving with inexorable intention, despite their teasingly slow descent. Down past his naval, his breath caught sharply, but she could not guess the true cause. She had expected such a reaction, believing it was a sign of his enjoyment of her actions. Then her fingers passed below his belt, hoping to find his arousal to be as intense as her own was. It was so wrong, lying as they were in the park, supposedly listening to the last of the free performances.

Other couples lay upon blankets nearby, but none were so bold as to lay beneath their covers. Families had attended the concert also, children playing tag in the gloom of the park's gas lamps, while their parents enjoyed the free music. There was more than one pair of eyes that noticed the couple, pressed so closely to one another, even though the blanket hid much of what Adolf and Helga were so scandalously engaged in.

Thoughts of propriety occasionally rose like wraiths of his mind, interrupting his enjoyment of Helga's affections, until she found another way to arrest his attention. As her hand moved below the band of his beltline, Adolf suddenly recoiled, startling both Helga and him. All the pleasured sensations that had been building to that moment were obliterated by a memory of a feeling he had long thought to be buried and forgotten.

Perhaps it was the brandy Adolf had imbibed with Helga's father. He did not like to drink. His father had drunk and smoked, and Adolf wanted nothing of his father's life. At least, that was the reason he had given himself. Now he understood the truth better.

The brandy had warmed his cheeks as much as his belly, relaxing him. Up until that moment, he had hardly noticed the alcohol's influence. Being with Helga always made him happy. He had not considered the fact that the one drink with Otto might have affected him so strongly.

But Adolf did not normally drink, and brandy is much stronger than Friar Roald's church wine. That memory of a feeling . . . it was sickening, twisting his stomach into a stone-sized knot. His arousal, every thought of intimacy, was banished by the memory of a feeling his mind had labeled *wrong*.

Helga could not have known her hand had come to rest where

Friar Roald had first put his hand when instructing Adolf on how to breathe properly. She was startled by his sudden reaction as he twisted away from her touch. He had almost moved out from the blankets entirely, and she instantly felt shamed by her own intentions. She had gone too far, surely. Having heard Elise recount her various experiences with men, Helga had thought Adolf would enjoy her actions.

Adolf had. Were it not for the sudden remembrance of Friar Roald's hand, Adolf would likely be ascending in the feelings of intimate bliss. Instead, he was nearly out from under the blankets, panting and looking at Helga's surprise and shame with a wild-eyed fear and confusion. He could hardly explain his reaction to himself— how could he ever explain it to Helga?

They spent the rest of the evening just lying next to another in silence. Helga returned her head to Adolf's chest, though closer now to his shoulder, allowing a sliver of distance between them where before they had been pressed hip to hip. Adolf was no longer worrying about controlling his breathing; he was too busy controlling the thoughts that whirled like a tempest inside his heart and mind.

The concert ended. Helga had apologized time and again. Adolf answered with apologies of his own, but he had not thought of the way to explain why he reacted as he had. So Helga continued apologizing, saying she was sorry over and over again, sometimes in pleading whispers, sometimes in contrite looks, and while she convinced herself that she had been too bold, that she had disappointed his expectations of a proper lady, he struggled to find the words that would help him explain himself.

He never found them. Instead, Helga's apologies enhanced his own feelings of guilt, which, coupled with the stress of remembering Friar Roald, relegated him to an uncomfortable silence. They lay beneath their blanket while others began to leave the park. Adolf redid the buttons on his shirt and tucked the shirttails back into his pants, pressing his hand beneath his belt as he did. His cold shiver had nothing to do with the night's temperature.

He walked her home in that same chilled silence, the heat of their intimacy gone, leaving them both feeling hollow. Nothing could be colder than the emptiness that persisted in the absence of conversation. Adolf's eyes were intense as ever in their gaze, but they did not find Helga. He kept his posture straight, his eyes fixed forward. He was not man enough to look at her. Even when she glanced at him with more apologies on her lips, he kept his eyes forward as he willed himself to keep his thoughts facing forward, too.

His efforts were futile; his childhood in Lambach refused to be forgotten. He had learned to cope with his father's beatings by asserting control in his relationships, but right now, he had no control at all, unless his silence could be considered such. Their footfalls echoed loudly in the evening. With autumn's chill keeping most folks at home, the streets were empty and wasted. Warm lights shone in many windows, and the smell of wood-smoke drifted from chimneys.

As they approached her home, Helga tightened her grip on Adolf's arm. It was enough to force him from his thoughts. She was afraid of what he had been thinking. This was all her fault, after all. She had gone much too far, and he was too much a gentleman to want that sort of attention. She had thought she was nothing like Elise, but now she wondered if she had judged her sister too harshly.

Adolf, absorbed by his own issues, gave very little thought to what Helga must be thinking. He had no idea she was still blaming herself. Her tightened grip on his arm drew him out of his frigid isolation. He looked at her cerulean eyes and found that they were still anxiously apologetic. He could have cried.

Instead, he took her into his arms and hugged her tightly. He must have disappointed her entirely. She was still whispering apologies, and he still could not give voice to an explanation for his response. Instead, he held her there at the edge of the cold street, held her at the precipice of his shame, unable to leap forward and admit the reason for his reaction.

"Thank you for taking me out, Adolf. And for dancing with me . . ." Her voice was tenderly soft. She looked up from their embrace, meeting Adolf's hard eyes at last. "I . . . I hope I will see you again . . . soon."

Her voice held uncertain fear, her honesty and ability to expose her weakness returning to Adolf a sense of his power. He felt control returning at last, though he still battled his guilt over letting Helga feel as though anything that happened was her fault. But he still could not speak. He could not admit her to his thoughts, for she would see his own weaknesses. She would see his guilt, and his shame, and it was too much. So he kissed her.

Tentative sweetness, entirely absent of passion or, a soft reconnection after so many steps that he felt as if they had walked in opposite directions, rather than arm in arm. She kissed him back, just as softly, and she knew she loved him. "You do not have to thank me. It was my honor." His voice was tight with emotion, for the contact of that kiss was transcending the night's stresses. When his lips met Helga's, thoughts of Abbey Lambach, of Friar Roald's lessons, or anything else all vanished. He wished he could kiss her forever, but the air was still growing colder, and even if Helga's father had not stayed up to witness their farewells, it did not mean that a neighbor would not see—and

note—how long Helga lingered in Adolf's arms. "I'll write, soon. You'll understand then."

Helga furrowed her brow at those words. "Understand?"

Adolf took a deep breath, wondering how he might explain his intention to write an apology . . . but the words stuck on his lips. Instead, he kissed her again, even lighter and quicker than before. "Yes." he offered lamely. "But now I think it is time I said goodnight. I wouldn't want to test your father's warning, and I still have a long walk ahead of me."

She nodded, and gave him another good squeeze. "Goodnight, Adi. I will miss you. I'm sorry if . . ."

Adolf laid his index finger across her lips. "Stop. You have nothing for which to apologize. As I said, you will understand." He took his finger from her lips and pressed it to his heart. "I'll write soon and see you soon again. I swear it. It is I who should apologize, and I do. You will understand. Good night, Helga."

She stared at Adolf, wondering what he could possibly mean. Well, she would understand someday. He had promised that much. It was enough to satisfy her. She kissed him one last time, on the cheek this time, then turned and entered her home.

Adolf was left standing in the cold emptiness, with the air chilling the spot of moisture on his cheek where she had kissed him last. He remained standing as he was, transfixed by thoughts, feelings and deeper emotions. There was nothing else to do, but he found it hard to even walk away from her house.

As he walked, he could not help but analyze his gaffe earlier that evening. The hurt and disappointment in Helga's eyes as he recoiled from her had been nearly as difficult to endure as his half-remembered feeling of *wrongness*. Or was it something that just happened? Something that could be ignored, and then forgotten? Could he just tell her he had felt a pinch, or perhaps a cramp? Could he lie to Helga? Would it be easier to simply say what needed to be said?

She needed to know that she had not hurt him. He did not understand himself what he had felt—a memory, just a memory of an uncomfortable sensation. Unnatural, awkward and embarrassing, a feeling suppressed and shaming that had been forgotten for so long, as his parents had hoped such an experience would be. How could he explain that? She had not made him uncomfortable at all. Friar Roald had made him uncomfortable.

His preoccupied steps eventually took him home. Engrossed as he was in his pondering, the long walk had shortened drastically. He felt as though he had just left Helga. He could still feel the press of her lips on his cold cheek.

So late in the evening, he had not expected anyone in his family to be awake; it had to be well past the tenth hour. Even on a

Saturday, his mother, sister and aunt should all be long asleep, and yet from the street, Adolf saw the glow of an oil lamp in his mother's window, its yellow light a foreboding omen. Adolf, finding the front door unlocked, grew concerned. Why was it unlocked? Had someone merely forgotten to latch it? Had there been a burglar? Or something worse?

His blood was pulsing by the time he walked into the house, toward his mother's bedroom window, the source of the light he had seen outdoors. Seeing her door was ajar, he grew very afraid. He was about to enter the room when he heard a familiar voice, one that he dreaded more than any burglar. The doctor.

"She should rest a little easier now. The laudanum will help her sleep."

Knowing that Dr. Bloch must be talking about his mother, Adolf's heart clenched.

"Will she be better in the morning?" Johanna's voice drifted from the room. Adolf should not have been surprised that his aunt was present. He should be grateful anyone at all was there for his mother. Paula was still young and would have long since been tucked into her bed.

"Rest will surely help, but I cannot guarantee the pain will be alleviated. It is something we will monitor closely. It may only be a particularly stubborn cold, but these symptoms have now lingered for nearly a month. We must wait to see if she improves."

Adolf heard Dr. Bloch's voice gaining volume as the man finished gathering his various tools and instruments and made his way toward the bedroom door.

The doctor was about to bid Johanna Poltz a good evening when he caught sight of Adolf lingering in the hallway's shadows. "Adolf! Dear boy, you cannot frighten an old man that way. I see enough ghosts without you appearing as one." The Jewish man looked quite startled. His rectangle-framed glasses sat slightly askew on his nose, eyes opened wide and glaring.

"Adi?" came an airy voice from the bedroom, hoarse for the

dryness of Klara's throat. Klara should be soundly sleeping from the laudanum. Hearing her son's name must have been too much even for the opiates to overcome.

"Dr. Bloch, I am terribly sorry. I had just come in and noticed the light in Mama's room. Is she all right? Is she well?" What's wrong?"

Softly now," the doctor said. "Settle yourself. We have already woken your mother. Come inside so that she can see you, and then perhaps go to sleep."

Adolf did not hesitate. He had heard the weakness of his mother's call, and he hardly waited for Dr. Bloch to stop speaking before he was past the man and at his mother's bedside. He went to his knees, reaching out to take his mother's hand. The laudanum had already begun to make her palms sweaty.

"Mama, what's wrong?" Adolf was nearly trembling with anxiety.

Klara looked at her boy through half-lidded eyes, a slightly slack smile on her face. "It is all right Adi." Her voice was like feathers scratching ice, faint and chilling. "I will—" she paused to yawn deeply, "I will be better, in the morning." Her eyes were inching closed, and her grip on his hand went lax.

Adolf remained on his knees for a moment, waiting and watching as if to ascertain that his mother was only sleeping. Once he was convinced, he rose and kissed his mother's forehead. Dr. Bloch was waiting in the hallway, watching through the door. Johanna remained in a chair on the other side of Klara's bed, still waiting for Adolf to acknowledge her. His concern was for his mother's welfare, and so he turned back to Dr. Bloch first.

"What ails her, Doctor? She has been sick a month, you said? Why has no one told me she was ill? What is wrong?" Adolf's tone was coldly demanding, quiet so as to not disturb his mother's respite, but calculated and controlled, evidenced by his precise enunciation of each word and the formal inflection he used in his speech.

Dr. Bloch was impressed as much by the lad's compassionate concern for his mother as he was by the boy's demeanor. At sixteen, young Adolf spoke with a maturity that eluded men twice his age.

The doctor turned on the light in the hallway and beckoned for Adolf to follow. Without so much as a backward glance for Aunt Johanna, Adolf begrudgingly left his mother's bedside.

Johanna snuffed the oil lamp's flame.

The doctor paused before the coat rack beside the front door. By then, the hour was close to midnight, and good Dr. Bloch had stayed at the Hitler residence far past his bedtime.

"Your mother has been suffering from chronic pain in her back, just behind her left shoulder blade, although she complains the pain comes from deeper than the muscle itself." The doctor furrowed his brow at that statement, as if it were something through which he was puzzling even as he spoke.

Adolf only nodded.

"After my first examination nearly four weeks ago," the doctor continued. "I believed that your mother may have simply strained an unfamiliar muscle. When the pain persisted into the second week, I thought perhaps that she had a touch of pneumonia. I examined her with various instruments, but with none was I able to ascertain a viable diagnosis. I can say with some fair certainty what is *not* wrong with her."

Dr. Bloch shrugged and adjusted his glasses. He waited for Adolf to voice any potential questions or comments, but the boy only looked directly into those spectacled eyes with an intensity that suggested the boy was trying very hard to will the doctor into giving hopeful news. Dr. Bloch had encountered such looks before, but never from a person as young as Adolf. However, despite the young lad's force of will, Dr. Bloch could only speak the medical truth.

"As of now, I can only monitor her condition. While she has yet to show signs of improvement, she does not seem to be getting worse. Apparently the pain is most frequent at night, which is why I am still here now, but I am uncertain as to why that should be. In any case, the laudanum I administered just before you arrived should make certain that she at least gets a very good night's sleep. Perhaps that alone will improve her. Whatever the case, it is nothing she would want you worrying over." The doctor continued, although now he had taken on an almost grandfatherly tone. "Now what has you coming home at such a late hour, anyway? You are too young to be missing sleep."

The question caught Adolf off guard. He was too focused on his mother's condition and suddenly felt exposed and guilty for what had occurred in the park earlier. His defensive instinct took control, and he resumed his rigidly formal tone and manner. "I thank you for your advice, Dr. Bloch, but it is not my health for which you are currently being compensated. While I appreciate your concern, I would rather you reserved it for my mother. I will speak with her in the morning and learn why she did not tell me of this problem sooner. Perhaps I will learn something that will help you determine the cause of the ailment."

The doctor knew he had been rebuffed, but after seeing the boy's genuine concern for his mother and hearing the tension in the boy's tone, the good Dr. Bloch decided to take Adolf's instruction and reserve his concerns for Klara Hitler's health. "You are a good son, Adolf. Your mother raised you well. Look after her, and we will talk when I come to check in on her again. For now, please take my advice and get some rest."

Adolf nodded and opened the door for Dr. Bloch. "Thank you for helping Mama and staying with her until such a late hour. Good night, doctor."

Adolf watched the doctor as he made his way into the cold, clouded night. Then, fearing the cold would enter the house and worsen his mother's condition, Adolf hastily closed the door and locked it.

The late hour had amplified the day's difficulties, exertions and worries, so Adolf decided to take the doctor's advice and quietly made his way into his bedroom. He stripped off his clothes, too tired to take his usual care of folding and hanging his trousers and shirt. Instead, he tossed them into a corner, crawled beneath his covers and slept.

In the morning, Adolf woke to the smell of sizzling breakfast sausages. After washing and dressing, he made his way to the kitchen, where he was as surprised as he was relieved to find his mother standing in her apron in front of the stove. She stood straight and looked healthy enough, despite where the sleepless nights had darkened her eyes.

Seeing her son standing in her kitchen put a welcoming smile on her face. "Come and get your breakfast," she said. "Mama, you should not be up. You are feeling better?

Sit down, and let me do that."

Klara shook her head and pointed to Adolf's chair with her wooden spoon. "You sit. I am feeling better this morning. I am sorry you had to come home to such a scene last night. I did not expect Dr. Bloch to stay so late, but the pain is worse at night."

Adolf obeyed his mother and sat at his usual place at the table. "How long have you been sick? Why did you not tell me?"

His mother smiled at her son's concern, but shrugged gently. "Sometimes I cough, and there is a pain in my chest and back. Sometimes there is just the pain. It comes and goes. I do not think it is serious; it just keeps me from sleeping well some nights. Dr. Bloch's medicine should help. Do not worry Adolf, I will be just fine."

Adolf was entirely relieved to hear that. His family had dealt with so much loss over the years. His father, of course, as well as many of his siblings. Edmund had been so young when he died, it had been years since Alois Jr. had run away, not to be heard of again. The Hitler family had moved many times since Al had run away from their farmhouse in Hafeld. It was unlikely the boy could track down the family's current address if he tried. Adolf had other siblings who had passed away, but they had been born before him, and so he hardly thought of their existence at all. Only his mother did; perhaps the loss of those other children was why she had so much love for the two children that remained to her.

As if on cue, Paula came into the kitchen. Her eyes were red from rubbing the sleep from them with her pudgy fingers. She was nine years old now, but she still maintained much of what their mother called baby fat. She was a cute child, and although she would never achieve such beauty of a girl such as Helga, she was still kind and often made Adolf laugh.

"Adi! I did not know you were home." She walked over to give her brother as big a hug as she could manage.

Adolf smiled and turned in his chair to hug his sister back. She had been such a pest when she was younger. He had lost his patience with her on more than one occasion, but he still loved her, and she loved him. Instead of remembering when he had teased her by keeping dolly away from her or when he had struck her, she was just excited to see him home.

"My, you have grown. I think you must have gained another two inches on me!" Adolf was smiling and, after disengaging from his sister's hug, he tousled her light-brown hair. He was teasing her, as Paula was still short and petite, even for her young age.

"Sit down so you both can eat." Klara walked to the table, holding the frying pan, which sizzled with sausage grease.

"Have you been taking care of Mama?" Adolf asked Paula as she followed her mother's instruction.

Paula paused for a moment, as if she had to seriously consider her answer. At last she nodded and smiled. "Yes, Adolf. I try!"

"And you do a very good job," said Klara. "She has been a very good little girl."

Adolf nodded, feeling older as he realized that both Paula and his mother's answers were a relief. "Well, I am glad to hear that."

The three of them ate their breakfast. Aunt Johanna never came down to join them, and at one point Klara mentioned how her sister must have had a poor night's sleep. She had awoken this morning to find Joanna asleep in the chair next to her bed, where she had remained after the doctor had left and Adolf had gone to bed.

After breakfast, Adolf returned to his room, telling his mother that he had work he needed to finish. That much was true, although it was not any sort of academic subject that occupied his thoughts as he sat at his desk. With his mother's health no longer quite such a pressing concern, his attention turned back to Helga. He had a letter to write her.

What could he say? The virgin sheet of correspondence paper waited for his precise handwriting to stain its page with his explanation. His confession, perhaps. His stomach twisted into a sickening knot, and embarrassment flooded his normally pale features. What could he tell her?

A friar had once made him feel very sick and ashamed, and now, years later, he still reacted reflexively to someone touching him in the same place. The taste of Friar Roald's wine still lingered in his thoughts. Adolf had not sung since that fateful day, despite his love of music. Somehow he knew he would never sing again. None of that helped him with his letter to Helga.

Maybe he did not need to explain anything. Maybe he just needed to assure her that his reaction had been no fault of hers. But how could he say that in this letter? *It was not your fault that I flinched and stared like a wild animal. I am just sensitive there. You tickled me? No, I certainly was not smiling . . .*

Should he simply tell her the truth? He did not understand that truth himself—would she? That salty taste that had cloyed his throat that day still turned his stomach. No, he could never explain all that. Not to Helga or his mother, and surely not dear Gustl. He knew he would never tell anyone.

The longer he sat at his desk, the more he felt that a letter was not the right idea at all. After more than an hour with nothing written on it other than "Dearest Helga," Adolf snatched up the paper, crumpled it into a tight ball and threw it in an arc that landed it least a foot off target from the wastebasket. No letter could adequately explain what had happened. He would have to tell her in-person. Instead of writing the letter, he would visit her on his way back to Steyr. It meant he would need to leave his mother and sister's company much sooner than was usual, but he would explain that he had left an important book in his room at Frau Cichini's and could not continue his studies without it.

Before he knew it, the hour-long walk from his house to Helga's had passed, and he was standing on her broad front stairs. Throughout the walk, he had considered what he should say. Maybe he would not have to say anything. Maybe Helga would simply act as if nothing had happened.

The heavy brass knocker squeaked on its hinges as Adolf lifted the thick ring. His nervousness nearly paralyzed him, but at last the knocker fell. Once. Twice. A minute passed, and then another, and just as Adolf raised the knocker one last time, he heard the sound of locks snapping open through the thick door. Adolf let the knocker fall and stepped back as the door opened.

Helga had on a simple brown dress that was for casual wear around her house, was nothing compared to the stunning velveteen dress she had worn last night, but Adolf would likely not have paid much attention to her clothes if they were woven of silver and gold. He only had eyes for her face.

"Well now, this is a very pleasant surprise. Have you been waiting for Papa to leave, or is it coincidence that you arrive now?" Helga's tone was teasing, but she was obviously excited to see him.

Already nervous and embarrassed, the question caught Adolf entirely off-guard. "Waiting? No, not that. I . . . I just had to see you again before I go back to Steyr. I did not want to say in a letter what I want to tell you now."

Helga could tell he was nervous, which in turn made her nervous, too. "Well come in, and you can tell me whatever you would like. Papa went to a friend's home to help fix something, I do not know. He told me he might not be home for supper though. We have the house to ourselves for quite a while, I think."

"Ourselves?" repeated Adolf in almost a whisper. Adolf might very well have missed noticing Helga's father in the street, preoccupied as he had been with his own thoughts, but it was the thought of being alone in the house with Helga that truly unnerved him. What would happen?

"Yes. You are sure you have not been watching from behind a tree or something? He truly just left no more than a few minutes ago. I would not be surprised if you passed each other in the street." Helga looked up and down the street, and then shook her head, beckoning in Adolf. "Now stop standing there, and come inside so I can close this door, and you can kiss me without the neighbors gawking. I cannot believe you would surprise me like this!"

He stepped inside, his nervousness mounting as Helga closed the door behind him before turning to wait for him. He kissed her then, light and tenderly, and then smiled gently. At least half his anxiety seemed to have escaped in that kiss, for it was sweet. However, half of his anxiety still left him with the other half, and considering his anxiety had been great to begin with, he remained very nervous indeed. Helga's eyes were bright as they opened from the kiss, and her smile made them seem even brighter. "I am so glad to see you. I was afraid that I would have to spend the entire evening all alone in this house. With Elise gone, I have begun to notice how big and empty it can be. I wonder if Papa felt the same thing when Elise and I left him alone.

All those nights we were on dates, he probably sat there in his chair..."

She shook her head and smiled, amused by her behavior, an unconscious way of stalling for time. She did not know why he had recoiled from her last night in the park, but she had decided she would make up for whatever she had done. Although Adolf did not know it, Helga's thoughts were as preoccupied as his own with cares, concerns and fantasies for him.

"But he is not in his chair, and I am not alone." She grabbed the sleeves of his coat and pulled him into a far more mischievous kiss than the sweet tenderness with which they had met each other at the door.

Adolf was surprised by her forwardness. He kissed her back with equal enthusiasm, his hands snaking around to the small of her back. His thoughts of giving her explanations and apologies were soon exchanged with communication of a less conventional medium—still oral, although interpreted by touch and taste more than sound or sight. She was apparently trying to apologize as fervently and earnestly as he had planned to do. However, her method was far more enjoyable than a conversation.

"Come on," she said breathlessly. "Papa should not be home until dark, but that does not mean we should waste what time we have." She had stepped back, but now took his hand and pulled for him to follow, her golden curls bounced gently with her steps.

Adolf floated up the stairs behind her, her scent drew Adolf up as surely as her hand in his. As they reached the doorway to Helga's bedroom, she stopped and whirled to kiss the dapperly dressed artist that followed her—her Julien, perhaps, although she had had not yet proven to be a Louise. It had to have been fate that introduced them at that first opera, serendipity that she should notice him there. They had grown so close to one another since that chance meeting ...

She kissed him hungrily, her hand leaving his to instead reach up and press his cheek. His response was timid at first. She had surprised him again, but as always seemed the case, he was quickly becoming the aggressor. His hand closed tightly on the nape of her neck, deepening the kiss further. Her knees wanted to buckle in subservience. He was such a reserved boy, so constrained by his perspective of societal propriety that many would mistake him for being prude.

Helga knew better. Unfettered, Adolf's passion was dominant. It was aggressive, awesome, arousing Helga more than anything she had experienced with a boy. True, she was not nearly as experienced and knowledgeable as Elise, but Adolf would not be the first boy she had brought to her bed. Adolf had never asked, so she had never thought to tell him, but she was two years his senior, and with a sister such as Elise, it should not be any great surprise that she was not a virgin.

Adolf's eyes were wide and lusting. After all his anxieties of what he should say or do, this moment was the last he had expected. And yet, what better way to resolve last night's problem than to finish what they had started? That fleeting thought opened a whole separate door of anxieties. He knew what was expected of him, more or less. At fifteen, growing up in villages and towns as much as he had in a city, he knew at least as much about sex as did any lad his age.

He continued kissing Helga as they backed into her bedroom, nipping, pecking, pressing his kisses when those others taunts became too much. He was compensating for his inexperience with enthusiasm. As they neared Helga's bed, he abruptly grabbed her shoulders. He kissed her with mounting passion, felt her respond in his arms, and then he broke the kiss and threw her upon the bed, falling beside her.

"Adi! What a wolf you are! Your eyes are gleaming with hunger." Helga's words were breathless and full of her own lustful hunger.

"I have you," he said, staring through her clothing, his teeth clenched. "I am starved." Simple words, but such definitive statements.

Helga smiled coyly and began undoing the buttons and ties on the front her dress. "We are both famished, having skipped so many meals before. You do have me, though. What will you do with me?"

Adolf was not strong. Beneath his dapper dress was a skinny frame, possessing little muscle and less definition. He was not sculpted like the heroes of his opera, like Siegfried or Tristan. His strength was all in his eyes, in his manner. Even his speech was dominant. But seeing Helga beginning to undress provided Adolf with the courage to do the same. He began with his coat, taking his time to hang it on the back of a chair, along with his buttoned shirt. He was left to stand in the light chill of Helga's room, bare-chested and meager, his lank frame no longer hiding in his middle-class finery. He put a toe to heel so that he could step from his shoes and socks, and then finally came his trousers, one balanced leg at a time. He was no longer an aspiring Bohemian artist, nor an eloquent, persuasive young man with firm ideals. He was not the son of a customs official. He was a scrawny, nervous and nearly naked Adolf Hitler.

As he folded his trousers neatly and set them on a chair, Helga finished removing her own dress, although she remained in the light cotton shift ladies wore beneath their garments. It was the most revealing article of clothing Adolf had ever seen on a girl. His nervousness suddenly doubled, and another part of him doubled in size as well. Despite his dominant actions, he had never before felt so vulnerable. Well, almost never . . .

By contrast, Helga was utterly confident. She lay in her white, nearly translucent shift and stretched languidly across the bed, her golden curls fanning in a halo over her pillow. "Adi, let the clothes wrinkle, just this once. I miss you. Come here." She reached out and beckoned to him. Her voice was raspy and playful, and the way she looked at him only added to his own confidence and comfort. However, instead of obeying her command directly, he very deliberately set the trousers on a chair. Then, with a last deep breath, he turned and lay down next to his Helga.

She met him with a kiss that was more tender than the passionate kisses that had led them here. This kiss was slow. Lingering, and soulful, it broke so that Helga could then trail kisses across his narrow shoulders and hairless chest. He enjoyed her attentions as his resolve continued to stiffen. He felt as if the world was suddenly spinning wildly, as if time had both stretched out and sped up, making this moment of intimate passion surreal.

"I love you, Adi. I love you so much." The words were spoken between kisses, desperate and airy. She did not pause to hear him respond, but continued her trail of kisses, descending down his chest to cover the places her hand had quested under the blankets during the previous night's concert. His body may have been closer to that of a boy than a man, but he strained and excited her. He may not have the muscles of a boy like Johan, but she truly loved him. He was her Julien, and so much more.

Hearing Helga's admission, Adolf was overcome by a sudden wave of happiness and relief. He loved Helga, too. He had thought he had loved Elise, but that had been a boy's fantasy. This was real, and it was better than his wildest dreams. "I love you, too, Helga. I love you. I love you. I love you."

Adolf continued to repeat himself until he felt Helga pulling at his small clothes. Then her kisses became something more. They had talked in terms of hunger, and she was apparently famished. Moist warmth surrounded him, enveloped him in swirls and strokes of lustful passion. He could have fallen through the bed. He felt so heavy as he pressed himself up from it, stretching, straining to reach higher, to extend beyond himself, and into her. He wanted to be inside her, even as he experienced the blissful sensations of her tongue and lips alone.

She continued her slips and flickers of tongue as her savory attention to his arousal continued to mount her own desires. She wanted to make him larger than he ever guessed possible. She wanted him to feel ecstasy that would assure he would never flinch from her touch again. He would crave it. She wanted him to want her as much as she wanted him. She could feel herself trembling in anticipation. After only a few minutes of attempting to pleasure Adolf, she was moist and silky.

At last she could wait no longer. She wanted him inside of her, filling and stretching her so that she was complete.

Whole. She watched his expression as her hand guided him, feeling him linger for a moment beneath her, quivering as she kept him just on the verge of ... everything.

Everything in the world was suddenly there, surrounding Adolf as he gasped from the overwhelming sensation of wet heat and blissful closeness. Oneness, perhaps, for this union destroyed anxieties of friars or sick mothers or technical schools. This was bliss, and Adolf might have remained there forever if he could.

Helga felt the same, repeating in airy breaths her love for Adolf. She sat atop him, thighs spread to either side, her torso arching backward so that her breasts bounced gently as she pulled off her shift and began to rock gently atop him.

Adolf watched her in awe, for she was more beautiful than he ever imagined a woman could be. He soon felt himself responding to her movements. His dominant personality began to take over, and he started thrusting himself in a close rhythm to her rise and fall atop him. Helga's whimpers and occasional cries only encouraged Adolf's lustful urgency. The waves of pleasure began to mount, rolling over him as he watched Helga move over him, her trim abdomen flexing over her thick thighs and ample bottom.

It was quite suddenly that blissful pleasure shifted and became orgasmic ecstasy. All at once, following one of Helga's particularly inspired cries, Adolf felt fire filling the length of him. It gathered itself in a moment so intense that it treaded the borders of pain and pleasure. With an awkward groan, the first sound that he had contributed besides an occasional grunt, Adolf experienced the most incredible feeling of his young life.

Helga, feeling him strain so urgently already, smiled and slowed her oscillations. She had hoped for a more satisfying experience of her own, but she had expected worse. She knew Adolf's age and could be patient with him. It was the benefit of her own experience to know such.

"That . . ." Adolf had to swallow; he was breathing heavily, and the most ridiculous smile was affixed to his face. His young mustache glistened with hints of sweat, although he had not done much of anything at all except lie there. "That was amazing. Incredible. I love you. I love you so much, Helga."

Helga smiled tenderly and laid her head on his pale chest. "I love you, too, Adi. Rest a while, and perhaps we will try again. There is plenty of time before Papa returns." The mischievous look in her eyes aggravated Adolf somewhat. He felt so complete, so happy and content, but she still looked at him with more hunger than satisfaction. "Yes, rest. That is a good idea." His attitude was more a result of his own disappointment than for anything she had said.

The look in her eyes made it obvious enough that he had failed to please her in the manner she achieved for him.

Helga was surprised by the sudden cold distance of his tone. "Adolf?"

"Yes?" His voice was still cold, and now bordering on a tone of aggravation.

Helga thought about what she should say. Had she upset him so easily? She did not mean to say they would try again as a reproach. She thought to apologize, but decided it might be best not to say anything at all. Instead she fell back to something safe, something easy to say, now that they had admitted it to each other already. "I love you."

Adolf stroked a strand of her golden curls, stretching it out to tickle himself with its end as he circled his nipple in feathery strokes. Enjoying the distraction, he then thought to do the same to Helga. "I love you, too," he responded with less distance. And he did. "I am sorry," he said after a few moments of silence. "I was up late last night, and I must be tired. Mama was sick, and the doctor was still there when I arrived, and then I walked here. It has been a long day already."

Helga nodded on his chest, and then kissed him wherever her lips happened to fall. "It is all right, you have nothing to apologize for. After making you uncomfortable last night . . ." She paused to look up at him, uncertain if she should continue along this line. "I just wanted to make sure you were more . . . comfortable, this time."

Adolf could have laughed at the irony. As was usual, he had been worrying for nothing since he left Helga's company last night. He had not needed to tell her about Friar Roald or anything else. She was sorry for whatever she had done, but he could have left it at that. If this was how she apologized, he would have to let her be sorry more often.

More importantly, today he had learned that Helga could touch him wherever she pleased. The memory of Friar Roald had been horrible and unfortunate, but it did not mean he would remember that incident every time Helga's hand passed beneath his belt. That was perhaps a greater weight off his shoulders than anything.

He was still ashamed of himself for not lasting longer for Helga's enjoyment, but instead of dwelling on his performance and her lack of satisfaction, he closed his eyes, kissed the top of Helga's head, now resting on a pillow, and then let his own lingering sensations of satisfaction lull him to sleep.

Helga, upon feeling that gentle kiss press the crown of her head, smiled. Beneath the sheets she pulled over them, her finger was working toward what Adolf had not managed.

By the time she was biting against her own ecstatic cries, Adolf would be long asleep.

Perhaps she would wake him to try again, after she finished. Her hand was still so pleasingly cool, after all.

Chapter 13

AT LEAST ONCE a year, Klara made a point to visit her hometown of Spital. Even after her husband's death, Klara still packed up Paula, Adolf and Johanna and spent the late spring weeks in the cottage she had left behind when Alois asked her to be a maid in his second wife's household.

Returning to Spital was a tradition Alois had frequently found excuses to avoid. The first of his line to emerge from the stinking mud of the farm village and climb the social ladder, he seldom desired to see the same folks who knew him only as a bastard child.

Klara, however, felt it was important that Adolf and Paula know their heritage. So the Hitler family made the long trip in the last week of May, and Adolf did not want to go. He normally loved the open country and fresh air that surrounded the stink of the village itself. This year, however, instead of looking forward to the vacation, he could only think about how much he would miss Helga.

It had been months since the two had so intimately expressed their love for each other. Since then, they had only managed to create a few opportunities to repeat the act. It did not matter. Adolf was genuinely in love. His life had become a fantasy surely as dramatic as any opera. While they did not see each other as frequently as either would like, they did manage to keep close contact. He exchanged letters with Helga weekly, keeping them safe in the same leather script that held his sketches. What he felt for Helga had become more than puppy-love or even mere romantic love. She became his muse. She would compliment his drawings and encourage him in almost every interest he held.

Adolf had in Helga an invaluable resource, for she was a wellspring of positive energy. Whenever he felt tired or aggravated by schoolwork, he remembered his promise to his mother, but wanted more to please Helga. Whenever he looked at a sketch and decided it was good enough, he would pause and look through Helga's eyes.

Then he would breathe deep and set to perfecting the piece with stolid dedication. Although his true interests lay only in painting and drawing, he also improved in other subjects, such as German and history. He worked hard to earn their praise and affection, both of which he craved sharply.

Dear Gustl inspired Adolf, too, although for entirely different reasons and, of course, in different ways. The Kubizek boy was older than Adolf by nearly a year, but his deferring manner gave Adolf the chance to rant to an accommodating ear. This trip to Spital would be the first time he had been away from both relationships since having formed either.

So Adolf was not in a cheerful mood when the family packed into the coach Klara had hired for the trip. Although Adolf could rarely be described as cheerful, he was unusually stoic, staring with a listless gaze into the passing countryside. He soon discovered that the heartsickness he had felt when he first left home to lodge at Frau Sekira's boarding house was nothing like the intense, aching longing he felt for Helga. But his mother did not notice, too occupied with teaching Paula a new stitch as the coach bumped down the country dirt road.

Aunt Johanna was with them, her hunched back causing her to take not only her half of the bench seat, but also part of Adolf's space. He had remedied this intrusion by sliding tight against his window. Hanging one arm out, he was content to feel the winds of their passage as he contemplated the recent events of his life.

Helga's love was always new and fascinating, but it was also something he had grown accustomed to over the past several months. They had been dating for half a year. There were times when he wondered what life might have been like if Johan had wanted Elise to begin with, rather than intending Adolf for the girl. Then Adolf might have been with Helga for over a year now. It was a fleeting thought, as the more important matters were always closer to mind in times of stress, and Adolf certainly felt stressed by this vacation.

Klara had planned the trip for the same week as every year. The difference was that this year the family was once again moving. Although the family lived well enough off Alois's pension, Klara had decided that the Garden House was simply too large for the three of them. Adolf encouraged the idea because his mother had proposed relocation to a modest-sized apartment in Linz, which would give Adolf more opportunities to see Helga and August. Really, it was the best news he had received since Helga had proclaimed her love for him.

His issue was with the true reason for the move. Although Klara's illness had not worsened much in the past few months, it also had not improved. She still took laudanum at night to sleep and still pretended that nothing was wrong when morning came. By moving to Linz proper, she would be that much closer to Dr. Bloch's office. Alois's pension had left the family with ample funds, but bills for house calls that lasted until midnight were expensive.

So the Hitler family would sell the Garden House and move to an apartment at 31 Humboldtstrasse. First, though, there was this visit to the family in Spital to endure, and endurance it would be for Adolf, who was ashamed of his relations for a variety of reasons. His parents were second cousins, which meant he had only one set of great-grandparents, and his surviving relatives were poor cottagers mired in Spital's muddy streets. It was peasant country, and it represented everything Adolf hated.

Helga's lineage had not begun in a place such as this. Her line surely traced back to some queen or countess, at least. Well, perhaps nothing so royal—she supported the German nationalists, after all, not the monarchy. Still, her family was long removed from the farm life most of these villagers knew.

Wood smoke mingled with the scent of wet earth. In a few hours, women would begin cooking dinner on those hearths, savory stews whose flavorful odors would briefly replace the stench from the tannery, Spital's main source of commerce. Whoever had designed the town's layout had been a fool to place the tannery at the southwest corner; the northeast winds too often carried the smells across town.

Many other residents were simple farmers, but Spital was also home to several Jewish families. Alois never relished returning to visit with Klara and the children simply because he had realized his life dreams of rising from Spital's muck. He knew no appreciation for the hard lives these peasants lived. He was born in a wealthy inn. He had always lived in well-furnished apartments or comfortable houses. He had no understanding of the character it takes to rise each day with the sun or without it to feed animals and begin the day's work. So Adolf had no respect for the dirty faces and worn clothes of his own ancestral village

With his father dead, Adolf understood the man's shame; it mutated in Adolf, twisted from personal embarrassment to a sort of ignorant loathing. Alois had told Adolf how hard he had worked to become more than the town cobbler's apprentice, how he had studied for the civil service exam and risen out of Spital's mire. Only now, seeing the place after a long night of rain, did Adolf understand how his father must have felt. He saw the dispirited and the damned, and he pinched his nose at the smell of flesh rotting or curing at the tannery.

His shoes covered with mud as soon as he stepped out of the coach. How his mother and sister could navigate the puddles to reach the safety of their relative's porch was beyond Adolf's imagination. Aunt Johanna would surely have little choice but to tread through the muddy pools, as she had neither the grace nor agility of her sister or niece.

"Adolf, be a good boy, and give your aunt your arm," directed his mother.

"Of course, Mama," was Adolf's less-than-enthusiastic reply. He could not refuse his mother, although his skin crawled as he imagined Aunt Johanna leaning heavily on him as he guided her around some particularly fathomless puddle. It was all Adolf could do not to laugh at the thought of accidentally letting go of his dear aunt as they neared that sort of element in their path. He dutifully moved around the coach to open Aunt Johanna's door and help her climb down from the coach. He hardly managed to retain his own balance when his aunt added her weight to his thin frame, threatening to tumble them both into the puddle-strewn street.

With Adolf's arm on her left side and her short cane on her right, Aunt Johanna fussed and huffed at every labored step she made. Sitting in the coach for such a long trip had cramped her disfigured muscles, and so the sounds of her efforts were sincere, but Adolf had no sympathy for them. His own shoes were wet and cold from when his aunt's crippled path had forced him to walk through the very puddles into which he had imagined pushing her.

His patience thinned further when his aunt paused ten paces from the porch stairs. She had managed to hobble off of the street and onto the walkway in front of the small cottage before she had needed to rest—so close to their destination that waiting was agony for Adolf, who was left to stand in ankle-high grass and weeds that smeared the mud on his shoes. His aunt's breaths were deep and painful to hear, but her weight on his arm was becoming too much for him to stand beneath.

He was going to catch a cold standing in mud and water like this. In fact, he may already have caught one. The weather had been as damp and rain-soaked in Linz as it had been in Spital the past few days. His throat had felt itchy and aggravated all the morning, although the feeling had subsided as the day progressed. Now that he was out of the coach and standing with wet feet, the annoying itch was back in his throat as well.

"Come *on*, Auntie. It is not much further now." The impatient inflection was not the encouragement Adolf should have offered; it was good that his sister and mother had already gone inside. His grandfather greeted his favorite daughter at the door and was already beckoning Adolf and his aunt onward, but that was as much attention as the Polz patriarch was willing to give. Perhaps Adolf's impatience with the disabled was in his blood.

A short cough caught Adolf by surprise, leaving him without time to cover his mouth. His aunt took the gesture to be another indication of Adolf's impatience, and so she lost her own.

"Adolf, do not dare chivvy me on as if I were a head of livestock. I am not as spry as you, and it is not so easy for me to move. Just because I do things slower does not mean I will not do them with what dignity I can—and I will not lose that dignity to the impertinence of my nephew!"

Adolf pulled his arm away, wheeling to face his aunt. The suddenness of his movement pulled her off balance, so that she stumbled and put her foot in a puddle before she could regain her balance. Adolf at last lost his temper.

"I will not be spoken to thus by a disabled and disfigured woman, even if I must call her aunt! Impertinence? I had no intention of chivvying you anywhere. I have already walked through puddles to keep you out of them, and in your endlessly useless nature, you have now found yourself in one anyway. I coughed, Aunt. I apologize for the sudden tickle that seized me, but not every bodily function of mine is intended to insult you!" Adolf shook his head. "In fact, Auntie Jo, I think you have very much insulted me, and so you have lost the favor of my aid. Make your own way into this hovel from which you came." Without waiting for her response, he turned and walked into the house, coughing again, this time into his handkerchief.

Johanna had no recourse for offering a rebuttal. Adolf left her with one wet foot and an arduous set of stairs to climb. She could call for help, but if her father and nephew would not help her, she could not imagine whom to call. She did not want help from Klara, who was so perfect in her family's eyes. She gripped her cane tighter, leaned on it heavier and slowly made her way inside her childhood home.

Adolf already knew that this year's visit would be terrible. After the scene with Aunt Johanna, things had only grown worse. On the third day of their visit, Adolf's coughing had persisted and become increasingly violent, his spittle tinged with blood. Fevers and night sweats soon followed, and so the good Dr. Karl Kleiss was summoned from the neighboring town of Weitra.

"There is certainly fluid in his lungs," the doctor announced as his stethoscope traversed Adolf's chest. "Mucus or more blood, I could not say, but he should rest." The middle-aged doctor straightened and adjusted his circular, black-rimmed spectacles. "Consumption," Dr. Kleiss announced with a confident clap. "Lad has contracted tuberculosis," he added in a mildly apologetic tone.

Klara's hands tightened on the handkerchief with which she had been drying her tears. In peasant villages such as Spital, tuberculosis killed at least half the people who contracted it. "But I do not understand—he has been so healthy lately. How could he now be so ill?" Her question hung in the air as Dr. Kleiss merely shrugged.

"Has he been in confined spaces much?" he asked. "You say he has been healthy 'lately'... might I then presume that he has been sick in the past?"

Klara explained the series of ailments and illnesses that had plagued Adolf since the time he was born.

With that medical history revealed, the doctor frowned. "Well, I think it might be best if Adolf did not return to school this fall. If he survives this illness, he will be vulnerable to other maladies for some time to come. No, no, it will be best for him to avoid the public altogether. The lad will need plenty of air, although not this country air: He is not hearty enough for it. He will need to take antibiotics for a time, but he should recover." The doctor's tone might have been genuinely optimistic.

Adolf, contradictory by nature, answered the doctor with a vehement cough, wondering if his timing had been too perfect. Had the good Dr. Kleiss suspected his patient's symptoms were perhaps not as severe as they might seem? As soon as the doctor had prescribed a leave of absence from his classes, Adolf had known this was the opportunity for which he had so hopelessly waited. Only divine providence could have provided this chance. It was a manifestation of his self-proclaimed destiny to be an artist.

Although exaggerated, the illness was no less authentic; his cough still produced reddish phlegm. He should never have come to Spital. At one point, he wondered if his distance from Helga might have explained the sudden onset of this ailment. And yet, the sickness itself was the answer to so many prayers. If he were sick because of his distance from Helga, and the sickness provided the reason to at last leave school in Steyr permanently, then perhaps his love for Helga was beneficial even when they were apart. How strong that love must be!

"My poor little Adi." Klara sat on Adolf's bed, filling the space Dr. Kleiss had vacated when he finished his examination. The worried mother brushed his hair, made damp from the sweat of his fever, clear of her son's brow. "My poor boy. Rest now, rest, and you will be better soon enough."

Adolf, infirm as he was, obliged his mother by letting his eyelids sink shut. His mother was practically cooing at him, but his adoration for her kept him from feeling embarrassed, as other boys his age might have done. Instead, he smiled weakly, even with his eyes closed.

"Give him plenty of fluids," said the doctor. "Chicken broth and whatnot, but be sure he drinks slowly and is careful not to let any liquid go down wrong. There is enough fluid in his lungs as it is. I do not need to remind you how serious this illness can become, although he seems to have a mild enough case of it right now. All the same, I would keep him mostly indoors for the next few weeks. If it becomes cool at night, close his windows. Be sure he takes it easy, even as soon as he begins to feel better. I am sure he will seem ready for classes when they start, but so many bodies in the confined space of a classroom might simply be too much for his immune system."
"Immune system?" Klara asked. "Doctor, when would Adolf be able to resume his studies? Certainly he must go
back to school at some point or another."

Klara had tried to listen to the doctor's instructions as he finished packing his medical instruments into his black leather bag, but she did not understand what an immune system was, and her thoughts were scattered by her worry over Adolf's health. So many of her children had already been taken by sicknesses. She sometimes wondered if Adolf had any memories of his younger brother, Edward. Paula certainly would not. Mumps, diphtheria and now tuberculosis threatened her last surviving son.

Dr. Kleiss finished pulling on his light coat and hat. Summer in Spital was not particularly hot, being so close to the mountains, but it was a very sunny village, and the doctor had a long walk back to Weitra. Answering Klara's question, he said, "His immune system is comprised of the parts of the body responsible for fighting off diseases and infections. His constitution, if you will. From the medical history you have given me, I would say his immune system is naturally weaker than other lads his age. He will be weaker still once he recovers from this, and he will need to gather strength for some time to come. Perhaps by Christmas his body will have recovered enough for him to resume his studies."

Klara was grateful to the doctor for speaking with confidence that Adolf would recover at all. "Thank you, doctor, for coming all the way here to see us."

The good Dr. Kleiss smiled kindly. "Glad to be of service, Frau Hitler. Relax before you worry yourself sick as well. Keep the lad in bed for a few days—maybe so much as a few weeks, depending on how he feels. Certainly for the duration of your visit here in Spital. Once you return to Linz, I recommend you have the lad checked out again. If his condition should worsen significantly while you are still here in Spital, do not hesitate to call on me again. Not for a rise in his fever, mind you—that is to be expected a few times before it breaks entirely. No, I mean that you should call if he begins coughing up more blood or if his breathing becomes heavily labored."

Dr. Kleiss paused then and smiled, "But I am sure you know all this. You were smart enough to call when you first saw hints of blood. Many folks would have waited until their lungs were half full with blood. What am I expected to do for them then? And people wonder why the disease is so deadly . . ." He shook his head sorrowfully.

Klara listened intently, nodding when appropriate. "Of course, doctor. Thank you again for everything." She then rose and left

Adolf's bedside only long enough to show the doctor to the door. Once he had departed, Klara returned to Adolf's room, where she would spend the majority of her remaining vacation there in Spital.

Adolf, not yet sleeping, but daydreaming behind closed eyes, exulting in the plans the doctor had just made possible, smiled imperceptibly as his mother sat in the chair beside him. His mother loved him, and Helga loved him, and now he was free of school. His head was throbbing, and his chest burned, but he had salvaged a great victory from the relative misery of this trip to Spital.

The summer of 1905 passed, and Adolf did indeed survive his illness. In fact, he recovered far sooner than expected. Dr. Kleiss had been right in that Adolf's strain of the illness was mild and that they diagnosed and begun treating the illness early enough to end it all the more quickly.

The family's time in Spital had given the movers time to transfer the Hitler belongings from the Garden House, to their new apartment in Linz. As soon as Adolf was able to convince his mother he had the strength to travel again, Klara packed up their things and arranged for a coach. She was as anxious to return to Linz as her boy, although for very different reasons. Klara wanted to evacuate her son from the source of his illness, which she believed was Spital itself. Consumption and diseases like it were all too common in the poorer villages, even those that enjoyed such wonderfully fresh mountain airs.

Once back in Linz, the first thing Klara did was send for Dr. Bloch. It had been Dr. Kleiss's advice that Adolf be reexamined by a physician in the city, and despite the medical expenses that continued to mount, Klara did not think twice about sending for the Hitler family doctor.

When Klara had first contacted his office, he had feared the woman's own condition had deteriorated. He still was not certain what was causing Klara's chronic discomfort, but it did not seem to respond to any treatments the doctor had yet tried. Perhaps the pain had been particularly intense, and her laudanum dosage needed to be increased proportionally. The doctor decided to include a spare vial of the opiate in his medicine bag before he left the office, just in the event Frau Hitler was doing worse.

When Dr. Bloch arrived at the new Hitler residence, he was not surprised to find it decorated with the same modest taste as the Garden House. Klara greeted the doctor at the door, but quickly led him into Adolf's room without exchanging common pleasantries.

Soon the doctor's stethoscope was lifting from Adolf's chest. "Well, there is still some fluid in his lungs." Dr. Bloch announced as his stethoscope passed from one side of Adolf's pale chest to the other. "I am sure it will rattle itself out within another week's time. Remain in bed until then, Adolf. If you overexert yourself, you could rupture a lung and hemorrhage fresh blood. Then you will either be dead, or we will be starting over with you in bed for weeks again. Would not want that, would we boy?"

Adolf considered the question and recognized that although he certainly did not want to be dead, it perhaps would not be as unpleasant as remaining in bed longer. He had passed the time thus far by painting, reading and writing meticulous letters to Helga. He had to tell her his wonderful news regarding the end of his formal schooling, but knew he could yet not make the walk to her home. She would have come to him, straight away, but these were not the circumstances under which he wanted to introduce his girlfriend to his mother. Now that he thought of it, he did not want Helga to see him at all in this state.

In his first letter to her, he explained the reason for their shortened stay in Spital, and included specific instructions that she was not to try to visit and to only contact him by post. He would not risk Helga accidentally contracting his tuberculosis, and when he did see her, he would be robust and well again, not enfeebled and infirm.

He had learned that spending time away from Helga was not altogether bad. He held a fantastic image of her in his mind, an ideal to which his thoughts turned on frequent occasion. Thinking of her was a panacea, for he was happy when he thought of her, and so he thought of her often.

And his excusal from classes? Well, he did not make mention of that. It was a wonderful secret. A glorious secret.

It was a triumphant secret, and he wanted to be with Helga when told her that all his dreams were coming true.

"The fever is gone," announced Dr. Bloch. "Your blood pressure is good. Aside from that rattle in your chest, I think you have almost made a full recovery. You should know how lucky you are. Take it easy for a few more weeks, but start getting a little air. Short walks and such, nothing too strenuous."

Adolf nodded and began pulling his undershirt back over his head. He did not enjoy exposing himself for anyone, even doctors. Girlfriends were perhaps the only category absent from that particularly list. Well, Helga, specifically.

"I do, sir. I know I must be marked for something, surely." Surviving this illness had not only marked him for greatness—as a painter, he knew—but also provided the means by which he could now begin traveling on the road toward his destiny, rather than having to continue skulking and straggling along for years, no doubt winding up in the civil servant role of his father's dreams.

"Just continue to watch after your mother, young Adolf," the doctor said. Remember how she cared for you while you have been ill. Love saw you feel better as much as any destiny might have." The doctor readjusted his spectacles and turned to Klara. "Do not let him strain himself, and he should be out and about before the summer's end."

Klara smiled brightly. "Thank you, doctor. That is wonderful news." Her smile then tightened, and concern returned anew. "And what of his schooling? Do you agree with Dr. Kleiss's advice? What will the boy do if he cannot attend school?"

Dr. Bloch understood his colleague's reasoning; Adolf's health would be at greater risk in the confines of a crowded classroom. "If the boy had not been sick so often in the past,

I might say that he could certainly return if he wore a mask, a simple kerchief over his nose and mouth, perhaps. Adolf, however, prone to respiratory ailments . . ."

Adolf coughed on cue, as he had with Dr. Kleiss. He had refined his acting skills by that point, and the effort sounded genuine.

"He should perhaps take a sabbatical from his scholarly pursuits," said the doctor slowly. "Perhaps he could be privately tutored? Whatever the case, he will need the rest of the summer to recuperate."

The news frightened Klara. What sort of life could her son lead if he did not finish his education? And yet, what good was an education if he risked contracting another illness to get it? Perhaps she could afford a private tutor, if she found an even smaller apartment. Her boy coughed again, and her heart gripped in terror.

How could she know Adolf coughed only to hide the smile of satisfaction that had threatened his gaunt, pale face?

"Thank you Dr. Bloch. Your wisdom is always appreciated." Klara's tone was full of worry, as she absently patted Adolf's hand to calm his coughing.

"And what of yourself?" the doctor asked of Klara. "How have you felt lately?"

Klara blushed at the suddenness of the question, for she had wanted to lie for Adolf's sake, but the doctor had caught her off guard. "I have been feeling better. Some times I do not feel anything at all."

The doctor, having decades of experience with patients and their proclivity for lying about their health around other family members, only nodded. "I am very glad to hear that. Well, then, if you do not mind, could we step outside?

I would like to discuss my bill, and Adolf should get his rest."

Klara nodded, and then bent and kissed Adolf's forehead before following Dr. Bloch out of the room.

With the doctor and his mother beyond his door, Adolf allowed the cough to become a smile again. He was so very pleased with his performance and its outcome that all his thoughts went to what his next step should be. He thought of Helga, and then he thought of Vienna, for in his mind, he had decided that he needed to make a pilgrimage of sorts to that most bohemian of Austrian cities. He had no true plan beyond getting to Vienna; it had only been a dream. But to his delight, this dream was actually becoming true thanks to his sheer will and determination. Now it was time to think of what would happen next after he reached Vienna?

After walking Dr. Bloch a few steps down the hall from Adolf 's bedroom, Karla admitted to Dr. Bloch that the pain had not in truth subsided. It lingered now through the night and into the late morning, as well. No, she had not begun taking larger doses of her medicine, but she had wanted to. Badly.

Adolf had no idea that while he feigned the severity of his illness, his mother suppressed and disguised hers. In fact, since falling sick himself, Adolf had not heard his mother mention her own pain. She had cared for him just as she always had. Everything seemed so right. So . . . *good*. Helga was his, and he would soon be free of the chains his father had wrapped about his spirit. He would not be forced into a life of service. He was free to pursue his talents, and he had no idea:

Dreams that came true— Were still only dreams.

Chapter 14

ALMOST TWO WEEKS had passed since Adolf returned from the country. His illness was still present. He would hack and rattle in coughing fits, raising his blood pressure with the strain of his efforts to expel the fluid in his lungs, which lingered in a much smaller volume than his violent coughs suggested.

Adolf was indeed ill, but he had been sick many times in his young life. Those experiences provided him with ample opportunity to learn the symptoms he had been using to make his condition appear much worse than it truly was. Since arriving home, Adolf had artfully managed his illness. He remained in bed for most of his days, and when he did rise, it was to walk about as though he had risen from his deathbed.

He made one mistake on his second day home. His mother had come into his room and found her patient sitting upright at his desk, frantically trying to hide that he had been penning a letter. He flipped open his sketchbook and set it on top of his correspondence to Helga.

His mother paid no mind to whatever her son was so obviously trying to hide; her concern was that he was out of his bed. "Adi, you know you are supposed to be resting. Get back to bed before you strain yourself. You will never recuperate if you push yourself too much."

Adolf did not argue with his mother. What could he do, convince her that he was feeling better? The truth was no help to his cause. So he rose with a feigned effort and shuffled back into his bed.

Klara came and sat on the edge of her boy's bed, brushing his dark hair off his brow, and playfully pinched his pale cheek. "There, that is better. You will be well soon enough. Now, to whom were you writing?"

His mother's question surprised Adolf. He had been so sure that he had covered his letter to Helga in time. He used a fit of coughing to forestall his answer. Should he lie to his mother? Explaining who Helga was might take more effort than he could muster; it would be difficult for him to speak of the lady and sound anything but love-struck. No, the truth would not serve in this situation, either. It was the problem with fabricating realities. You still had to play by their rules.

"August, mother," he said after he regained his breath. "I was writing to dear Gustl, since he does not yet know of my illness. I would hate to worry him, otherwise. Would you mind mailing the letter if I feel well enough to finish it later?"

Klara was glad her boy had found such a good friend in August. She had met the older boy on several occasions, during which he always acted with the sincerest manners. "Of course I will mail it, but sit up in your bed, and write from here. Sitting at a desk is still too much for you, I think."

Adolf smiled at his small victory. "Of course, Mama." He would indeed write a letter to August. And in that letter, he would include his letter for Helga with instructions for August to forward it to her.

After a week passed without receiving a response, Adolf became anxious and suspicious. Had his friend lost the letter and told him he had delivered it? Had Helga and August secretly met while Adolf had been away in the country? He did not really believe either Helga or August would do that to him, but August had dated Elise—what if he had been interested in Helga all along?

No, no, that was all foolish. His anxiety was getting the better of him. Helga was probably writing to him now. Perhaps it was taking a few days before someone used the kitchen door, and she was just now finding the letter. He should have had August drop it in the front-door mail slot. Attempts at romance only complicated things, it seemed.

Now he waited, and as the count of days without response grew, so did Adolf's anxiousness. As a result, he began acting as if he were getting better, well enough to allow him his freedom, but not well enough to return to the classroom. It would be a tight rope to walk, but if he could reach the other side, he would have Helga and his freedom, the next steps in achieving his ultimate goal of being an artist in Vienna. That life was his destiny still. Ever since his father had so suddenly passed, Adolf had known that it would only be a matter of time before he achieved his dream of living the cultured life.

He could not wait to share his news with Helga. It had been a constant torment to remain patient, to remain in bed as long as he had. Would she come with him to Vienna? Would it be proper for them to live together?

Social mores were often at the forefront of his thoughts; he never ceased to worry about society's perceptions of him, not only in his personal appearance, but also in his public relationships. He knew it would be wrong for Helga to move in with him. It would be wrong, but in this case, he very much wanted to rebel against society's norm. He did not have enough money from his father's pension to support the both of them, and if he were going to be an artist, he certainly could not get a normal job. Even if Helga wanted to be Louise, as things stood, Adolf could not afford to be Julien.

But none of that really mattered. Helga could stay in Linz, and Adolf would travel by rail to visit her with the same frequency he had managed while living in Steyr. It would not be an ideal arrangement, but a necessary one— and ultimately worthwhile. Adolf had no doubt that Helga would understand completely; she might not like it at first, but she would soon come to see his way of thinking.

It was another day before Adolf convinced his mother that getting some fresh air would do him good. By then, his lank frame seemed wasted by the weeks Adolf had spent in bed. He dressed himself as meticulously as he ever would have, but his clothes hung poorly, making him feel self-conscious. He would have his mother alter the clothes later—or perhaps his stepsister, Angela, could find time to do the work while her husband got drunk again. His thoughts returned to Helga. What would she look like after all this time? It had been nearly a month now since he had left her bed to vacation with his family. Thinking back brought a blush to his pale cheeks—or perhaps it was a flush of a more lustful design. Before he became sick, Adolf had spent his daydreams either in remembering or recreating his last time with Helga. On their way to Spital, he had gazed at the passing countryside and instead of picturing a landscape scene he might paint, he thought of Helga.

When the illness had been at its worst, and there was no acting in his ailments, his thoughts were less carnal and more spiritual. Helga still remained at the forefront of his thoughts, but she was an angel, a beacon of hope—a thought of pure comfort. His mother had previously been the source of such feelings before, but something had changed. Even as his mother sat at his bed, lightly stroking his forehead, Adolf's thoughts centered on Helga.

Now that he was recovering, Helga became less of a balm. Thoughts of her no longer soothed him, but inflamed him. He felt smoldering desire mixed with anxiety—he had not seen the girl for a month, and, worse, she had neither responded to his letter nor written him one of her own.

Just walking again through Linz itself helped to restore a certain vitality. He needed to see Helga and dispel all his negative thoughts. The prevailing belief that had sustained Adolf for all those weeks apart still held true: Being with Helga would make everything all right.

There was nothing particularly different about the city since Adolf had last stridden its cobbled streets. Linz in midsummer was bustling with pedestrian traffic. The open market vendors were selling vegetables and cheese to housewives out shopping for dinner fare. Uniformed soldiers occasionally rode by on horseback, the sound of iron shoes on cobble was more than enough warning for pedestrians to make way for them.

Adolf's legs began to cramp. He had spent weeks in bed, and this was by far the longest walk he had been on since before he had become ill. Luckily his anxieties had been good for one thing—they had occupied his mind while he walked. He was already at the top of Helga's street. Seeing her house sent an entire squadron of butterflies into evasive maneuvers within his chest. More than one crashed: His lungs were burning as if they were filled with liquid fire. A rough cough reminded him that while he might no longer be acting sick, he was still not fully recovered.

He took a moment to straighten his appearance, shifting his shorts so that they lined up with the buttons down the front of his collared short-sleeve shirt. Linz was not particularly hot in the summer, but the air was comfortably warm; Adolf wiped his brow with his handkerchief. He then coughed into that same cloth and returned it to his pocket.

He started taking the last steps toward Helga's house.

Would she answer the door herself? What if her father answered it? Had he found out about Adolf's last visit? What if he had found the letter and, breaking Helga's privacy, read it himself? It certainly contained lines that would be outright damning if read by the wrong eyes.

He lifted heavy brass knocker affixed to the Faveshra's front door once, and then twice. Adolf stepped back and waited, his heart racing. Weeks of separation were spawning a flurry of rational concerns and absurd possibilities. What would Helga look like after all this time? What would she think of his own appearance? What if she had met a new boy in his absence? What if she begrudged his extended absence? Had Johan come calling again?

What if someone had discovered his letter? Josef might have been the first to find it, and what younger brother would not read something so secretively delivered and obviously intended for his sister? Adolf might have opened such a letter to Angela, had he ever found one, and she was only his half-sister!

Too many possibilities presented themselves to Adolf's emotional mind. He hated feeling so completely powerless. Anyone could be waiting beyond the heavy front door to the Faveshra home.

Adolf 's excitement crested as the door swung inward. A joyous swell of relief and excitement clashed against his remaining apprehensions, which had nothing to do with Otto or Josef, but rather with Helga's perception of him.

His anxiety vanished when at last the door opened enough to reveal her. The moment he saw her, he again felt the connection between them that had been dormant in their separation. He had worried for nothing.

"Adolf?" Helga looked shocked and excited. She paused a moment, and then hurried through the door with her arms open.

Smiling and laughing with relief, he held her tightly to him.

She hugged him back with equal intensity, crying joyful tears and saying nothing distinguishable beyond his name, over and over again, until her voice was little more than a whisper.

As he held her, Adolf was certain their reunion was making a fine show for passersby. For once, Adolf could care less what society thought. Old women could gossip if they liked. All that mattered was that he was holding Helga in his arms.

At last, Helga moved back slightly so that she could lean up and kiss him tenderly. The kiss was eternal: It lasted only a moment, but he knew he would remember it forever. It was an affirmation of their love's survival. It was a confirmation that his dreams were still his destiny.

"I missed you, Adi. I missed you so very much." Helga wiped tears from her cerulean eyes. "Come, come inside. We have so much to talk about, and I do not have very much time. Come in, and I will explain."

He heard sadness in Helga's voice, and his heartbeat accelerated again. His mouth dry and his thoughts filled with new anxieties, he followed Helga into her home. What had happened?

Once the front door was closed behind them, the house was dark and quiet inside. Adolf frowned. The furnishings and décor had not changed, but something felt different. Adolf looked more carefully and noticed a light layer of dust covering the tables. The floors were somewhat dirty, too. He wondered what had happened to the housekeeping in this normally fastidious house.

As if following his eyes to his thoughts, Helga led him into the kitchen and explained, "You must excuse the state of our home. Josef became ill not long after you left for vacation. He has been in the hospital all this time now. When father comes home from work, we leave straightaway for the hospital to see him. When father is not home, I spend so much time worrying about Josef—and you—that I have let the housekeeping go. She sighed, looking around the room. "I suppose I have a lot to catch up on."

"I am sorry, Helga, both to hear about your brother's illness and to have given you cause for worry myself. Did my letter at least find its way to you?"

"Not soon enough." Once the words had left her mouth, Helga blushed. "That was not fair. I apologize." She rubbed her eyes and smoothed her hair. "Things have been so difficult, but hardly easier for you, I am sure. I am so relieved to see you, Adolf. Knowing that you and Josef were both sick taxed me. I wrote you letters, but you never replied."

"I never got any letters." And why would he? His mother had found the family a new apartment when they returned from the country. The Garden House was sold, and he had not thought to specifically include his new address in his hastily written letter. "I am very sorry, Helga." What else could he say?

"Well, you are here now. That is better than any letter. You could not help being sick yourself. I am just glad you did not decide to run off with some country girl!"

Adolf blushed at Helga's teasing.

Helga's smile at Adolf's embarrassment did not remain on her features long; nor did her tone remain playful. Her voice again sounding said, she said, "I was waiting for father to come home so that we could go visit Josef together. He is working late tonight, and it will be dark by then. The nurses never let us visit with Josef long after dark. Would you take me? I can leave a note for father to join me when he can. You would not have to stay long. I know how you dislike the hospital. I would appreciate your company walking there, though."

Adolf hesitated for a moment. He had not intended to stay so long as he had already. His mother believed he had gone to visit August; he had all but promised to be home before the night's chill settled on streets. And yet, how could he say no? "Of course I will escort you."

"Wonderful!" Helga kissed him lightly. "Thank you, Adolf. It will only take a moment to write father a note."

Once Helga had penned a brief explanation to her father, she and Adolf set off to see poor young Josef.

As they walked, Adolf had a number of thoughts. How would he explain his tardiness to his mother? She would be so worried. And when should he tell Helga the incredible fortune his illness had afforded them? The secret he had harbored so closely to his heart pressing against his chest, even as his pulse quickened from the simple exertion of walking again after being bed-ridden for so long.

For the first block, Helga enjoyed his company in silence as they made their way through streets that were beginning to empty as the sun sank lower in the sky. Finally, she said,

"You are better now, right? This is not too much of a strain for you?"

Adolf was startled by the question, "Better? Yes, much better, really. I am weaker than I am used to feeling, but this air and exercise will see me right again soon enough."

"I am glad. The doctors warned us how deadly tuberculosis can be. When I read that was your illness, I was terrified. That is what Josef has. His case is much worse, I think. The doctors . . ." Helga paused and shook her head sadly, "They do not know what the outcome of this illness will be—only God knows."

Adolf squeezed Helga's hand gently and wondered if revealing the triumph of his plans was wise when the sickness that made his dreams possible was the same illness that could claim her dear brother's life. He did not want to raise hope in her that all would be as well with her brother as it had been for him. Instead, he said simply, "Josef has endured much in his young life. I am sure he will be well."

Helga squeezed Adolf's hand in return. "Thank you. Your words are heartening."

Adolf smiled and paused in his steps. "Come, there is a shortcut to the hospital. I remember Johan showing me this alley. We can save ourselves at least ten minutes if we go this way. Just mind your step, people tend to use alleys for . . . well, you will see—and smell, I'm afraid."

Helga did not wait for Adolf to lead the way. "If it gets us to my brother faster, I am sure I will navigate it carefully enough."

Adolf admired Helga's courage as much as her dedication to her brother. The alley was long and full of deep shadows and piles of refuse, but she held her head high. The sun by now had descended behind the city's buildings. Twilight seemed darker in the confined alley, and the smell of garbage made the detour far from pleasant. What the pair gained in time would certainly be compromised for comfort.

The end of the alley was marked by a street lamp. As Adolf and Helga were almost at the end of the narrow passage, a stranger obstructed their past. It was a man, tall and gaunt in the long shadow of the street lamp. He was muttering something to himself, words that Adolf could not quite understand, but spoken with an accent. Slavic, perhaps? He felt Helga squeeze his hand tighter.

Adolf paused in his steps and led them from the stranger's path. He pressed himself against the side of the alley, and Helga did the same, keeping her grip on Adolf's hand as tight as ever.

The stranger seemed to pay them no attention. His short, sometimes faltering, steps continued to echo dully in the confined space. He was still muttering, but he did not look twice at Adolf; nor did he give a second glance at Helga's beauty.

Adolf thought the man must be opium addict. The sunken eyes with their dark bags were a strong indication of drug usage. Such men were dangerous, and Adolf felt himself tensing as the man came ever closer. Helga's grip on his hand was almost painful as the stranger continued inexorably toward the couple.

The stranger never looked toward them, but continued his shambling steps. In a moment, he would be past them. "Money," said the stranger. The words were hardly distinguishable from the rest of his accented ramblings, but distinctive all the same. He pivoted and strode directly toward Helga. Adolf tried to put himself in the man's path,

but the stranger was faster.

Helga screamed as the man grabbed her, drawing a small pistol his tattered coat. He pressed the weapon to her and the soiled index finger of his other hand against her lips, silencing her cries.

"Money," the man repeated, his Slavic accent thick and slurred.

"Leave her alone!" said Adolf in the most menacing tone he could manage amidst his shocked terror. "Here!" he began digging in his pockets. He had no money, but he did have an old pocket watch. "Take this and leave us be! Please!"

Helga had stopped screaming and struggling. She knew from the look on Adolf's face how dangerous the situation was.

"Money!" said the man fiercely, ignoring the watch Adolf offered.

"But I only have this—" Adolf's breath caught as the small pistol left Helga's side and elevated to instead to level its barrel at his head. The robber's arm trembled as he held weapon, his sunken eyes staring wildly from their hollowed sockets.

The man was breathing down on Helga, suffocating her with his fetid breath. When the man waved his gun at Adolf, she took a dangerous chance.

Before the man could blink, Helga dipped her head, and then snapped it back into the robber's pox-pestilent chin. Even her golden locks could not cushion the impact of her skull against the robber's face. She stumbled away from the stunned assailant, gasping.

Adolf ran forward even as Helga escaped the assailant's grasp. There was no time for anything but instinct, and even as weakened as he was, primal adrenaline gave him a sublime sensation of slow motion. He had to wrestle that pistol free of the man's grasp. There was no course but the one his momentum carried, and he tackled the man violently in a collision that hurt Adolf as much as the man.

The impact of Adolf's shoulder folded the man in half as Adolf tackled him to the ground. The pistol fired only a moment after Adolf's impact with the man, its sudden crack resounding in Adolf's ears. Outside the alley, cries and screams erupted from the few folk who had remained out in the deepening twilight.

The man lost his grip on the weapon as Adolf's momentum carried them both to the ground, and for a moment they wrestled until the larger man ultimately overpowered Adolf. The man could have throttled Adolf then, but the witnesses were moving toward the alley. Without looking for his pistol, the man climbed over Adolf and ran away into the deeper darkness of the alley.

For a heartbeat, Adolf lay in the alley's filth. He sat up slowly, gaining his bearings in the deepening darkness. People were hovering just at the edge of the alley's mouth. He looked for Helga, and the missing gun.

Helga was leaning against the wall, one hand rubbing absently at her chest, where the man had grabbed her dress. "Adolf?" she said, her voice breathless, "Adolf, it hurts."

Helga took one step toward Adolf, before she stumbled and fell. The empty despair that already opened in Adolf's stomach stole his breath. She had been shot.

"Helga!" he cried hoarsely. Raising his voice, he screamed, "Someone help her! Someone help!" He gathered Helga to him, drawing her onto his lap. "Oh, God, help her!"

He pressed his hand to her wound, trying to staunch the flow of blood. The warmth of her blood in his hands mingled with that hollow sense of hopelessness that grew within him. He was powerless.

"Adolf, I . . ." Her voice was so soft. Helga began to shake as shock overcame her, and she fell unconscious.

Men and women still shouted in the night, calling for the authorities, for doctors, for help, even as bystanders edged closer.

Even as people came rushing to help, Adolf sat numbly in the alley's darkness. Helga was still breathing. Thank God, she was still breathing, but her breaths came shallow and faint. She could not die. She *would* not die.

He should have gone home. He should have visited Helga, and told her his wonderful news, and then gone home. He had no business escorting her to see Josef so late at night. His own constitution was not hardy—he had not been strong enough to protect her.

"Make way! Move, you louts! Clear a path, and let me through!" Adolf heard commands echoing in the alley, but his attention remained on Helga, still pressing his hand against her wound.

A doctor made his way through the crowd of gawkers. "Cloth, boy," he called. "A clean cloth will staunch the wound better than your hand." The doctor removed the white scarf he was wearing.

Adolf at last noticed him. "Who are you—?"

The doctor cut the question short. "Not important. This scarf is." He folded the silk cloth into a thick square pad and handed it to Adolf. "Press that firmly, and hold it there until we reach the hospital. I already spoke to the owner of the tavern across the street. He keeps a cart for transporting kegs that we will borrow to transport your young lady there."

"But how did you know?" Adolf said as he followed the strange doctor's instructions and pressed the cloth to Helga's wound.

"How did I know we would need a cart? There was a gunshot, and screams, and a boy calling for help. Requisitioning a cart seemed a prudent step."

The weight in the doctor's words gave Adolf the chills. "Ah here we are," the doctor announced at the sound
of the cart rattling over the cobblestones. "The man did say it would take only a few minutes to have the horse hitched. Good man! Well, we had best move her now. There is no time to waste if she is going to survive. Here, I shall carry her if you can maintain the pressure on her wound."

Adolf did as he was told, and soon Helga was loaded onto the cart as carefully as haste allowed. The doctor jumped up into the seat beside the cart's driver, Adolf remaining at Helga's side in the back of the cart, pressing the doctor's scarf to Helga's chest. Her dress was now stained a deep red.

"Hold that pressure as evenly as you can boy," the doctor called back. "We shall try and warn you of bumps and ruts as best we can, but you must keep that wound staunched so that her blood pressure does not drop further."

Adolf listened intently to the man's every word. He spoke fluent Austrian, but his manner was odd. Most doctors were tempered men, stoic and reserved in their demeanor. This fellow was animated, talking with his hands even as he spoke with the gravity of a man who possessed the educated mind of a doctor.

"A horrible tragedy." The doctor had turned in his seat and was watching Adolf. "Senseless and stupid, really. When will mankind learn that violence is not the answer?"

Adolf hardly heard the man's question as he continued to stare at Helga's pale features. All the color had left her creamy skin, the vitality of her natural beauty subdued.

Why had he taken her down that alley? Why had he taken her out so late at all? Her father would have had more sense. Her father would have intimidated the Slav and protected his daughter better than Adolf.

Adolf said nothing as the cart arrived at the hospital. He did not know how long the trip had taken, but only the darkest shades of twilight lingered as the stars grew brighter overhead.

When the nurses rushed to bring Helga into an operating room, the doctor right behind them, Adolf was at last forced to leave her side. Another nurse showed Adolf to a waiting room before he had a chance to thank the good doctor.

It was late into the night before a nurse informed Adolf that Helga was out of her surgery and that he might visit her briefly if he promised to be quick and quiet. By then, Adolf was exhausted and barely able to keep his bloodshot eyes open, but nothing would stop him from remaining by Helga's side.

The long hours he had spent in the waiting room had provided ample opportunity for Adolf to recreate the entire day in his mind, beginning with the lie he had told his mother, to meeting Helga at her door, to how wonderful it had felt to walk with her on his arm, and then, finally, to the poor decisions that had led to the tragedy. He thought about how worried his mother would have been, how worried Helga's father would be when Helga could not be found. He thought about how he had never had a chance to tell Helga his news.

His regrets had mounted to a state of supreme apprehension as he drew closer to the recovery room, hearing the frightening sounds of various medical instruments and apparatuses, a low whirring punctuated by the sound of air pushing through something thick and heavy.

Helga's room Helga was far from hospitable. The whitewashed walls of the horsehair-plastered room were already yellowing from the cigarette smoke of family members visiting their sick relatives. Everything smelled of soiled linens and bleach. At last Adolf took a deep breath and entered the room.

She was lying on the bed bed, affixed to a ventilator that kept her unconscious self breathing. Her gold-spun hair was fanned on her pillow, looking dull and lusterless. Her naturally rosy complexion had turned pale like caulk from the blood she had lost.

Her hand was cold, so cold to his touch. Each beep, every air exchange when the ventilator's pumps circulated, did nothing to ease his fears, nothing to convince him that Helga could recover from this state.

He wanted to speak to her, but found that he had no idea what he should say. He was too self-aware and embarrassed. He did not like it when the nurses and doctors passed the room's open door. He did not like that none were stopping in to check on Helga. He did not like that this situation was as hopeless as it seemed. His frustration over his lack of control was elevating his blood pressure. He could hear his heart pounding in his ears.

"I am so sorry," he found himself whispering through his tears. Could she hear him? Was she listening somewhere in her dreams?

He sat with her, holding her hand, as her chest continued to rise and fall within the confines of her bedcovers. He wanted little else than to kiss her, like Prince Charming, to wake her, but her lips were covered by the mask that allowed her to live.

When would she wake? How could he care for her? The machines seemed to be doing more for her than he certainly could, but there must be something he could do.

She was his Louise, and he had hoped she would offer to run away with him when he told her he was free from secondary school. He hoped she would follow him to Vienna, but even if she could not, he could visit her on weekends if she remained here in Linz. Now, as he held her too-cool hand, he could not help but wonder if he would visit her anywhere besides this hospital room ever again.

He suddenly thought of his mother. He had been with Helga now for at least three hours, waiting through her surgery and then sitting with her as he fought his own conscience. His mother would be worried sick about him. He would have to leave Helga, and he could not help but selfishly hope that she would not wake until he returned again. He wanted to be there when she woke, to be the first person she saw when she opened her eyes.

He was just gearing himself to rise and leave her bedside when her body suddenly convulsed. He jumped up, knocking over the chair he fell backward and caught himself against the wall. Her ventilator pumps continued to whine as her body thrashed and racked under her blankets.

"H-help," said Adolf, shock muting his first cries, until at last he found himself shouting, screaming, "Help! Someone! Doctor! Nurse! Somebody HELP!!"

As he screamed, watching Helga in horror, she continued to convulse, coughing violently into her ventilator mask, which was filling with the same fluid in which her lungs were drowning. There was too much of it; even the machine could not help her breathe any longer. She was dying.

As her body continued to shake and strain for air, doctors, nurses and attendants came pouring into the room.

One of the orderlies took Adolf by the arm as he continued to scream for someone to help her. The last image Adolf would have of his Louise, his Isolde, his Helga, would be of her body, finally falling limp again as doctors injected her and called directions to the nurses.

It was the most horrific moment of Adolf's life.

Hours passed, but Adolf had no memory of them. After the doctors informed him of Helga's passing, he had left the hospital in a numb state, wavering between shock and outright denial.

Adolf at last found himself at home. He had never told his mother about Helga. Now his mother would never meet his first true love. Now she never would. She would never see Helga's cerulean eyes or her angelic, gold-spun hair. She would never hear the intelligence in Helga's speech or the warmth of her laughter. That thought was unbearable.

When Adolf opened the door to his family's still-new apartment, he felt outside himself, surreal, as he walked woodenly to the stiff-cushioned couch. There was a buzzing in his ears, a great cacophony of chorusing banshees. Well, perhaps only one banshee—Aunt Johanna, yelling at him for causing so much worry.

"Where have you been? You have worried your mother half to death! She and Paula are out looking for you! That Kubizek boy is looking too! A fine friend you are—you never were going to see him. He told your mother and me that he never expected any visit from you. Where have you been?"

Adolf sat heavily and tried to catch his breath as his Aunt's chastisement continued. He was still detached from the moment, disconnected at the brink of consciousness, for he was aware of everything that happened, but was in a kind of stasis. Everything was too intense, too real, coming too fast.

"You know your mother is supposed to be resting," Aunt Johanna scolded. "She has been scarcely better in health than you ... and her having to care for you certainly taxes her. Yet you go off gallivanting for hours without giving any thought to her poor soul."

As Aunt Johanna's words registered with Adolf, he suddenly felt himself centered and focused back into that moment, his grief suddenly synthesizing with defensive anger that arose from his aunt's accusations. He did not need to speak; he did not yell or argue. He simply focused his gaze, bearing all the wild emotion of Helga's death and the cruelty of that loss, and leveled a look of tormented fury at his deformed and disabled aunt.

The ferocity of that grievous stare was enough to startle the old woman into stumbling backward. She slipped as her cane caught on the edge of the hallway carpet. Adolf's eyes followed the hunched woman's descent until she crashed into a chair, breaking it before falling into a heap on the floor.

For a moment, the surprise and shock of what had just happened replaced his grief and anger. He did not feel guilty; nor did he find any humor in the event. He only watched with curiosity as his aunt struggled to rise.

This woman, like Josef, was completely worthless; therefore any chastisement that came from her must also be worthless. It was true that he had worried his mother half to death. He was certain of that, but that certainty was spawned from the certainty of her love for him. He would have done the same for her, had she gone missing for hours. Once she returned and learned the reason for his absence, she would console him, not scold him. His aunt, though, was a useless creature. If she loved him, she would have been out searching, too— and if her disfigurement had kept her from leaving the house, then what good was her worry? All his rage and grief focused into the dark eyes that watched his aunt's heavy struggles to regain her feet.

His feeling of detachment had returned. He was not only observing his aunt, but also himself, as if he were a third person in the room. In that moment came a sudden sense of dread and embarrassment, a unique and genuine shame, for he thought of

Helga. If Helga ever saw him behaving like this toward his aunt, she would hate him. She would hate him forever.

Just as suddenly as that thought flickered through his mind, Adolf felt himself return to himself again, and instead of just sitting on the couch, watching his poor aunt struggle, he rose and crossed to her.

"Here, Auntie, take my hand," he said softly, his voice contrite. His meager frame was hardly strong enough to lift his aunt, but he was able to provide support enough for her to come upright again.

She was breathing heavily, and there were tears in her eyes, although whether they were from a pain or a shame of her own, Adolf would never know. "I am sorry, Auntie," Adolf said quietly, but with definite conviction. "I am sorry for a lot of things."

His aunt paused for a moment, her eyes weighing him with intensity akin to Adolf's own. She smiled softly and said, "This is the good boy my sister always brags about. Sometimes, Adolf, 'I'm sorry' is all a person needs to hear." She appeared thoughtful for a moment. "Most of the time, it is *all* people can hear. Come on, help me into the kitchen. I can at least make sure there is something hot for when your mother and sister return from their search. They will be so relieved to find you here."

Adolf now understood that what his aunt lacked in charisma or physical ability, she made up for in wisdom. He helped her make her way to the stove with slow steps. By the time she was halfway there, she was walking in her shuffling step, using her cane again. Exhausted, Adolf sat in his chair at the table.

"Just where had you been, Adolf? What kept you out so long?"

But Adolf didn't hear his aunt's question. Helga was dead, and although he was free of school and could live out his dreams in Vienna, he would never be truly happy again.

Epilogue

IT WAS NEARLY three years before death again touched Adolf Hitler's life. This time it was expected, although Adolf 's grief was no less because of it.

Christmas was less than a week away, but the Hitler apartment was not decorated this year. Paula had thought to hang a wreath on their apartment's front door, but even that felt too festive. Klara Hitler had been sick for years now. The doctors had pronounced her condition as terminal when the cancer continued to spread even after her mastectomy. There was nothing to be done.

Adolf had returned from Vienna, where his dreams of being an artist had so far been realized only by frustrations and failures. Now that he was home, his every waking moment was spent at his mother's bedside.

Yesterday August had come to pay his best friend's mother a final visit. She had whispered something to him, something Adolf had not quite been able to hear. August had looked at him quite seriously before nodding and patting Klara's hand in assurance.

Adolf wondered what his mother had said to dear Gustl. He wondered many things as he sat solemnly in a chair, eyes flickering from the page as he meticulously sketched the portrait of his mother in her final repose, tears rolling silently down his drawn, pale face. His pencil had grown short with the effort: He was constantly erasing or shading or sharpening it to the finest of points. His mother's death felt different from Helga's. His mother's was expected; her impending death was almost as much a mercy as it was a source of grief. But Adolf had learned to cope with grief. He had already had years to master that skill. So he sat and drew a final and lasting tribute of his beloved mother's beauty.

The good Dr. Bloch would later comment on Adolf 's attentiveness to his mother's every care or need. How he would sit morosely, mournfully, for days at her bedside, watching her attentively, almost desperately, or else he would stare listlessly at the sky through a nearby window. Never for long though; his gaze always returned with care or concern if his mother so much as shifted in her sleep.

For the first time, Adolf felt truly alone. He would still have August as a friend. Paula was still his sister, and Angela still his stepsister, but without his mother or Helga, he had no more love.

There was a girl, or at least, an ideal, for she was very much like Helga. They were both beautiful, crowned with golden-blond hair. Her name was Stefanie, and he and August would watch for her each day as she strolled in the park with her mother at dusk.

He had never approached her—*could* never approach her, for she could never live up to what he had lost when Helga had died.

And so he sat alone, drawing his mother's death portrait.

He did not know what he would do tomorrow. Little had gone his way. He had fulfilled his dreams of burning books and pencils, but what were his dreams today? He had failed the entrance exam to art school in Vienna. Failed it once, and then failed it again. He was no more an artist than he was a bohemian, but he drew his mother's portrait, expressing grief he could not otherwise convey.

He had been a boy, like many others, but he was not a boy any more. He was Adolf Hitler, and his future awaited him.

www.ingramcontent.com/pod-product-compliance
Lightning Source LLC
LaVergne TN
LVHW040133080526
838202LV00042B/2888